Contents

T0075589

Online extras

This manual includes a series of downloadable forms that accompany the chapters. These forms are available from the BSAVA Library.

- **How to identify the forms in the text:** in the selected chapters, each form is identifiable by a 'download' symbol in the top right corner.

- **How to access the forms:** the forms can be accessed via QR codes, which can be found at the end of each chapter containing forms. You will need a QR code reader on your smartphone or tablet – a number of QR code reader apps are available. The forms can also be accessed by typing the web address provided at the end of the chapter into a web browser.

Contributors

Heather Bacon
OBE BSc(Hons) BVSc CertZooMed SFHEA MRCVS
School of Veterinary Medicine,
University of Central Lancashire,
Preston, Lancashire PR1 2HE

Penny Barker
BVetMed BSc DipCoaching MRCVS
VDS Training,
4 Haig Court, Parkgate Estate,
Knutsford, Cheshire WA16 8XZ

Carolyne Crowe
BVetMed(Hons) MSc BSc(Hons) DipCoaching DipStress Management
and Wellbeing FRCVS
VDS Training
4 Haig Court, Parkgate Estate,
Knutsford, Cheshire WA16 8XZ

Kelly Deane
FdSc CertVNES RVN
Beaumont Sainsbury Animal Hospital,
The Royal Veterinary College,
Royal College Street,
London NW1 0TU

Jo Hinde-Megarity
RVN
LagoLearn Ltd

Lisa Howe
A1 Cert Pet Bereavement (BC) RVN
Pet Bereavement Services Ltd

Becky Jones
DipAVN(Surg) RVN
Langford Vets,
Langford House, Langford BS40 5DU

Carrie Kearns
ACC DipPBC VCA Cert Pet Bereavement(BC) MACCPH AdvDipBCT
Animal Bereavement Counselling with Carrie Kearns,
151 the Rock, Bury BL9 0NB

Rachel Lumbis
MSc BSc(Hons) PGCert(MedEd) CertSAN FHEA RVN
WSAVA Global Nutrition Committee member,
Former Lecturer in Veterinary Nursing,
Royal Veterinary College

Jim Mackie
The Zoological Society of London,
Regent's Park, London NW1 4RY

Amy Martin
BSc(Hons) DipAVN DipHE CVN NCert(BusDev) DipCoaching and
Mentoring MBVNA RVN
Holly House Veterinary Hospital,
468 Street Lane, Moortown,
Leeds LS17 6HA

Anne McBride
BSc PhD FRSA
School of Psychology,
University of Southampton,
Highfield, Southampton SO17 1BJ

Chirag Patel
BSc(Hons) PGCert(CAB) CPBC DipCABT MAPDT(00923)
Chirag Patel Consulting,
7 Edward Road,
Chadwell Heath, Essex RM6 6UH

Matthew Rendle
RVN
Association of Zoo & Exotic Veterinary Nurses,
PO Box 10637,
Market Harborough LE16 0HG

Craig Tessyman
RVN
Rutland House Veterinary Hospital,
Abbotsfield House, 4 Abbotsfield Road,
Reginald Road Industrial Estate,
Saint Helens WA9 4HU

Adina Valentine
CertVNES VNCertECC NCert(Anaesth) RVN
Origin Vets Clinic,
The Coachworks Centre Unit,
30 Dynea Road, Pontypridd CF37 5DN

Molly Varga Smith
BVetMed DZooMed MRCVS
Rutland House Veterinary Hospital,
Abbotsfield House, 4 Abbotsfield Road,
Reginald Road Industrial Estate,
Saint Helens WA9 4HU

Hayley Walters
MBE RVN
The Jeanne Marchig International Centre for Animal
Welfare Education,
The Royal (Dick) School of Veterinary Studies,
University of Edinburgh,
Easter Bush,
Roslin EH25 9RG

Chloe White
RVN
VetzPetz UK

James Yeates
BVSc BSc CertWEL DipWEL DipECAWBM(WEL) MBA PhD FRCVS
World Federation for Animals,
25 Chestnut Square, Boston
MA 02130 USA

BSAVA Manual of Practical Veterinary Welfare

Editors:

Matthew Rendle
RVN
Association of Zoo & Exotic Veterinary Nurses
PO Box 10637
Market Harborough
LE16 0HG

Jo Hinde-Megarity
RVN
LagoLearn Ltd

Published by:

British Small Animal Veterinary Association
Woodrow House, 1 Telford Way,
Waterwells Business Park, Quedgeley,
Gloucester GL2 2AB

A Company Limited by Guarantee in England
Registered Company No. 2837793
Registered as a Charity

A catalogue record for this book is available from the British Library.

ISBN 978-1-910443-78-1

The publishers, editors and contributors cannot take responsibility for information provided on dosages and methods of application of drugs mentioned or referred to in this publication. Details of this kind must be verified in each case by individual users from up-to-date literature published by the manufacturers or suppliers of those drugs. Veterinary surgeons are reminded that in each case they must follow all appropriate national legislation and regulations (for example, in the United Kingdom, the prescribing cascade) from time to time in force.

Save 15% off the digital version of this manual. By purchasing this print edition we are pleased to offer you a reduced price on online access at www.bsavalibrary.com
Enter offer code 15PVW922 on checkout

Please note the discount only applies to a purchase of the full online version of the *BSAVA Manual of Practical Veterinary Welfare* via **www.bsavalibrary.com**. The discount will be taken off the BSAVA member price or full price, depending on your member status. The discount code is for a single purchase of the online version and is for your personal use only. If you do not already have a login for the BSAVA website, you will need to register in order to make a purchase.

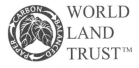

Printed in the UK by Cambrian Printers Ltd, Pontllanfraith NP12 2YA
Printed on ECF paper made from sustainable forests

Carbon Balancing is delivered by World Land Trust, an international conservation charity, who protects the world's most biologically important and threatened habitats acre by acre. Their Carbon Balanced Programme offsets emissions through the purchase and preservation of high conservation value forests.

Titles in the BSAVA Manuals series

Manual of Avian Practice: A Foundation Manual
Manual of Backyard Poultry Medicine and Surgery
Manual of Canine & Feline Abdominal Imaging
Manual of Canine & Feline Abdominal Surgery
Manual of Canine & Feline Advanced Veterinary Nursing
Manual of Canine & Feline Anaesthesia and Analgesia
Manual of Canine & Feline Behavioural Medicine
Manual of Canine & Feline Cardiorespiratory Medicine
Manual of Canine & Feline Clinical Pathology
Manual of Canine & Feline Dentistry and Oral Surgery
Manual of Canine & Feline Dermatology
Manual of Canine & Feline Emergency and Critical Care
Manual of Canine & Feline Endocrinology
Manual of Canine & Feline Endoscopy and Endosurgery
Manual of Canine & Feline Fracture Repair and Management
Manual of Canine & Feline Gastroenterology
Manual of Canine & Feline Haematology and Transfusion Medicine
Manual of Canine & Feline Head, Neck and Thoracic Surgery
Manual of Canine & Feline Musculoskeletal Disorders
Manual of Canine & Feline Musculoskeletal Imaging
Manual of Canine & Feline Nephrology and Urology
Manual of Canine & Feline Neurology
Manual of Canine & Feline Oncology
Manual of Canine & Feline Ophthalmology
Manual of Canine & Feline Radiography and Radiology: A Foundation Manual
Manual of Canine & Feline Rehabilitation, Supportive and Palliative Care: Case Studies in Patient Management
Manual of Canine & Feline Reproduction and Neonatology
Manual of Canine & Feline Shelter Medicine: Principles of Health and Welfare in a Multi-animal Environment
Manual of Canine & Feline Surgical Principles: A Foundation Manual
Manual of Canine & Feline Thoracic Imaging
Manual of Canine & Feline Ultrasonography
Manual of Canine & Feline Wound Management and Reconstruction
Manual of Canine Practice: A Foundation Manual
Manual of Exotic Pet and Wildlife Nursing
Manual of Exotic Pets: A Foundation Manual
Manual of Feline Practice: A Foundation Manual
Manual of Ornamental Fish
Manual of Practical Animal Care
Manual of Practical Veterinary Nursing
Manual of Practical Veterinary Welfare
Manual of Psittacine Birds
Manual of Rabbit Medicine
Manual of Rabbit Surgery, Dentistry and Imaging
Manual of Raptors, Pigeons and Passerine Birds
Manual of Reptiles
Manual of Rodents and Ferrets
Manual of Small Animal Practice Management and Development
Manual of Wildlife Casualties

For further information on these and all BSAVA publications, please visit our website:
www.bsava.com

Foreword

As understanding of animal sentience and its implications is coming to the fore – the evidence for animal pleasures, pains, needs and wants, and what this means for the ethical use and treatment of animals – so the veterinary professions are moving to help create a better world for animals. Prioritising animal welfare has been a longstanding obligation towards animals under our care, but we now recognise that our professional duty is wider; it includes identifying and facilitating solutions to the root causes of welfare problems.

While some advocacy for improved animal welfare is through national policy and lobbying, it also finds expression in the daily actions of practising vets and vet nurses and their wider teams. A culture of animal welfare advocacy is as much about, for example, minimal-stress handling, informed quality of life assessment, and ethical decision-making, as it is about seeking new laws. The publication of this latest BSAVA Manual underscores this and supports delivery.

Fittingly, this is the first BSAVA Manual to be led by veterinary nurses. While animal welfare advocacy is a shared veterinary responsibility, veterinary nurses are well recognised for being particularly effective and motivated animal welfare ambassadors. I have known and admired the Editors, Matthew Rendle and Jo Hinde-Megarity, for several years, and they have gathered a team of similarly eminent chapter authors. Along with a host of resources to support animal welfare advancement, the Manual also covers the critical importance of self-care for veterinary teams and the One Health links between animals, people and the environment.

Implementing animal welfare policies and activities in a range of settings including clinics, zoos, research and education facilities, and more can improve patient welfare, client satisfaction, staff morale, staff health and safety, and professional reputation. This valuable book will make a significant contribution to helping ensure all of these benefits are realised.

Dr Sean Wensley
BVSc MSc FRCVS
Past President, British Veterinary Association
Chair of Animal Welfare Working Group, Federation of Veterinarians of Europe

Preface

Awareness of animal sentience and welfare continues to grow in parallel with that of human mental health. The BSAVA Manuals aim to provide practical information; this new title joins their ranks as part of a trend in recognizing the importance of a holistic approach to animal health and how this is symbiotic with the One Health movement.

As experienced veterinary nurses that have worked and volunteered in various roles where animal care has been provided, we were deeply concerned by the apparent lack of regard given to the importance of welfare and found that the differences between welfare and ethics were generally not well understood. Having identified this knowledge gap, we contacted the BSAVA who were thankfully very supportive of the idea to create a manual that focuses on both the theory and the practical ways that welfare can be improved.

When we started scoping the topics to be covered in this manual it very quickly became apparent that as well as the obvious areas such as One Health, training and enrichment, it would be essential to cover areas that are not often associated with animal welfare such as nutrition, and human health and wellbeing.

It was important to us to provide practical ways of assessing welfare that can be documented in a quantifiable and non-emotive way that ensures optimal care is provided at all life stages for all species. Sadly, often non-evidence-based opinions and time pressures result in animals' welfare being repeatedly compromised. All too quickly this suboptimal care can become normalized, which then has profound detrimental effects on not only the animals, but the care givers too.

Undertaking welfare assessments should always be at the forefront of the care we provide regardless of the environment, species and resources available. It is also vital to understand that just providing environmental enrichment does not mitigate poor welfare. A wealth of theoretical information is already available, but compromises are often made in its practical application. This manual includes essential evidence-based information that enables readers to provide a truly holistic approach to the animals under their care, their colleagues and themselves.

We would like to give a heartfelt thanks to all the amazing authors we have collaborated with on this manual. Their diversity, passion and dedication has helped our initial vision come to life and will have a long-lasting positive effect on welfare.

Being in a position to care for animals is a huge honour and responsibility. We recognize that the levels of welfare we can provide are not always perfect; however, we must strive to improve our understanding, interrogate misconceptions and challenge beliefs as this will always lead to the improvement of welfare for all.

Matthew Rendle and Jo Hinde-Megarity
July 2022

Chapter 1

Animal ethics and welfare

James Yeates

Introduction

Context for readers

This manual is about 'practical veterinary welfare'. By being practical, it is all about ethics, which is best characterized as 'practical wisdom' (with some disagreement over what is 'wise'). Veterinary clinical work is practical insofar as it is all about making decisions to achieve some good. More precisely, the purpose of veterinary practice is arguably all about animal welfare, insofar as we make (and implement) decisions to make animals better (with some disagreement over what is 'better' and what is 'welfare'). This purpose is achieved alongside a whole raft of other considerations, including what is good for clients, what kind of professionals we should be and concern for nature.

Given these multiple concerns, veterinary staff are sometimes (perhaps often) faced with circumstances that are morally challenging. For example:

- An owner asks us to put a healthy animal to sleep or refuses to allow us to euthanase a suffering patient
- An owner asks us to provide a treatment that we think 'goes too far' (e.g. chronic case management or surgery) or is unwilling to fund optimal or even basic treatment (e.g. pyometra surgery)
- We are presented with problems that owners have caused or could have prevented (e.g. dystocia or fear-related aggression)
- The best treatment option for a patient could also perpetuate wider problems, such as inherited disorders or antimicrobial resistance
- We disagree with colleagues or our boss about what is the best treatment for our patient
- Our practice rules prevent us from providing emergency treatment without payment
- Our professional rules appear to forbid us from reporting owners we suspect may have committed criminal offences
- We are asked to officially give an opinion about matters of which we are unsure.

Such circumstances can be clinically and technically difficult, requiring sophisticated medical and communication skills. They can be emotionally difficult, causing us (and others) stress, anger and guilt. They can also be ethically difficult, in the sense of working out what one should do. Fortunately, while ethics most obviously helps with the last point, developing one's ethical skills and understanding can help with all three.

Ethics *versus* welfare

Ethics (and morality) relate to standards or norms ('normative'). It involves the word 'ought' or 'should' more than 'is' (somewhat like law, logic and grammar). Ethics is thinking about what one should do (and when, how and to whom). This includes what one should say, how one should judge oneself and others, and how one should live one's life. In working out the 'what', 'when', 'how' and 'to whom', it often focuses on, and ideally clarifies, the 'why' – what facts and reasons should prompt us to live and behave in certain ways. So ethics is about the meaning of life.

Animal welfare is essentially about what is good (or bad) for animals. The term is somewhat contested, with multiple definitions of what is welfare and/or good for animals (Hetts et al., 2005; Nordenfelt, 2006; McMillan and Yeates, 2019). These definitions cover various broad approaches, particularly in relation to the relevance of animals' subjective mental states and naturalness (Barnard and Hurst, 1996; Duncan and Fraser, 1997; Fraser et al., 1997; Appleby and Sandøe, 2002; Appleby and Stokes, 2008). Nevertheless, we can state that animal welfare is about what is important for animals, from their point of view. (It is, therefore, not what is important about animals, i.e. for their owners.)

Health is an overarching individualistic concept incorporating many aspects of an animal's genetics, physical state and mental state. In comparison to 'welfare', veterinary professionals seem not to worry too much about the nuances of what 'health' means, although it can be understood in many different ways (e.g. as what is statistically normal or in terms of particular valued functions). There could also be cases where some short-term impacts on health seem good overall (e.g. a mild infection may lead to subsequent immunity). Health is not a separate concern to welfare. Certainly they are related, and often the best approach is to consider health as part of welfare. In practice, there is no real need to define the relationship between the two concepts so long as: (a) one is considering health in a way that relates it to the animal (rather than, say, reproductive health); and (b) one does not then convert concern for welfare into concern solely for health. We should avoid considering them both together and then only focusing on health.

Ethics and welfare are two different, if inter-related, ideas. Ethics is about decisions and actions; animal welfare is about states. Both relate to questions of what has value: animal welfare concerns what has value for animals; ethics concerns what has value *per se*. Of course, they also combine. Put simply, we should be morally motivated to improve animal welfare. How they combine is a more complicated question. There is a risk of assuming that concern for animal welfare inevitably goes with some aim for moderate, incremental improvements or some utilitarian approach – as opposed to 'animal rights' views (and this assumption comes from both animal welfarists' and animal rights theorists' camps). This assumption is wrong: one could think animals have rights based on welfare (e.g. to avoid extreme suffering or torture).

Legal, professional and moral responsibilities

Types of responsibility

Veterinary nurses and surgeons face a variety of potential legal, professional and ethical responsibilities linked to a variety of relationships (Figure 1.1).

Party	Relationships
Veterinary staff	• Patient (animal in hospital) • Client (person procuring services) • Other veterinary surgeons/nurses (colleagues) • Practice owner (partner, employer) • Other people (fellow members of society, provide licence to practice, legislators)
Patient	• Veterinary staff, practice owner (provider of care) • Client (owner)
Client	• Patient (property/companion) • Veterinary staff, practice owner (providers of services) • Other people (fellow members of society)
Practice owner	• Patient (animal in hospital) • Client (person procuring services, customer) • Veterinary staff (partners, employees) • Other people (fellow members of society, owed corporate social responsibility)

1.1 Relationships encountered by veterinary surgeons and nurses in practice.

Criminal obligations

Criminal obligations concern what a given country's legislation prohibits (e.g. stealing) or mandates (e.g. taking reasonable steps to ensure animals' needs are met). They are often framed as negative prohibitions (i.e. 'Do not...') – even many laws that seem to mandate actions are actually prohibitions insofar as they proscribe doing something without also doing something else; for example, keeping an animal without caring for it, serving clients without protecting their health and safety, or earning money without paying taxes. Criminal laws tend to be minimalistic in that they leave a wide range of freedom as to what one does, within the legal parameters. Non-compliance can result in punishment (e.g. fines or imprisonment).

Civil obligations

Civil obligations tend to be related to particular relationships. In a veterinary context, these tend to be employment (i.e. with colleagues, employers and employees) and 'commercial' relationships (i.e. with clients and suppliers). Examples of areas that civil obligations address include negligence, battery, contract breaches and unfair dismissal. In many cases, civil law is about redressing balances if one person harms another or fails to fulfil an undertaking. Non-compliance consequently often leads to compensation to rebalance those harms.

Regulatory requirements

Regulatory requirements concern compliance with the veterinary profession's rules or codes of conduct. Sometimes these rules underscore legal obligations, although they may alter them somewhat; for example, a professional rule on consent goes beyond redressing any financial harm and makes treating an animal a risk of potential sanctions. Regulatory rules can vary from very precise rules (e.g. prohibiting kidney transplantation) to broad principles to consider. As such, their implications can seem more or less restrictive and more or less clear. These rules could be seen as mere 'etiquette' or 'club rules' (i.e. conditions of membership), which are more self-protective than moral *per se* (but hopefully not immoral). Alternatively, they might be seen as ways to make morality pay (or, more accurately, make immorality risky) because those who create risks for the whole profession (e.g. reduced public trust) thereby also face personal risks (e.g. professional sanctions).

Professional undertakings

Professional undertakings are those to which we subscribe on becoming, or remaining, part of a profession (e.g. by making a declarative promise to follow certain rules or authoritative bodies). This could be because society gives us exclusive licence to practice on the expectation of us meeting certain standards in how we treat animals and clients. This could also be because coordination, consistency and reliability would help all veterinary surgeons (veterinarians) overall (even if it means individual clinicians foregoing some benefits in particular cases; for example, by reducing competition, introducing minimum standards of care or prohibiting practices such as devocalization or declawing.

Absolute moral duties

Absolute moral duties may relate to rules that one should always follow in every case to which they are relevant. In one sense, all ethical approaches have at least one rule (i.e. 'Thou shalt use this ethical approach'); for example, one might apply the single rule: 'Always do whatever leads to the most valuable outcomes overall for everyone affected'. Other theories apply multiple rules directly and explicitly. These can be positive ('You must') or negative ('You must not'). One might consider such duties imply others' rights (e.g. a duty not to kill corresponds to a right not to be killed). Moral duties can be adopted by following an ethically authoritative source (e.g. God), defined by logical analysis (e.g. it is paradoxical to lie), or they can be self-imposed rules (e.g. by making a promise).

General moral principles

General moral principles may be less prescriptive than absolute moral duties insofar as each person should have some flexibility in their decision-making (e.g. everyone who can afford it should give to charity, but each person may choose which causes). Some principles may be rules of thumb, which each person has to balance in each case. For example, Beauchamp and Childress (2009) suggested four principles that should be applied in every case:

- Beneficence (doing good)
- Non-maleficence (not harming)
- Justice (being fair and respecting rights)
- Respect for autonomy (respecting others' ability to make independent decisions).

Interpersonal undertakings

Interpersonal undertakings occur when practitioners agree various obligations with others, such as contractual relationships with clients, employers and employees. More widely, one could argue that veterinary professionals have an agreement with the rest of society to protect animals and public health, in return for the privilege of a licence to practice veterinary medicine. One should arguably fulfil those expectations (unless it is otherwise immoral to do so). However, this approach on its own does not necessarily provide any direct moral responsibilities to animals (or humans) who cannot make such agreements. Indeed, many ethical responsibilities can be framed as responsibilities to someone (e.g. patients, clients, employees or colleagues).

Personal development requirements

Personal development requirements suggest that we should be trying to be the best we can, as individuals. This goes beyond any single action, into considerations of wider character or broad virtues. Some ethical responsibilities are negative: for example, not to harm any patients, regardless of the benefits to other animals, clients or oneself. Other responsibilities are positive: for example, to monitor and mitigate pain in hospitalized patients. These requirements might be reframed as responsibilities to others (e.g. the responsibility to ensure one is competent to provide treatments is essentially a responsibility to future patients and/or to current patients who need treatments beyond one's abilities).

Prudential requirements

Prudential requirements perhaps cover what is good for oneself. These can be considered morally irrelevant in as much as morality relates to other people, and normally concern avoiding being overly biased towards one's own self-interest. Alternatively, these could be considered ethically relevant insofar as veterinary surgeons and nurses are stakeholders as important morally as anyone else and, at the least, should not be expected to be self-sacrificial martyrs or saints, depriving or harming themselves in all cases. In addition, the clinician's own interests may align with ethical responsibilities; for example, gaining a specialist qualification might mean they can help patients better, while losing their ability to practice (e.g. through practice financial unsustainability or loss of licence) could mean many patients do not receive needed veterinary care.

Ethical *versus* professional responsibilities

Legal and regulatory obligations do not capture everything that we might think ethically important. For example, they often miss out concerns such as lying (outside of specific cases of fraud or perjury), infidelity and being offensive, obnoxious or ungrateful. Furthermore, legal and regulatory duties do not necessarily take precedence over ethical concerns (e.g. one might think it morally right, but legally wrong, to exceed the speed limit *en route* to an emergency call-out, or one might think it morally right to give a patient the necessary treatment and risk having to compensate an absent or irresponsible owner for 'damage' to their property; although it should be noted that this does not constitute legal advice or sanction to do so).

Professional responsibilities can be thought of as a combination of our legal and regulatory duties, our ethical responsibilities to one another as colleagues, and a presumption that we will fulfil the moral expectations of society. One can also think of professional responsibilities as duties to make expert ethical judgements in cases, rather than simply following predetermined rules set by someone else. At the same time, being a professional goes beyond each individual's personal moral views, and involves living up to a collective set of norms. Perhaps most of all, it involves relinquishing some opportunities to benefit personally in our interactions with our clients, in ways that arguably do not apply to 'non-professional' trades and services, where market forces might be thought to ensure everyone benefits from mutually beneficial transactions, and where principles of *caveat emptor* ('buyer beware') may have some justification.

Challenges

This variety of interacting responsibilities presents a whole set of challenges for veterinary surgeons and nurses in practice.

Justification

We should be able to explain convincingly why particular responsibilities apply and should be followed. This requires that we think they have a good basis; for example, they are based on some form of authority, logic, fundamental values or social construct. It also requires that they are not outweighed by other responsibilities (except as part of a wider ethical approach). Furthermore, the responsibilities need to be justified themselves, and that justification also needs to be justifiable – one cannot just use any weak argument to back up an ethical view; it must be one that can be defended (*ad infinitum*).

Interpretation

All responsibilities need interpretation, in terms of when they apply (i.e. to whom and to which cases) and how to apply them. For example, does a duty of confidentiality apply to all client data; does it prohibit sharing information with colleagues or other practices; does it apply to sharing anonymized or pseudonymized data; does it exclude informing authorities about suspected offences and, if so, which ones? We need to consider the scope of application of each responsibility, what it means in various cases, what exclusions it has, and whether (and when, and how) it can be overridden by other responsibilities.

Filling in the gaps

Many types of responsibilities do not tell us what to do in every case (especially legal, regulatory and moral rules), answer every question of what we should do in practice, or include adequate consideration of everything that is important. There might, therefore, be cases where particular rules, if taken alone and/or applied inappropriately, could make us disregard important ethical concerns. For example, a professional rule about confidentiality or consent, if considered alone, could be taken to imply that we should do nothing about suspected animal cruelty.

Conflict

One challenge for veterinary nurses and surgeons is what to do when different rules or principles conflict so that one faces a choice of which to break. We could try to limit the scope of our principles so they do not conflict (e.g. limit our respect for clients' or colleagues' autonomy so that it does not include allowing them to harm animals). However, this could require very complicated rules to cover every possible exception. Alternatively, it could be said that one should balance the different principles (e.g. client confidentiality and patient protection). However, one then arguably needs some overarching rule to follow to do such balancing (e.g. do whatever will best protect patients) – in which case, perhaps one should just use that rule as a single rule anyway.

Veterinary nurses and surgeons may perhaps face a particular type of conflict where no option seems morally right. Such moral dilemmas can cause genuine moral distress (in addition to the unease and stress of merely complicated and high-pressured decisions that we need to make every day). It might be argued that such dilemmas demonstrate the limitations of ethics: if it cannot decide what to do in every case, then what is the point of it? Alternatively, one might argue that there are no real moral dilemmas insofar as every case has a right or best option – except where previous action has eliminated the acceptable options and we are left only with bad ones.

Indeed, there is an argument that many of our morally difficult cases are due to our previous decisions. For example, if one promises a client a treatment and later thinks it may be harmful, one then faces a choice between breaking a promise to the client and harming a patient. Many difficult cases are due to the previous actions of others, in particular owners (e.g. breeding dogs at risk of dystocia). Regardless of one's views on whether moral dilemmas are possible, one might still choose the 'lesser of two evils' in each situation. Indeed, veterinary practice is arguably all about making the best of bad situations. In addition, by predicting these cases, they can sometimes be prevented or avoided.

Making ethical decisions in practice

How should a veterinary professional work out what to do in a given situation? There are various methods.

Moral intuition

This might be based on feelings (e.g. pity, distaste) or intuitive conscience. This approach can be fast, efficient and authentic. The key challenge is to ensure that these intuitions are based on all relevant concerns and environmental cues and avoid bias due to morally irrelevant cues (e.g. prejudicial presumptions), contexts (e.g. overall mood that day) or excessive self-interest, partiality or pressure from others (e.g. clients) – suggesting that a degree of emotional self-control and intelligence are required. Intuitions and emotions are also hard to justify or discuss with others who do not share the same emotional response profile.

Doing what someone else wants

One could follow instructions from someone considered to be morally authoritative in the particular issue (e.g. boss, legislators, regulators or clients). The challenge here is to determine why that authority is morally valid (which is itself a moral question that, ideally, should not be answered by asking someone else). Another challenge is what to do when an instruction seems otherwise immoral.

Consistency across cases

A veterinary professional's decision could be based on what they, or someone else, has (or should have) done before. Consistency across cases may be impartial and fair, which might be right for similar species (e.g. no tetrapods should be caused pain or fear without justification). It also allows some idea of reciprocity (i.e. I should treat others how they should treat me). However, it can be challenging to determine which similarities and differences between cases justify or preclude such comparisons (e.g. when is species or relationship relevant?), especially since a case or action could be described in many different ways (e.g. 'euthanasia of a suffering animal', 'killing a living being', 'murdering someone who does not want to die' and 'injecting some blue liquid'). So some rules are needed to determine which comparisons to draw (which can be copied from other cases, but at the risk of infinite regress). In addition, different comparisons or consistencies might seem fair or unfair, depending on individual definition (Figure 1.2). Whatever has happened before, it is better to change than to keep consistently treating more people or animals wrongly.

Broad definition	Examples	Challenges
Equally	Identical pay for male and female employees	This seems impossible (especially on a global, cross-species scale) Different people and animals have different needs, so what does 'equal' mean in this context?
Above minimum standards	No animal should undergo severe suffering or have a life worth avoiding	Which minimum standards and how should they be set? What about when going beyond this minimum standard would have very significant effects on others?
According to some consistent and impartial processes	Fair criminal trial Performance-related pay	Consistency could be consistently wrong Sometimes perhaps one should not be impartial (e.g. loyalty to family and colleagues)

1.2 Definitions of the terminology used in some approaches to fairness.

Logically applying criteria

Categories could be defined and each situation assigned to the category that it 'fits'. For example, start with identifying the situation, i.e. 'stealing' or 'murder' and then work out if taking some money or killing a patient in a given case would fit that category. This approach can avoid emotional bias, and some have argued that ethics is all about logic. The challenge for this approach is to come up with a coherent, comprehensive and practical set of criteria that covers all possible cases.

Conforming to type

One could try to conform to particular archetypes: for example, the ideal human or the perfect veterinary professional–client relationship. This approach is perhaps best known in virtue ethics, in which one tries to embody particular character traits (e.g. courage, temperance, wisdom and justice) and avoid others (e.g. pride, greed and sloth), as well as employ technical veterinary skills (e.g. clinical reasoning, welfare assessment and communication). This approach can be a useful, if vague, way to think about our lives holistically – and perhaps to avoid the 'inhumanity' of more prescriptive approaches. However, it is not necessarily easy to agree what combination of virtues is ideal for different people (e.g. veterinary surgeon *versus* nurse) and contexts (e.g. work *versus* home), in particular when different virtues would suggest different actions (e.g. when kindness to a patient would cause embarrassment to a client). It could be assumed that all extremes should be avoided (e.g. dogmatism and weakness), but this does not necessarily help find the ideal balance. Developing a particular skill (e.g. wisdom or praxis) could help to make such balances, but this needs careful definition. Virtuous people could be emulated, but criteria would be needed to choose them. Such balances, traits and role models could be defined in terms of something else (e.g. what outcomes they achieve or whether they fulfil our 'purpose'), but then decisions could just be made directly using that premise.

Predicting outcomes

Another important basis is what positive and negative outcomes could be caused or allowed to happen (Figure 1.3). One could try to calculate what would achieve the best overall outcome (e.g. maximal enjoyment and minimal suffering) across everyone affected (regardless of species,

deservingness or relationship with them) so that harms to one individual may be 'outweighed' by greater benefits to others. A challenge with this approach is that it may seem unfair (e.g. it might be right to help owners exploit their animals, or steal from one owner to help another) or inhuman (e.g. in coldly calculating outcomes). Another challenge is the sheer complexity and uncertainty of such predictive evaluations (see below).

Bringing it together

Philosophers have generated a number of ethical theories that are based on many of these ideas (Figure 1.4). In most cases, these theories apply one idea, or a restricted selection, from each section to all cases. For example, classical (hedonic) utilitarianism considers all stakeholders, thinks only mental experiences matter, infers experiences from the animal's behaviour and physical measurements, and makes evaluative comparisons using implied scales – thereby predicting outcomes and calculating their overall value. However, applying theories 'off-the-peg' in every case can seem overly inflexible or run contrary to our intuitions, which might consider multiple states matter. We might, therefore, use methods that draw on multiple theories or concepts. For example, the ethical matrix considers the four principles of respect for autonomy, non-maleficence, beneficence and justice with regard to all stakeholders (Figure 1.5).

Ways one affects outcomes	Examples
Apportion (take from or give to)	• Remove body parts and fluids from patients • Administer medicines and diets • Take money from clients and employers • Pay employees and provide them with facilities • Provide knowledge and guidance
Alter (damage or enhance)	• Change animals' anatomy, physiology and behaviour, altering their functional performance • Change clients' and colleagues' (and our) minds and intentions
Effect (cause or prevent)	• Cause or prevent patients to suffer or to experience enjoyment • This causation may be indirect, for example through the inputs one provides
Regulate (improve or restrict agency)	• Improve animals' capability to exercise or interact socially (e.g. by repairing fractures) • Restrict their opportunity to move or make choices (e.g. by hospitalization) • Improve clients' capability to help their animals (e.g. through training) • Restrict colleagues' freedom (e.g. through regulation or practice policies)
No active impact (do nothing)	• Doing nothing may still have an impact • For example, not treating a patient may have an impact on their suffering or quality of life

1.3 Impacts of our actions on patients, clients and colleagues.

Theory	(Approximate) description
Direct/act utilitarianism	Doing whatever leads to the optimal outcomes in each and every case, based on the effects on affect (hedonic utilitarianism) or motivations (preference utilitarianism) or some more objective value (ideal utilitarianism) (from 'utility')
Indirect utilitarianism	Following whatever moral approach would overall lead to the best outcomes (even when another act could lead to better outcomes in a particular case)
Rights theories	Respecting actual or theoretical claims (and secondary claims in relation to those claims) of individuals to be treated in particular ways
Deontologies	Following particular rules on what actions to perform (from the Greek 'deon', meaning duty)
Contractarianism	Adhering to social, historical or metaphorical reciprocal agreements between people on how they will treat one another
Virtue ethics	Trying to live by particular moral character traits
Relational ethics	Determining ethical decisions based on interpersonal relationships
Casuistry	Case-based reasoning, using paradigms or precedents

1.4 Ethical theories that can be applied to making decisions in small animal practice.

Stakeholder	Principles			
	Respect for autonomy	*Non-maleficence*	*Beneficence*	*Justice*
Patient	Improving ability to achieve motivations; allowing animals to fulfil their 'purpose'	Avoiding iatrogenic harms	Preventing or curing disease or other suffering; allowing enjoyment (e.g. from longer life)	Not harming one animal to help another; ensuring animals' lives are not worse due to their different owners; ensuring all animals are above minimum standards
Client	What client wants for their animal and money	Not lying, stealing or reporting	Improving wellbeing, enjoyment or profit	Not harming one client to help another; helping the financially worst off clients
Colleague	Allowing clinical autonomy; improving technical abilities	Not bullying or competing	Helping with work–life balance; helping career development; pay	Avoiding gender pay gaps; avoiding discrimination; performance-related pay
Practice owner	Respecting practice management decisions	Not lying or making false claims; not stealing	Working above one's job's worth	Ensuring adequate returns on an investment

1.5 Applying the ethical matrix to the various stakeholders that may be encountered in veterinary practice.

What matters to animals and others?

Types of outcomes that matter

Ethics requires the consideration of other people who might be affected by our actions. Veterinary practice involves a three (or more)-way moral relationship between the veterinary professional, patient and client. (In comparison, in human medicine, the client and patient are the same person.) In addition to these primary stakeholders, others who may be indirectly affected by our treatment decisions might be considered (Figure 1.6). Others that might be conceived as stakeholders include 'society', 'the profession' and 'the environment', although these could be thought of as aggregates of millions of individual stakeholders.

A useful starting point is to determine what is important to those stakeholders: what should we (all else being equal) try to positively achieve or negatively avoid? For each stakeholder, there are various states of events that could be considered worth avoiding or achieving (Figure 1.7). Some states are directly important in themselves; others are important because they cause, contribute to, or are symptoms of others' states.

Outcomes for stakeholders depend on their environment, as this can affect their emotional experiences, their physical and mental capabilities, and their behavioural opportunities. Environmental factors can be beneficial or harmful (or irrelevant, e.g. hair colour, and sometimes species, breed, sex and age). This can depend on the context, the individual and the combination of factors (e.g. the balance of novelty and predictability), which can interact with one another (e.g. the presence of conspecific competition may reduce the availability of resources to an individual). Indeed, animals and humans and their

Stakeholder	How they may be affected
Patient	• Relieved of suffering • Caused iatrogenic harms
Client	• Improved relationship with their animal • Property protected • Fees charged
Veterinary surgeon or nurse	• Satisfaction, stress and guilt • Pressure from clients and others
Colleague	• Camaraderie, support
Practice owner	• Profit and equity growth

1.6 How stakeholders can be affected by treatment decisions.

Factors	Examples
External inputs	• Physical and chemical environment • Microbiological environments • Social environment • Diet, veterinary treatment
Internal factors	• Genotype, epigenetic and ontogenetic factors • Immune status • Personality and preferences
Observable biology	• Functioning (including stress) • Physical and mental health (capabilities) • Survival • Behaviour
Mental experiences	• Negative affective states (e.g. pain, frustration) • Pleasant affective states (e.g. pleasure)
Agency	• Fulfilment of preferences/motivations (including choice and control)

1.7 Factors that are important for patients as key stakeholders.

environments are constantly affecting one another (so it is an oversimplification to argue of animals and their socio-physical environments as two separate factors).

Individuals can often achieve outcomes for themselves by fulfilling their preferences or motivations (in clinical practice one can use various closely-related concepts such as motivation, volition, preferences and desires). This can depend on:

- What motivations an individual has. Some motivations may be inappropriate in particular conditions: for example, if they are maladaptive (e.g. a desire to fight or breed can risk injury or infection) or immoral (e.g. a desire to harm one's pet)
- Whether the animal has a meaningful opportunity to make a choice and exercise some control
- Whether the animal has the capability to perform their behaviour and achieve their aim.

Human autonomy (the ability and freedom to make and fulfil decisions) tends to be respected more than that of domestic animals, for example in terms of client consent for treatment and the veterinary surgeon's clinical autonomy. Clients often do want to be able to exercise autonomous choice and control over what happens to their pet, lifestyle, money or other property. However, sometimes, clients may prefer not to have to make decisions, or implement them. Owners' motivations may be affected by their capabilities and opportunities (which can also affect their behaviour directly, as above), which one can sometimes improve.

In many cases, as well as the individual themselves, stakeholders' inputs are also affected – or almost completely determined – by the behaviour of others (e.g. the standard of care provided by owners or veterinary professionals). These, in turn, may depend on those individuals' opportunities, capabilities and motivations – which need to come together in the right combination (e.g. 'loving' motivations can be harmful if they prevent necessary euthanasia). So what happens to our patients depends on their motivations, capabilities and opportunities, which in turn depend on their environment, including their owners' motivations, capabilities and opportunities, which depend on their environments.

One can also think of how well an animal or person is faring in terms of whether it is flourishing. This not only goes beyond 'coping' but suggests some objective (if not easily measured) concept of what an ideal life should be like. This might be in terms of naturalness, or in terms of morality (i.e. an immoral life is bad for that person, however enjoyable it might be). In a similar vein, one might think of the integrity of an animal or person, both physically (e.g. not having body parts removed) and morally (e.g. having consistent moral views and behaviours). For example, one could argue that our clients' flourishing is not simply (but arguably includes) each individual's aggregated subjective emotional experiences, but also some idea of whether they are 'doing well' or being a 'good person'. Similarly, one could argue that to flourish as a veterinary professional is not to make money or publish papers, but to maximally help animals (perhaps unlike other private or research enterprises), thereby fulfilling our public undertakings.

It could be argued that being moral, in itself, matters to us: to be a good person, to act ethically, and to make a difference in the world. Being virtuous and doing good is necessary for our flourishing as humans. It could be argued that our actions are sometimes more important than the outcomes; for example, if it is less bad to let someone else hurt an animal than to do so oneself – perhaps even if the latter suffering would be less severe. Alternatively, one could argue that our morality should be more pragmatic – doing whatever leads to the best outcomes – but this could feel like one is 'sacrificing' one's standards or integrity (unless, of course, one's moral standards are to be pragmatic). As such, it could be argued that client or clinical autonomy is good only when it allows freedom to perform morally acceptable actions.

It is, therefore, particularly helpful to decide how much we should consider our own interests. One could argue that ethics is about doing right by others, potentially prioritizing helping (or not harming) others above doing what is best for ourselves (i.e. veterinary surgeons should decide what is best for clients and patients, with income being a fortuitous side effect). However, one could also argue that we should ensure our decisions do not (normally and/or overly) harm ourselves, at least above some limits of self-sacrifice, as we are as deserving as anyone else providing professional services. We might think we should factor in concerns such as health and safety, and our mental health and wellbeing, but not factors such as profit, feeling 'heroic' or popularity.

Forms of animal welfare assessment

Broadly speaking, we might then make assessments in one of three forms:

- Criteria-based assessments
- Relative comparisons
- Cardinal measures.

Criteria-based assessments

Sometimes we assess a state as 'x' or 'y', usually according to some predetermined criteria, such as whether they are over a benchmark (e.g. target bodyweight). A key challenge with this approach is, where we are using categorical approaches to continuous data, there are no 'natural' cut-off points (Mendl, 1991).

Relative comparisons

Another approach is to assess each animal's state by comparison with another state. One could compare an animal's state with previous states of the same animal (e.g. growth rate or habituation) to identify improvement or deterioration; this can ensure the assessment is suitable for each individual's idiosyncrasies (e.g. preferences or comorbidities) and can be particularly useful for species for which there is limited knowledge, or individuals that are abnormal to start with. Alternatively, an animal's (or group's) state could be compared with that of other animals (e.g. assessing abnormal behaviour or tachycardia). However, this approach risks us jumping to conclusions. All one can conclude from a difference or abnormality is that an animal's welfare could be different or abnormal – it could be better or worse off (or the difference could be irrelevant). This approach also runs the risk of normalizing problems that are common (e.g. breed-related conditions).

Cardinal measures

Numerical scales can be employed for some measures, including physical parameters (e.g. biochemical concentrations, bodyweight and longevity), or numerical scores can be used to record subjective assessments (e.g. Likert continua). One might try to score animals' experiences based on their perceived intensity, duration, frequency and probability. However, while the last three arguably have natural quantities, scoring the intensity of another's experiences is perhaps impossible. Furthermore, one might argue that, since not everything that matters can be measured (or at least we have not yet developed methods to do so), this approach risks missing important states.

Challenges

The plethora of ways in which one can make assessments and decisions can be daunting. It should make us more humble about our own moral views and more tolerant of others'. However, it is important to not give up on ethics just because it is complicated (any more than we should wash our hands of difficult clinical cases).

One key challenge in assessing welfare (in addition to those associated with working out what matters and observing whether it has occurred) is bringing all observations, inferences and assessments together. The main challenge is that what matters seems to include multiple types of state (Figure 1.8). Furthermore, an overall assessment requires the comparison of positive states (e.g. pleasant feelings) with undesirable ones (e.g. pain) (Dawkins, 1990). Given this complexity, one can argue that there is no perfect single method for assessing welfare.

An aggregative approach presents particular challenges concerning how to meaningfully combine different domains that could involve very different concepts (e.g. how to relate a given experience of pain with a loss of bodily integrity) or very different assessment methods (e.g. measuring bodyweight *versus* behavioural latency).

Source	Definition of animal welfare
Broom (1986)	[An animal's] state as regards its attempts to cope with its environment
Dawkins (2006)	Is the animal healthy; does it get what it wants?
Duncan and Dawkins (1983)	The animal in complete mental and physical health, the animal in harmony with its environment, the animal able to adapt to an artificial environment provided by human beings without suffering, with the animal's feelings, somehow, taken into account
Mench (1998)	High level of biological functioning, freedom from suffering, and positive experiences
OIE Terrestrial Animal Health Code (2018)	Healthy, comfortable, well nourished, safe, is not suffering from unpleasant states such as pain, fear and distress, and is able to express behaviours that are important for its physical and mental state
Webster et al. (2004)	Fit and feeling good

1.8 There are a variety of approaches that can be taken for evaluating animal welfare.

This approach also presents challenges in how to compare the value of different factors (such as which is better: time spent playing or a cosy bed?) or different intensities or durations (such as which is worse: a week of mild pain or a day of severe pain?) – when there are no common 'units' for measurement. One approach is to use relative assessments of what would be acceptable or desirable trade-offs across quantifiable states (e.g. is a week of mild pain equivalent to a day of severe fear?). However, this approach still struggles to take into account the effects of interactions between different factors and cumulative effects over time.

An additional challenge for ethical approaches trying to predict welfare outcomes is that the future is uncertain: any given treatment could have multiple different sequelae (except perhaps euthanasia) and many of the 'facts' on which one bases predictions are statistical measures of frequency (e.g. incidence and mortality rates), so it cannot be known which subpopulation any given patient will be in. Furthermore, it can be difficult to predict what others will feel or want. Even if this approach is agreed upon, one faces the challenge of the sheer complexity of making such calculations, especially when one's predictions are uncertain (one could also factor in probability to our calculations, but this makes it more complicated still). Nevertheless, this approach could be useful when dealing with relatively simple cases (e.g. which analgesic agents would be better) or, conversely, really wide-scale problems (e.g. determining which veterinary policies would best protect animals). In such cases, veterinary surgeons and nurses can draw upon available evidence, but may still need to base some predictions on a more subjective 'confidence'.

Making animal welfare assessments

Broadly speaking, welfare assessments can be made in a number of ways (it should also be noted that the various methodologies can be combined):

- Direct observation
- Personal empathy
- Relating to oneself
- Inferring from behaviour and context
- Ask the individual
- Ask an expert.

Direct observation

Assessments can be based on pure observation of biological parameters (e.g. glucose concentrations or maintenance behaviour). However, this approach either assumes that such physical parameters are valuable in themselves, or requires (or implies) an additional step relating observations to what is important (e.g. animal's experiences).

Personal empathy

We could make intuitive assessments based on our emotional responses to observing animals. This approach sounds unscientific, but is very useful and powerful (and common) in practice. However, this approach may risk us using irrelevant or misleading cues (e.g. the aesthetics of a vivarium or visible blood). More importantly, this approach is probably insensitive to problems where people lack visibility or interspecific empathetic ability, or are insensitive to noticing normalized problems (e.g. common pedigree conformational issues). So veterinary professionals should endeavour to develop empathy (to empathize with wider ranges of emotional states in various circumstances, in people and animals who are very different to oneself).

Relating to oneself

As an extension of personal empathy, one could try to analogize from one's feelings and needs to those of other people and animals – to put oneself 'in their shoes'. This approach might be the basis for any inferences of others' mental states, and most domestic animals plausibly share somewhat similar feelings and needs (at a sufficiently generic level). However, it risks uncritically assuming similarities across individuals (and species).

Inferring from behaviour and context

Assuming that all domestic animals' behaviour is linked to their motivations, we can observe animals' contexts, neuroanatomy and behavioural responses and infer their preferences, needs and evaluation of current (e.g. 'pain-related' behaviours) and potential (i.e. depending on whether they appear to want to achieve or avoid them) outcomes. Indeed, we could give clients, colleagues or patients opportunities to fulfil those preferences directly, where this appears safe (for themselves and others) given our knowledge.

Ask the individual

Assuming some analogy that allows us to infer evaluations from other humans' verbal behaviour, we can of course ask people what they like, need and want. For most clients and colleagues (unlike animals), we can ask them to tell us how they are and what would be good for them, particularly in terms of mental experiences, agency and quality of life. One simply asks them, and takes their word for it. While veterinary nurses and surgeons can claim expertise in making such assessments for animals (at least relative to other humans' proxy evaluations of those animals), there is no similar basis to claim that 'we know best'. However, concepts of 'flourishing' that go beyond an individual's perception may allow some external objective assessment (e.g. we do not rely on an individual's assessment regarding whether they are acting morally).

Ask an expert

One could also ask other people to make proxy assessments, in particular clients and specialists. It could be argued at length as to who is best placed to assess patients' welfare. In general, we would expect owners to know what is individual, idiosyncratic and historical; while veterinary professionals will know what is general, normal and abnormal. One could try to assess patients' welfare together, drawing on the knowledge of the whole team: veterinary surgeon, nurse and owner. Alternatively, one could try to improve owners' assessment (e.g. by informing them about species-specific needs or behaviours) and then using their evaluation or *vice versa* (i.e. forming one's own assessment informed by owners' observations of the individual animal's preferences and normal behaviour).

Bringing it all together

All veterinary staff should use multiple methods to assess what matters to others. Several animal welfare frameworks consider multiple facets (e.g. Five Freedoms and Five Opportunities (Figure 1.9); for information on the Five Domains, see Chapter 2) and can help provide an overview. However, these qualitative approaches do not necessarily help us to make one overall evaluation of an animal's or a group's welfare, taking into consideration multiple individuals and/or multiple factors, except by using an intuitive view; one needs to construct or aggregate an overall evaluation (of the whole) based on multiple evaluations (of particular factors, domains or subpopulations). This still involves some subjective assessment (e.g. in making comparisons or scoring). Indeed, we would do well to remember that all our assessments, including for health, rely on some subjective and evaluative elements, either implicitly in the construction of the method or explicitly in its application. One can 'objectively' measure some aspects of some states, but for these to have importance, they need to be combined with some axiological assessments.

Five Freedoms and provisions	Five Opportunities and provisions
Freedom from hunger and thirst – by ready access to fresh water and a diet to maintain full health and vigour	Opportunity for (satisfaction of) dietary preferences – by provision of a varied diet from which to choose
Freedom from discomfort – by providing an appropriate environment and a comfortable resting area	Opportunity for control – by allowing the achievement of motivations that alter the animal's environment
Freedom from pain, injury and disease – by prevention or rapid diagnosis and treatment	Opportunity for pleasure, development and vitality – by providing enjoyable and beneficial interactions
Freedom and Opportunity to express normal behaviour – by providing sufficient space, proper facilities, and the company of the animal's own kind	
Freedom from fear and distress – by ensuring conditions and treatment which avoid mental suffering	Opportunity for interest and confidence – by providing conditions and human interactions that allow mental enjoyment

1.9 The Five Freedoms and Five Opportunities that form the basis of various animal welfare frameworks. Red = physical and mental biology; Green = experiences; Orange = agency; Blue = inputs.
(Adapted from Yeates, 2019)

How domesticity/captivity compromises welfare

Species and individual suitability as pets

Humans have kept companion animal species for at least 12,000 years for various reasons, including aesthetics, sport, hunting, profit, assistance, luck, status and companionship. During this time, animals have bred amongst themselves (and sometimes with wild conspecifics) with varying degrees of deliberate and unintended selection pressures from humans. Natural and artificial selection have altered the phenotypes of several species (or subspecies) kept as companion animals, including (but not limited to) dogs, cats, rabbits, pigeons, koi and goldfish. These selection processes have 'domesticated' several species to varying degrees, sometimes creating what can be termed 'subspecies' (as the animals are very different to their wild counterparts, although they can still interbreed). One might define 'domestic' as those species that have adapted from a welfare perspective to life with humans.

'Domestication' is different from 'taming' through habituation or conditioning methods (usually as juveniles), both of which could increase animals' ability to tolerate (or even enjoy) human interactions. Indeed, these processes may interact inasmuch as the species originally domesticated, and/or the populations selected for, may be more easily tolerant or tameable. If so, then species that have only been recently kept, or even bred, may be less suitable as pets than subspecies domesticated many years ago (even though some visible phenotypic changes might suggest that more recently kept species have already undergone changes, this does not mean that they are 'domesticated' in a welfare sense). At the same time, individuals who have not undergone training (and, in particular, if they have missed the juvenile developmental stages most conducive to taming) may be less suitable as pets.

This does not mean that tamed individuals or domestic species are able to tolerate human lifestyles without any welfare compromises (or even that humans can). Firstly, both processes probably need to happen (i.e. you probably cannot really tame non-domestic species to enjoy company, and domestic species still need positive experiences, especially during 'socialization' periods). Secondly, many needs and motivations (which were naturally selected prior to domestication) have not been significantly affected by selected breeding and remain maladaptive in home environments (indeed, many long-kept species, such as rats, rabbits and pigs, were selected for functions other than as pets). Furthermore, artificial selection itself has introduced many welfare compromises, in particular due to the concentration of deleterious genes and harmful phenotypic morphological, physiological or behavioural traits.

If one defines companion animals as 'companions', then many animals may be unsuitable as companion animals because they cannot enjoy or provide genuine human companionship (although they might still fulfil other roles, such as ornamentation). Some animals may be unsuitable to keep as pets because they do not find human company rewarding (with the exception of learnt associations) or may even find it stressful. Others may be unsuitable because they cannot enjoy the environment in which they would be kept in order to interact with humans (i.e. human homes usually cannot accommodate sufficient ranges, hiding or group size). Some animals may be dangerous to humans due to aggression (e.g. primates), predation (e.g. large snakes), accidents (e.g. very large animals) or zoonotic disease (e.g. salmonellosis).

Supply chains

Some animals are caught from the wild (as eggs, juveniles or adults). This can create risks for the wild population in terms of sustainability (e.g. orange clownfish, *Amphiprion percula*) or collateral damage (e.g. to coral reefs). Wild-caught animals may also not be 'tamed' adequately, and the international supply chain can involve significant morbidity and mortality rates.

Some companion animals are unintentionally bred by unneutered animals within pet (e.g. cohabiting rabbits) or stray (e.g. cats) populations. This can sometimes involve mis-mating (with possible dystocia) or inbreeding through the mating of close relatives, particularly when this occurs over several 'generations' (e.g. in some multi-cat hoarding cases). More commonly, it can lead to unwanted progeny, which may not receive adequate care as juveniles (e.g. kittens born outside may not be exposed to humans in early life) or later in life (e.g. if they are taken on by owners relatives or neighbours without adequate commitment).

Many companion animals are now captive bred. This might be by 'hobby' breeders or small businesses for various reasons, including enjoyment, profit, show competition success, or identification and perpetuation of a breed. Pedigree and purebred breeding has led to the creation of:

- A wide variety of 'fancy' breeds, sometimes with extreme or exaggerated morphologies or predispositions to abnormal behaviours (e.g. brachycephalic dogs, tumbler pigeons and bubble-eyed goldfish)
- Inbreeding either to 'fix' physical or behavioural traits or due to restricted gene pools, inadvertently increasing incidences of various inherited disorders.

Breeding of some species also occurs in medium- or large-scale commercial units, including dogs (i.e. 'puppy farms'), rodents, rabbits, reptiles and fish. These may provide unsuitable environments (e.g. impoverished environments, the presence of stressors and risk of infectious diseases). They can run the risk that pressures for cost efficiency limit standards, for example through low staffing ratios. The conditions are also likely to be different to the animals' future home environment, limiting opportunities for habituation, potentially increasing fear and undesirable behaviours later in life. Such units are not necessarily worse than some smaller-scale operations (which can also fail to meet the needs of breeding animals or progeny), but they have the potential to harm large numbers of animals (and their future owners).

Trading may also involve long-distance transportation (of both wild and captive-bred animals), suboptimal pet shop environments, mixing of individuals and species, poor diet, and a lack of discrimination in which owners are able to obtain animals.

At the population level, numbers of animals bred, imported and sold may be somewhat self-contained by market forces. However, some suppliers may aim for an over-supply to compensate for losses and avoid opportunity costs. In addition, the supply may show slow or poor reactivity to market forces due to lag periods involved in breeding (e.g. gestation periods) and the fragmentation of the industry.

Home environments and owner care

Owners determine most aspects of an animal's diet, environment and life. Being in a home environment can limit animals' resources and expose them to stressors, including:

- Captivity – limiting the opportunity to range, socialize or utilize resources
- Environmental factors that are set up for human comfort (e.g. thermoneutral zone and lighting cycles)
- Exposure to aversive stimuli (e.g. ultrasonic noise or predators)
- Exposure to harm (e.g. nutritionally inappropriate food, toxins or reverse zoonoses)
- Lack of control – pets are unable to directly control much of their environment or resources
- Lack of opportunity to perform motivated behaviours (e.g. hunting, foraging, scratching or digging).

Human interactions can also affect companion animal welfare in many ways, including:

- Direct harm – owners can, accidentally or deliberately, cause positive or negative punishment (e.g. electric shock collars)
- Resource control – owners choose the diet, company and environment for their animal
- Behavioural restrictions – owners may (or try to) prevent the expression of motivated behaviour (e.g. barking and digging)
- Behavioural manipulation – owners may train animals to perform maladaptive or unmotivated behaviours
- Fear – animals may be fearful of humans or specific human behaviours
- Existence – owners (using veterinary professionals) can keep animals alive when they otherwise would have died.

Key legislation applicable to small animal veterinary practice

A variety of legislative obligations apply to veterinary surgeons, nurses and practice owners (see 'Selected legislation'). These obligations usually apply to a range of actions (rather than omissions), particularly how we interact with other people and animals. Many legislative obligations are arguably based on ethical concerns, crystallized into rules that can be enforced by the state or other governing bodies. Many obligations have overarching legislation with subordinate rules and regulations, which may have been created by other bodies that are often themselves created by legislation, such as the Royal College of Veterinary Surgeons (RCVS).

Every country has its own laws, which differ both in content and in form. The legislation included in the 'Selected legislation' at the end of the chapter relates to the UK and is not exhaustive; readers are advised to consult legal expertise relevant to their jurisdiction and area of work as required. Clinicians practising in the UK must also be aware that this information on legislation applied at the time of publication, but may change as the UK leaves the European Union. In the UK, the Animal Welfare Act (2006) states:

"A person commits an offence if:
  a. An act of his, or a failure of his to act, causes an animal to suffer
  b. He knew, or ought reasonably to have known, that the act, or failure to act, would have that effect or be likely to do so
  c. The animal is a protected animal
  d. The suffering is unnecessary."

Given that this rule only applies once an animal has already suffered, there is a separate offence for someone who does not take such steps as are reasonable in all circumstances to ensure that the needs of an animal for which they are responsible are met to the extent required by good practice. In this case, an animal's needs include:

* The need for a suitable environment
* The need for a suitable diet
* The need to be able to exhibit normal behaviour patterns
* The need to be housed with, or apart from, other animals
* The need to be protected from pain, suffering, injury and disease.

Key ethical issues in small animal veterinary practice

Euthanasia

Intuitively, many people are used to death being considered 'bad'. However, it could be argued that life is 'good' or 'bad' depending on whether the animal's life would be otherwise 'worth living' or 'worth avoiding' (i.e. continued existence can sometimes be worse than non-existence).

Euthanasia can be considered as death in an animal's interest. In particular, euthanasia avoids a life of such poor quality that it is worse than death (or, more accurately, that a shorter life is better than an extended one). For this to be the case, the method of euthanasia generally needs to be sufficiently humane (i.e. avoidance of pain, fear and distress). One could also distinguish passive euthanasia (letting patients die) and active euthanasia (death via some direct action).

One difficulty is that, while death has predictable outcomes, it can be hard to predict and evaluate the life that the animal would otherwise have lived. Diseases are unpredictable, as are treatments (except euthanasia). Assessing whether death is better than life effectively requires us to predict, and evaluate, all possible sequelae and their value. For example, one would need to factor in all possible experiences of suffering, as well as the relative intensities, duration, frequency and probability. Euthanasia also evokes emotional responses, particularly from owners who worry that it is irreversible or 'playing God', or who are hoping for a miracle. Nevertheless, euthanasia is often the only reliable way to avoid suffering for many animals.

See Chapter 8 for more information on euthanasia.

Overtreatment

Veterinary treatment is intended to help patients (and clients). However, many treatments involve significant short-term suffering and all carry some risks of unintended side effects. There is, therefore, a risk that treatment causes more harm than good for our patients. This is of particular concern for treatments that involve greater suffering (e.g. 'invasive' surgery or long-term hospitalization), lower predictability (e.g. novel treatments) and those that extend life without curing the condition (e.g. management of chronic medical cases). It is also of concern where other motivations (e.g. research or profit) could bias our decision-making. However, any treatment could be overtreatment if the benefits are outweighed by the risks.

This does not mean that treatments that turned out badly were overtreatment. It depends on the predictions at the time, not on whether the patient was lucky or unlucky. One could define overtreatment as any treatment where the net 'gamble' is worse than: (a) no treatment; (b) more conservative treatment; or (c) euthanasia. One can therefore try to avoid it by structuring our decisions to minimize pressures and biases. For example, rather than trying to estimate all possible outcomes, identify the probability, duration and overall quality of life of set periods (e.g. post-operative recovery and rehabilitation). Similarly, differentiate research and clinical roles (i.e. the clinician has no professional, reputational or financial role in the research) so that clinical decisions are made based on what is best for our patients, without any prejudice or (perceived) conflict of interest.

Consent

Clients have relationships with their pets as companions and as their property (as well as sometimes for financial or entertainment reasons, such as breeding and showing). Ownership could confer positive rights so that owners can use and dispose of their animals as they see fit. Ownership could also create negative duties for others not to interfere with other people's animals. Of course, ownership is primarily a legal protection, but one could argue there are ethical concepts that correspond. How can one defend such ethical rights? One way is to say that the owner 'created' them (or bought them from someone who did). Another is to say that animals are protected by being someone's property, since otherwise anyone could interfere with them.

Legally, this can allow owners to refuse treatment of their pet. This means that veterinary surgeons should strive to obtain consent for treatment. Consent is essentially an owner's autonomous permission to perform procedures and administer medication. It needs to be 'valid' – this means that the owner needs to be informed and understand what they are consenting to (e.g. the associated risks), they need to be competent to make that decision, and must be able to make the decision freely (i.e. without coercion). Whilst consent does not necessarily need to be written, it is common practice in many countries to use a template form to record such permission (Figure 1.10). Since consent is only a permission (and not a mandate or a justification), its being granted certainly does not mean one must provide the treatment (i.e. one could decide not to do so; for example, if it would harm the animal). In addition, as consent is only one source of legitimacy (e.g. one could also justify treatment based on animal welfare grounds), its absence does not morally preclude providing treatment.

Gaining consent is sensible in cases where owner funding or compliance is needed (and where legally required). However, owners may sometimes refuse to give permission for treatment to prevent avoidable suffering. It could be argued that in some circumstances one may (or even should) provide treatment even when owners do not explicitly permit it. Some owners are unable to give their views (e.g. in emergency cases or with stray animals), whilst others may be unable to make medical decisions (e.g. if they lack the competence or understanding). More generally, one could argue that owners should not have the same rights to control their sentient animals that they have over their own bodies or insentient property, and should not have the autonomy to harm their animal (e.g. by refusing reasonable treatment that could otherwise have been provided).

Admission form

Owner name: ....

Owner address: ....

....

....

Home/landline telephone number: ....

Mobile telephone number: ....

Animal number:	Date: ....
Name:	Colour: ....
Species:	Sex: ....
Breed:	Date of birth: .... Age: ....

Details of operation and related procedures where appropriate: ....

....

The cost of the procedures described above will be: £............................... OR within the range: £............................. to £...............................

I hereby give permission for the administration of an anaesthetic or sedative to the above animal and for the surgical or other procedures detailed on this form together with any other procedures which may prove necessary.

The nature of these procedures and of other procedures as might prove necessary has been explained to me.

I understand that there are some risks involved in all anaesthetic techniques and surgical procedures.

I accept that the likely cost will be as detailed in the estimate above and that in the event of further treatment being required or of complications occurring which give rise to additional costs, I shall be contacted as soon as practicable so that my consent to such additional treatment and costs may be obtained.

In the event that the veterinary surgeon is unable to contact me on the numbers provided, I understand that the veterinary surgeon will act in the best interests of my animal.

Blood test required: [ ] Yes   [ ] No

Signature of owner/guardian: ....

All fees are due at time of collection

Admission

Weight: ....

Vaccinated:	Cage/basket/box:	Last eaten: ....
Blanket:	Last heat:	Collar/lead/choke: ....
Check sex:	Admitted by:	Other preparation: ....
Microchip: [ ] Yes [ ] No	[ ] Microchip today	Date: ....
Admitting Temperature:	Pulse:	Respiration: ....

Medication: ....

Notes: (including diet, toilet behaviour, exercise behaviour) ....

....

....

Booked by:

A downloadable form is available for this manual from the BSAVA Library

1.10 It is common in practice to use a form to record written consent from the owner to perform procedures on and administer medications to their animal. Species-specific consent forms are recommended.

Confidentiality

Another important concept is not revealing private information about clients (or patients) to other people without their permission or other justification (e.g. legitimate sharing of clinical information amongst practice colleagues). The principle of not sharing information may be defended directly in terms of the interests of the individual client, insofar as sharing data could embarrass or otherwise harm them. It can also be justified by a wider concern for outcomes, insofar as fewer owners would perhaps seek veterinary care if they were worried that their data would be shared (leading to untreated animals suffering). It is good for clients to have confidence in the veterinary team and confidentiality is an integral part of creating this trust.

However, it is surprisingly unclear exactly what confidentiality clients (argue they) should have. Most clients may plausibly think that a veterinary surgeon's duty of privacy should not prevent any disclosure of data in any circumstances. Indeed, it could be argued that clients would expect (and, in general, want) veterinary surgeons to pass on information where necessary to protect animals or public health, or where a criminal offence has been committed. The RCVS Code of Professional Conduct outlines these legitimate reasons for breaking client confidentiality.

Of course, if we are basing our duty on what clients would need to have confidence in us, this is a factual question. In the absence of strong evidence that all clients believe that one should never share data, then we should not base our actions on false hypotheses. In addition, maintaining confidentiality is one principle amongst many (e.g. not allowing suffering) and, therefore, should not necessarily override all our other moral responsibilities.

Practices should be up to date with the General Data Protection Regulation (GDPR) and ensure that all staff are trained and aware of their legal responsibilities around confidentiality, as well as their ethical duties. A specific example of ethics and client confidentiality clashing dealt with by the RCVS is a client presenting with an animal that is registered on their microchip to another person. The 'Client confidentiality and microchipped animals' flowchart walks veterinary staff through the steps to take in this situation to ensure that an animal is with the rightful owner without compromising their client confidentiality responsibilities (see 'References and further reading'). Veterinary surgeons should also be aware that by an owner registering their dog with the Kennel Club, this gives the veterinary surgeon permission to report any Caesarean section or conformation alteration to the Kennel Club.

Charging

An important ethical question (which is less often discussed) is how to charge for veterinary work. Arguably, owners should fund treatment for their animals – private practices need to be sustainable – but that still leaves questions as to how to set prices above cost. This could be left to market forces; however, this risks some animals not receiving veterinary care (through no fault of their own) if their owners will not (or cannot) pay or if they are unowned. Some work could be subsidized, but this effectively means that some clients fund the treatment of other clients' animals (although this does not seem unfair when considering *pro bono* care of unowned animals and wildlife). One could rely on charities, but their resources are limited (and they often need to procure veterinary services from private practices, which could be seen as veterinary practice owners 'profiteering' from charitable donations). It could be argued that veterinary practices should be not-for-profit, but this seems unfair for practice owners when compared with owners of other private firms (and still leaves questions about setting staff salaries, which affect service prices). This question has received little attention in veterinary ethics and each practice owner and manager may make a decision about what is 'reasonable', either informally or (in the future) within corporate social responsibility (CSR) policies.

Animal advocacy

What is animal advocacy?

It could be argued that every veterinary nurse and surgeon, and each profession as a whole, has a responsibility to inform, advise, encourage and, where necessary, correct others to look after animals well and avoid causing harm. Collectively, these responsibilities might be described as animal advocacy.

This duty arguably comes from:

- Our undertaking that we are knowledgeable and compassionate about animals
- An implicit or explicit desire and expectation of other people that we will do so.

As individuals, we receive fees from clients in order primarily to (help them) look after their animals. On occasions an owner might want something that would be harmful for their animal, but (in most cases) these owners still look to us to check that it is acceptable and that there is not a better way to achieve their aim. As professionals, we claim that we are particularly knowledgeable about animals (all aspects of animals, not just health) and that we care about them. Arguably, this is the basis for our licence to practice (similarly, the legal prohibition of others who are less knowledgeable to provide veterinary services is based on the risks that treatment by laypersons poses).

This undertaking, expectation and exclusive license means that failing to speak up for animals does not merely have an opportunity cost. Rather, since we have claimed that we speak for animals, our silence on a matter (be it a patient's obesity or a structural abnormality associated with modern pedigree dog breeding) implies that these practices are not harmful to animals.

Animal advocacy in clinical decisions

Veterinary surgeons and nurses have specific responsibilities towards patients and clients (Figure 1.11), which are taken on when we take animals into our care, make promises to owners or accept their money. For example, it is reasonable to assume that one should provide food and analgesia to any hospitalized patients who need them, but not to go around our neighbourhood looking for starving or injured animals. This is our duty of care for our patients, to ensure they each have acceptable welfare, and to monitor that welfare and take any reasonable steps needed to avoid suffering (a duty of care towards certain humans also exists; for example, with regards to client health and safety).

In clinics, animal advocacy is part of welfare-focused practice. This involves focusing on what is best for our

Moral principle applied to our patients	Example	Example of where this duty may not apply to other animals
Provide basic care to our patients	Ensure hospitalized animals are fed	No moral duty to send money to help starving animals in Sub-Saharan Africa
Give our patients treatment to prevent suffering	Should give first aid to wildlife brought in (even if it costs us money)	No moral duty to send money to fund wild animal rescue centres in Asia
Do not use our animals to benefit others	Experimenting on patients	Experimenting on animals in a laboratory
Helping our patients may involve harm to others	Using drugs developed/tested in a laboratory on patients Releasing a dog with leishmaniosis Feeding carnivorous patients with farmed/caught meat	

1.11 Moral principles that it could be argued should be followed for our patients but not for other animals.

patients, regardless of self-interest (e.g. profit, career or reputation). Welfare-focused practice includes six key elements:

- Honest and full disclosure (albeit tactfully) to owners about how well they are caring for their animals, in order to encourage and reinforce good practice
- Informing owners about the benefits and risks of different options (including the continuation of the *status quo*)
- Encouraging and supporting owners to choose the best option(s) for their animals (providing relevant professional judgements where appropriate; we are not paid fees just to reel off facts that the owner could have found elsewhere)
- Not providing (and not offering) harmful treatments (e.g. unnecessary or risky treatment)
- Discussing matters that go beyond the problem for which the patient was presented (e.g. diet, environment and behaviour)
- Taking action when owners are failing to care for their animal adequately.

In most cases, this is exactly what the owner wants and is paying for. Indeed, many owners explicitly ask for opinions (e.g. 'What would you do?'). However, such advocacy can feel difficult, especially as it can involve, or occasionally lead to, difficult conversations. It can be embarrassing to bring up concerns that could be perceived as critical of the owner or their lifestyle. One might be fearful of confrontation or practice complaints, especially if there is a perceived risk of litigation or complaints to the regulator (which can be stressful even if the regulator encourages members to be concerned with patient welfare). Animal advocacy requires us to step up resolutely and take responsibility.

Animal advocacy means not washing our hands of difficult cases (or wringing our hands in impotent frustration), finding excuses for inaction, or blaming other people when we could change their behaviour. However, it is still expected to operate within legitimate constraints, such as the criminal law, regulatory obligations and financial limitations.

Animal advocacy in practice management

Veterinary surgeons and nurses can also act as animal advocates in discussions and decisions on how the practice is run. This means ensuring that practice policies, facilities and staffing optimize patient welfare. This includes:

- Ensuring fees are set to help animals (and gain fair remuneration) rather than to maximize profit at the expense of some animals (who might otherwise not receive treatment and/or not be insured)
- Ensuring practice protocols are designed to avoid delays, overtreatment and any unnecessary suffering (e.g. transportation)
- Ensuring practice facilities are designed to promote animal welfare (e.g. reducing stress in waiting rooms and hospital wards)
- Ensuring unowned animals receive adequate basic care (e.g. stabilization, analgesia or euthanasia) without delay.

This means foregoing some self-interest (e.g. equity owners' profit). As for clinical decisions, this does not mean jeopardizing practice financial sustainability or employee wellbeing; these are significant constraints (insofar as veterinary nurses and surgeons should not be expected to undergo unreasonable self-sacrifice) and, in any case, these concerns are equally important for animals. It means ensuring that practices are managed to fulfil their primary purpose in the community, namely to look after the animals of clients.

Animal advocacy within the profession

Veterinary nurses and surgeons are all members of a profession. Each member has a role in ensuring that all members (i.e. themselves and others) are acting collectively and individually in ways that fulfil the profession's purpose of helping and protecting animals. This includes encouraging, educating and advising one another not only with regard to technical skills, but also on other skills to improve effectiveness (e.g. communication skills), decision-making (e.g. clinical reasoning) and moral virtues (e.g. compassion).

Animal advocacy within the profession helps individuals from becoming jaded or losing sight of the reasons why they entered the veterinary profession in the first place (students can play a particularly useful role in this regard, holding older members to account and reminding them of their more hidden and cluttered passions). Animal advocacy also involves ensuring that our professional regulations (which are often set by elected veterinary nurses and surgeons) are met (see 'Selected legislation').

- Encourage or require members to do what is best for animals (in particular to be advocates for patients).
- Do not force members to harm animals, or unnecessarily or unjustifiably prevent them from helping animals (e.g. excessive restrictions on when treatment can be provided).

In regulatory policymaking, animal advocacy is not simply about ensuring the clinical autonomy of members. Firstly, it is about ensuring autonomy to help animals – members should not be free to harm animals. Secondly, there can sometimes be cases where limiting an individual's clinical autonomy is for the greater good (e.g. prohibiting declawing may mean that some cats are euthanased but means that many others avoid undergoing the surgery). Professional advocacy should be concerned with what is best for animals as a whole across the population.

It should be recognized that animal advocacy is different to client advocacy (e.g. promoting consent and confidentiality). These need to be balanced or prioritized. However, they are not mutually exclusive because:

- Most clients want what is good for their patients
- Protecting animals, in general, needs clients to trust the profession to adhere to basic moral standards and not to cause harm (without good reason)
- The general expectation or desire of clients or society is not necessarily to do whatever every individual client wants (e.g. people might expect veterinary professionals to protect the interests of animals above those of clients).

Veterinary professionals have a role to play in identifying possible neglect, abuse and non-accidental trauma. Such trauma can have obvious direct welfare impacts on patients, but also indirect effects (e.g. increasing fear responses or anxiety). Non-accidental trauma may indicate that harm is being done to other animals (e.g. other pets in the household, or animals harmed in fighting or wildlife crime) and people. While these cases may be challenging, there is an ethical argument that our duties to our patients should (and most people would expect them to) outweigh our duties to our clients in such situations, or that owners have effectively "forfeited" the right to confidentiality on such matters through their abuse, and that taking appropriate action is morally justified or even required. Nonetheless, such cases can still be difficult (see Chapter 9), and the suspicion of abuse does not justify unprofessional behaviour (e.g. breaching confidentiality publicly in a "name and shame", rather than informing authorities).

Animal advocacy in campaigning

More widely still, as veterinary professionals, one has a relationship with all non-human animals. Society expects us to be the voice advocating compassionate treatment of animals (whereas one does not have an especial responsibility to advocate compassionate treatment of humans). This view could be based on our knowledge of animals, the public's trust that one cares about animals, and our own professional claims and undertakings. Indeed, it could be argued that our specific duties to patients are, partly, an application of our general duty not to harm any animal since, by taking animals into our care, one effectively stops other people (veterinary professionals and non-veterinary professionals) from caring for that animal or the animal meeting its own needs (or dying), so one should meet those needs as well as they would otherwise have been met. This is also true at a societal level – by privileging the licence to practice veterinary medicine, which stops others from providing such services, this means that we should provide as compassionate and knowledgeable care as other people would aim to (if given the same opportunities).

Veterinary nurses and surgeons, and the professions in general, also have the opportunity to advocate for animals at a societal level by advocating to improve:

- The behaviour of owners, vendors and breeders (e.g. how they care for their animals and make consumer purchasing choices)
- How society sees animals culturally
- Business models and products of industry stakeholders (e.g. pet retailers, pet food manufacturers, groomers, boarding establishments, animal shows, interaction/experience companies)
- Government legislation and regulation to improve how animals are treated (e.g. animal welfare, veterinary legislation)
- Other societal actions and legislation that directly affect animals (e.g. trade, environmental protection).

This applies to each individual and to the professions as collective groups (e.g. affiliative and specialist organizations). Indeed, insofar as individuals may feel powerful to affect significant change on their own, each individual might focus on ensuring their professions do advocate, supporting that advocacy and not damaging it (e.g. by muddying the waters).

Arguably, veterinary nurses and surgeons have a responsibility to take at least some of these opportunities. This responsibility might be based simply on the benefit that doing so would bring. It could be based on the fact that in terms of societal expectation and professional undertakings, silence or overly non-committal or socially conservative statements might be seen as implying there is no need for change (even if, simply, it is because professional bodies cannot reach a consensus for procedural reasons). It could also be based on the fact that, sometimes, veterinary clinical work has unintended consequences (e.g. perpetuating unhealthy genetics) or could make us feel complicit with irresponsible owners that we want to 'offset'. For professional bodies, this responsibility could also be based on the desires of members, who expect the professional bodies to work to help animals.

Advocating for animals societally needs to avoid an excessive concern for self-interest (e.g. professions should avoid overly protecting our own interests, especially when this is mixed up with advocacy for animals, as doing so risks losing our credibility). There is a concern that campaigning to change behaviour risks alienating clients, potentially affecting not only ourselves but also their animals. Indeed, there is a risk that such considerations bias our decision-making towards inaction. At the same time, advocating for animals may often improve our respect (and failing to do so may eventually damage public trust that we care about animals). We might, therefore, try to work collectively to minimize such effects and biases, for example, by campaigning via collective professional organizations (as long as these are adequately progressive).

Conclusion

Animal welfare and ethics are not sub-disciplines within veterinary science or medicine. They are integral to everything we do as veterinary professionals (whether we realize it or not). Emotional and intuitive assessments and decisions have their place, but often one can feel more confident when more structured and reflective methods are used.

References and further reading

Appleby MC and Sandøe P (2002) Philosophical debate on the nature of well-being: Implications for animal welfare. *Animal Welfare* **11**, 283–294

Appleby MC and Stokes T (2008) Why should we care about nonhuman animals during times of crisis? *Journal of Applied Animal Welfare Science* **11**, 90–97

Barnard CJ and Hurst JL (1996) Welfare by design: the natural selection of welfare criteria. *Animal Welfare* **5**, 405–433

Beauchamp TL and Childress JF (2009) *Principles of Biomedical Ethics, 6th edn.* Oxford University Press, New York

Broom DM (1986) Indicators of poor welfare. *British Veterinary Journal* **142**, 524–526

Dawkins MS (1990) From an animal's point of view: motivation, fitness, and animal welfare. *Behavioral and Brain Sciences* **13**, 1–61

Dawkins M (2006) A user's guide to animal welfare science. *Trends in Ecology & Evolution* **21**, 77–82

Duncan IJH and Dawkins MS (1983) The problem of assessing 'well-being' and 'suffering' in farm animals. In: *Indicators Relevant to Farm Animal Welfare*, ed. D Smidt, pp. 13–24. Springer, Dordrecht, The Netherlands

Duncan IJH and Fraser D (1997) Understanding animal welfare. In: *Animal Welfare*, ed. MC Appleby and BO Hughes, pp. 19–31. CAB International, Wallingford

Fraser D, Weary DM, Pajor EA and Milligan BN (1997) A scientific conception of animal welfare that reflects ethical concerns. *Animal Welfare* **6**, 187–205

Hetts S, Estep D and Marder AR (2005) Psychological well-being in animals. In: *Mental Health and Well-Being in Animals*, ed. FD McMillan, pp. 211–220. Blackwell Publishing, Ames, Iowa

Hubrecht R (1995) The welfare of dogs in human care. In: *The Domestic Dog: Its Evolution, Behaviour and Interactions with People*, ed. J Serpell, pp. 179–198. Cambridge University Press, Cambridge

McMillan FD and Yeates J (2019) The problems with wellbeing terminology. In: *Mental Health and Wellbeing in Animals, 2nd edn*, ed. FD McMillan, pp. 8–24. Blackwell's, Oxford

Mench JA (1998) Thirty years after Brambell: Whither animal welfare science? *Journal of Applied Animal Welfare Science* **1**, 91–102

Mendl M (1991) Some problems with the concept of a cut-off point for determining when an animal's welfare is at risk. *Applied Animal Behaviour Science* **31**, 139–146

Nordenfelt L (2006) *Animal and Human Health and Welfare: A Comparative Analysis.* CABI, Oxfordshire

OIE (World Organisation for Animal Health) (2018) Introduction to the Recommendations for Animal Welfare (Article 7.1.1.) *Terrestrial Animal Health Code.* Available from: www.oie.int

RCVS (2019) *Client Confidentiality and Microchipped Animals Flow Chart.* Available from: www.rcvs.org.uk/document-library

Webster AJF, Main DCJ and Whay HR (2004) Welfare assessment: indices from clinical observation. Animal Welfare 13, S93–S98

Wojciechowska JI and Hewson CJ (2005) Quality-of-life assessment in pet dogs. *Journal of the American Veterinary Medical Association* **226**, 722–728

Yeates J (2019) *Companion Animal Care and Welfare.* Wiley-Blackwell, Hoboken NJ

Selected legislation

Most legislation for the UK, Scotland, Wales and Northern Ireland can be accessed at www.legislation.gov.uk. Where important documents relating to the below legislation are found elsewhere, URLs have been provided.

Selected legislation relating to animals in the UK

- Animal Welfare Act 2006
- Animal Health and Welfare (Scotland) Act 2006
- The Animals & Wildlife (Penalties Protections & Powers) (Scotland) Act 2020
- Welfare of Animals Act (Northern Ireland) 2011
- The Dangerous Wild Animals Act 1976
- The Dangerous Wild Animals Act 1976 (Modification) (No. 2) Order 2007
- The Legislative Reform (Dangerous Wild Animals) (Licensing) Order 2010

Selected legislation relating to companion animals in the UK

- Animals Act 1971
- Animal Boarding Establishments Act 1963
- The Pet Animals Act 1951 (amended 1983)
- Consumer Rights Act 2015

Orders and Regulations

- The Non-Commercial Movement of Pet Animals Order 2011
- The Non-Commercial Movement of Pet Animals Order (Northern Ireland) 2011
- The Welfare of Animals (Transport) (England) Order 2006
- The Welfare of Animals (Transport) (Scotland) Regulations 2006
- The Welfare of Animals (Transport) Regulations (Northern Ireland) 2006
- The Animal Welfare (Licencing of Activities Involving Animals) (England) Regulations 2018
- The Consumer Protection from Unfair Trading Regulations 2008

Codes

- Code of practice for the welfare of cats (England) (www.gov.uk/government/publications/code-of-practice-for-the-welfare-of-cats)
- Code of practice for the welfare of cats (Wales) (gov.wales/code-practice-welfare-cats)
- Code of practice for the welfare of cats (Scotland) (www.gov.scot/publications/code-practice-welfare-cats)

Selected legislation relating to wildlife in the UK

- The Wildlife and Natural Environment (Scotland) Act 2011
- Wildlife and Natural Environment Act (Northern Ireland) 2011
- Wildlife and Countryside Act 1981
- Wild Mammals (Protection) Act 1996
- The Control of Trade in Endangered Species (Enforcement) Regulations 1997
- Pests Act 1954
- The Wildlife (Northern Ireland) Order 1985

Selected legislation relating to clients in the UK

- Health & Safety at Work etc. Act 1974
- Corporate Manslaughter and Corporate Homicide Act 2007
- Offices, Shops and Railway Premises Act 1963
- The Control of Substances Hazardous to Health Regulations 2002
- Consumer Rights Act 2015
- Equality Act 2010
- General Data Protection Regulation (GDPR) 2016/679 (www.gov.uk/government/publications/guide-to-the-general-data-protection-regulation)
- Data Protection Act 2018

Selected legislation relating to veterinary medicine in the UK

- Animals (Scientific Procedures) Act 1986
- Animal Health Act 1981
- Animal Health Act 2002
- The Veterinary Surgeons Act 1966
- Protection of Animals (Anaesthetics) Act 1954
- Protection of Animals (Anaesthetics) Act 1964
- The Mutilations (Permitted Procedures) (England) Regulations 2007
- The Mutilations (Permitted Procedures) (Wales) Regulations 2007
- The Prohibited Procedures on Protected Animals (Exemptions) (Scotland) Regulations 2010
- The Control of Substances Hazardous to Health Regulations 2002
- Misuse of Drugs Act 1971

Regulations

- The Veterinary Medicines Regulations 2013
- The Misuse of Drugs Regulations 2001

Codes

- RCVS Code of Professional Conduct for Veterinary Surgeons (www.rcvs.org.uk/setting-standards/advice-and-guidance/code-of-professional-conduct-for-veterinary-surgeons)
- RCVS Code of Professional Conduct for Veterinary Nurses (www.rcvs.org.uk/setting-standards/advice-and-guidance/code-of-professional-conduct-for-veterinary-nurses)

Selected legislation (civil and criminal) relating to employees in the UK

- Employment Act 2002
- Employment Rights Act 1996
- Trade Union and Labour Relations (Consolidation) Act 1992
- Employment Rights (Northern Ireland) Order 1996
- The National Minimum Wage Act 1998
- Income Tax (Earnings and Pensions) Act 2003
- Equality Act 2010

Regulations

- The Equality Act 2010 (Gender Pay Gap Information) Regulations 2017
- The Working Time Regulations 1998
- The Working Time (Amendment) Regulations 2003
- Employment Equality (Religion or Belief) Regulations 2003
- Equality Act (Sexual Orientation) Regulations 2007
- Employment Equality (Age) Regulations 2006
- The Maternity and Parental Leave etc. Regulations 1999

Selected legislation relating to campaigning in the UK

- Transparency of Lobbying, Non-Party Campaigning and Trade Union Administration Act 2014
- Defamation Act 2013
- Defamation Act (Northern Ireland) 1955
- Defamation Act 1996

 Online extras

- This chapter includes forms that are available to download and print from the BSAVA Library.
- Each form is marked in the text with a download symbol.

Access via QR code or: bsavalibrary.com/welfareforms_1

Chapter 2

Assessment and recording methods tool kit

Kelly Deane and Adina Valentine

Introduction

Ethics and welfare are similar concepts that are often confused with one another. Ethics has many branches and can be seen as a set of principles governing peoples' views of right and wrong. These principles can be taught by parents, teachers, magazines, movies, etc. and can lead to more philosophical discussions (Rollin, 2006). Welfare, on the other hand, refers to the actual state of an animal. The term 'welfare' is often used loosely in the context of human obligation to change the state of an animal; however, this is more accurately an ethical consideration. For example, a wild bird suffering from disease has poor welfare without human interaction, but whether interventions should be implemented to help alleviate that suffering can be ethically debated (Keeling *et al.*, 2011). The term welfare cannot be simply defined, either philosophically or scientifically; it encompasses the whole condition of the animal, including mental, physical and emotional health (Kagan and Veasey, 2010). See Chapter 1 for more information on the definitions of ethics and welfare.

Being able to assess welfare in a quantifiable way, recognize when intervention may be required and then implement the necessary changes is vital and a role for the entire veterinary team, including veterinary care assistants (VCAs), veterinary nurses (RVNs) and veterinary surgeons (veterinarians), as well as regular caregivers such as owners, zoo keepers, wildlife rehabilitators and primary care staff in other establishments.

The aim of this chapter is to provide different tools to allow welfare to be recorded in a quantitative manner, so that poor welfare can be 'flagged' and improved.

Welfare assessment

The assessment of welfare is an essential part of working with and treating patients. Welfare assessments encourage careful observation of the patient and critical thinking, and help facilitate provision of the best possible care. The welfare needs of individuals will change over time, so welfare assessments should monitor current patient welfare, allow potential future problems to be pre-empted and, most importantly, provide the evidence to encourage assessors to adopt changes in current routines and nursing support. Welfare assessments should facilitate changes in practice and not just be a 'box ticking exercise'.

The following stages are required for a meaningful welfare assessment:

* Stage 1 – Gather relevant information
* Stage 2 – Interpret the information
* Stage 3 – Evaluate the information and formulate a plan
* Stage 4 – Reassess and adopt any necessary changes.

Welfare assessments need to take into account more than just the basic requirements of an individual. By focusing on the idea of a 'life worth living', welfare assessments can help identify what an individual finds engaging and stimulating, enabling their quality of life (QOL) to be improved by ensuring positive emotional experiences. It should be noted that without regular welfare assessments, it is unlikely that subtle (or sometimes even obvious) poor practices will be recognized.

History-taking

Qualitative history-taking tends to form a large part of the initial consultation and although it is often unstructured it will sometimes highlight relevant information that may not be prompted by a quantitative questioning methodology. It should also be recognized that there are limitations with these assessment tools, inasmuch as there are always going to be changing variables that need to be taken into account, including:

* Each species will respond differently based on their natural behaviours
* Prey species will hide pain, illness and discomfort to avoid attention from predators
* Complex social species may have a hierarchy within the group (e.g. primates), which will need to be taken into consideration when developing treatment plans and reintroducing the animal following a period of hospitalization
* Co-dependence and life stage may change welfare requirements.

Human influences

It should be recognized that there are 'human factors' that can influence the evaluation phase of a welfare assessment, as well as the implementation of the changes that are identified as needed. These influencing factors should be borne in mind when conducting and interpreting welfare assessments and the aim should always be to keep the patient as the primary focus.

Speciesism

Speciesism is discriminating against one species and treating it with less care or morality than another. For example, some people may regard rats as vermin, whilst others recognize a complex, intelligent and altruistic animal, or food-producing animals may be treated differently to companion animals.

Bias

Assessors may have had a previous negative experience with a particular breed or species, creating an unconscious bias (e.g. a caregiver may have been bitten by a specific breed of dog and may now have negative feelings about interactions with different animals of the same breed).

Human–animal bond

The human–animal relationship can cause huge discrepancies in the assessment of animal welfare; a farmer who works with large herds or flocks may have a differing opinion on welfare needs to an owner who cares for a small number of animals.

Finance

Financial factors may affect the outcome of welfare assessments. For example, a theme park with a 'petting zoo' may not advocate for spending large amounts of money from the profits to improve animal welfare by building larger enclosures.

Personality

It is well documented that people have different personality types and traits, and that they interpret information and their environment, as well as react to stimuli, in very different ways. These factors may have a significant impact on welfare assessments (e.g. a surgeon may recognize a complicated comminuted fracture and formulate a plan to fix the physical problem, whereas a veterinary nurse may recognize an individual patient and aim to make all aspects of their care as comfortable and holistic as possible).

Five Freedoms

Many assessments are based on the Five Freedoms (see also Chapter 1), which were first established in the early 1990s by the Farm Animal Welfare Council (FAWC) in the UK, and are considered to be the absolute minimum in terms of welfare requirements:

- Freedom from hunger and thirst
- Freedom from discomfort
- Freedom from pain, injury and disease
- Freedom to express normal behaviour
- Freedom from fear and distress.

However, a marked increase in scientific understanding over the past two decades has shown that the Five Freedoms do not capture, either in specifics or the generality of their expression, the breadth and depth of current knowledge of the biological processes that are germane to understanding animal welfare and to guiding its management (Mellor, 2016). Thus, the principle of the Five Freedoms has been developed to form the Five Domains model.

Five Domains

The Five Domains model (Figure 2.1) features four physical or functional domains (nutrition, environment, health and behaviour), which are concerned with biological function and physical wellbeing, and a fifth domain that considers the mental state of the animal. The Five Domains model demonstrates that for every physical or functional aspect that is affected, there may be an accompanying emotional or subjective experience that also affects welfare, and recognizes that emotional needs are as important as physical needs when considering animal welfare.

Physical/functional domains	
1: Nutrition	
Restrictions on:	**Opportunities to:**
• Water intake • Food intake • Food quality • Food variety • Voluntary overeating; force-feeding	• Drink enough water • Eat enough food • Eat a balanced diet • Eat a variety of foods • Eat correct quantities
2: Environment	
Unavoidable/imposed conditions:	**Available conditions:**
• Thermal extremes • Unsuitable substrate • Close confinement • Atmospheric pollutants (CO_2, ammonia, dust, smoke) • Unpleasant/strong odours • Inappropriate light intensity • Loud/otherwise unpleasant noise • Environmental monotony • Unpredictable events	• Thermally tolerable • Suitable substrate • Space for freer movement • Fresh air • Pleasant/tolerable odours • Light intensity tolerable • Noise exposure acceptable • Normal environmental variability • Predictability

2.1 The Five Domains model was developed from the Five Freedoms and ensures that both the physical and mental state of the animal is taken into consideration with reference to welfare. (continues) ▶

Physical/functional domains	
3: Health	
Pressure of:	**Pressure alleviated by:**
• Disease: acute, chronic • Injury: acute, chronic, husbandry, mutations • Functional impairment: due to limb amputations, lung, heart, vascular, kidney, neural or other problems • Poisons • Obesity/leanness • Poor physical fitness: muscle deconditioning	• Lack of disease • Lack of injury • Normal function • Lack of poisoning • Appropriate body condition • Good fitness level
4: Behaviour	
Exercise of 'agency' impeded by:	**'Agency' exercised via:**
• Invariant, barren environment • Inescapable sensory impositions • Choices markedly restricted • Constraints on environment-focused activity • Constraints on animal-to-animal interactive activity • Limits on threat avoidance, escape or defensive activity • Limitations on sleep/rest	• Varied, novel, engaging environment challenges • Congenial sensory inputs • Engaging choices available • Free movement • Exploration • Foraging/hunting • Bonding/reaffirming bonds • Rearing young • Playing • Sexual activity • Using refuges, retreat or defensive attack • Sleep/rest sufficient
Affective experience domain	
5: Mental state	
Negative and positive mental states relating to nutrition	
Negative:	**Positive:**
• Thirst • Hunger • Malnutrition, malaise • Bloated/over-full; gastrointestinal pain	• Quenching thirst, pleasures of drinking • Pleasures of different tastes/smells/textures; masticatory pleasures • Postprandial satiety • Gastrointestinal comfort
Negative and positive mental states relating to environment	
Negative:	**Positive:**

• Forms of discomfort
  • Thermal: chilling, overheating
  • Physical: joint pain, skin irritation, stiffness, muscle tension
  • Respiratory (e.g. breathlessness)
  • Olfactory
  • Auditory: impairment, pain
  • Visual: glare/darkness, eye strain
• Malaise from unnatural constancy
	• Forms of comfort
	  • Thermal
	  • Physical
	  • Respiratory
	  • Olfactory
	  • Auditory
	  • Visual
	• Variety-related comfort

Negative and positive mental states relating to health	
Negative:	**Positive:**

• Discomfort of poor health and low functional capacity
  • Breathlessness
  • Pain: many types
  • Debility, weakness
  • Sickness, malaise
  • Nausea
  • Dizziness
• Physical exhaustion
	• Comfort of good health and high functional capacity
	  • Normal physiological parameters
	
	• Vitality of fitness

Negative and positive mental states relating to behaviour	
Negative:	**Positive:**
• Anger, frustration • Boredom, helplessness • Loneliness, isolation • Depression • Sexual frustration • Anxiety, fearfulness, panic, anger • Neophobia • Exhaustion	• Calmness • Engaged, in control • Affectionate sociability; maternally rewarded • Excitation/playfulness • Sexual gratification • Secure/protected/confident • Likes novelty • Energized/refreshed

2.1 (continued) The Five Domains model was developed from the Five Freedoms and ensures that both the physical and mental state of the animal is taken into consideration with reference to welfare.

Case example 1: Rabbits

Figure 2.2 shows what is widely accepted (and advocated) as an adequate set-up for a rabbit.

Five Freedoms

In terms of the Five Freedoms: food has been provided and water is available; there is substrate in the hutch to allow a resting place; there are bars on the hutch to prevent predators (such as cats and foxes) from coming into contact with the rabbit; the rabbit can see out and hear noises in the immediate environment, which will enable normal behavioural responses to be exhibited; and there is a covered area to facilitate hiding should the rabbit feel threatened. Thus, in terms of the Five Freedoms, this set-up would be considered adequate for the needs of the rabbit.

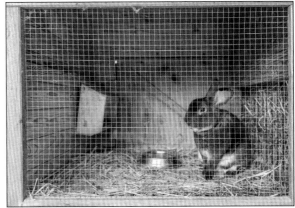

2.2 Rabbits require more space and enrichment for optimum welfare.
(Shutterstock.com/Kojin)

Five Domains

However, if a welfare assessment based on the Five Domains model is performed, it becomes evident that what is considered to be sufficient and acceptable based on the Five Freedoms actually falls significantly below what can realistically be called good welfare for the rabbit. It should be remembered that rabbits are:

- A crepuscular species (i.e. active predominantly during the early morning and at dusk)
- A social species that live in large family groups in a large space
- A fossorial species (i.e. burrowing animals) that live in intricate tunnels and warrens underground
- A grazing herbivorous species that eat regularly throughout the day to maintain essential gut movement
- A prey species that are always on 'high alert' for potential predators
- Fast sprinting animals that dash around quickly over short distances when threatened.

By applying these criteria to the set-up described above, shortfalls can be immediately recognized: the most obvious being a lack of space – 'a hutch is not enough' (Rabbit Welfare Association and Fund (RWAF); see 'Useful websites' at the end of the chapter).

Improving welfare

This basic form of welfare assessment (focusing solely on housing without taking any other factors such as illness or disease into account) provides a plethora of information that can be used to help implement better care for the rabbit (Figure 2.3).

Current welfare observations to be improved	Goals and objectives for improvement following basic welfare assessment	Achieving better welfare: actions
Small hutch	Large, multilevel enclosure to facilitate movement and stretching	• Suggested minimum sleeping enclosure dimensions (RWAF): 6ft x 2ft x 2ft tall (at least three hops in any direction) and must be permanently attached to a secure run of at least 8ft. (Total living space that includes sleeping and exercise areas should have at least a 10ft x 6ft footprint, not including any added levels) • A shed may be converted into a large enclosure with adaptations of tunnels coming out of it to mimic a more natural burrow-like accommodation, but providing a solid safe place to hide and relax • Ensure materials are easily cleaned to avoid damp and mould and secure enough to prevent predators entering
Elevated hutch on tall legs	Above ground level (good for access to maintain hygiene) Prevents flooding Abnormal living level (safer at ground level) At risk of toppling over if not secured	• Reduce height of legs so that the hutch is no more than 1ft off the ground (making it more stable but still should prevent flooding) • Consider placing the hutch inside a converted shed or aviary to increase enclosure size and reduce weather related risks • Permanently attach to suitable run(s) to allow access to tunnel systems and secure elevated platforms/levels
Multi-component concentrate food	Encourage a gradual change to an extruded pellet	• High quality, extruded pelleted food should compose only 5% of diet, 85% being a high quality hay or grass • The remaining 10% of the diet should be leafy green vegetables • High crude fibre diets reduce the risk of acquired dental disease and improve gut health

2.3 Assessment of the housing for the rabbit provides information that may be helpful for improving welfare. (continues) ▶

Case example 1: Rabbits *continued*

Current welfare observations to be improved	Goals and objectives for improvement following basic welfare assessment	Achieving better welfare: actions
Companion	Keeping solitary rabbits does not conform to good welfare practices	• Ideally rabbits should live in neutered, bonded opposite sex pairs. Trios and larger groups can work but can be hard to bond • Neutering is vital for all rabbits to prevent unwanted pregnancies, problem behaviours and maintain health
Water presentation	Clean water sources presented in a way which is accessible to the individual, whether bowl or bottle	• Many water bottles will quickly grow algae; daily cleaning is required and water replenished when low – hot days may require multiple water changes. Always ensure the spout/dropper and ball bearing are cleaned and working correctly. If using bottles, ensure there are at least two per rabbit • A heavy crock bowl is a better option as more natural for the rabbit to drink out of. Offer at least two water bowls per rabbit. Clean and fill with clean water at least twice a day
Exercise	No outdoor access seen	• Provide permanent access to a large run, which meets the RWAF minimum size of 8ft so this can be used as an exercise area and will also encourage natural 'happy' behaviours such as 'binkying' • Ideally place the run on patio slabs for ease of cleaning and increased predator protection
Enrichment	No toys or tunnels seen	• A range of rabbit safe toys and tunnels can be used to provide enrichment. These include digging pits, hard plastic stacking cups, willow balls and hard plastic tunnels. All items should be checked daily for signs of wear and tear and digging pits should only be used during direct supervision

2.3 (continued) Assessment of the housing for the rabbit provides information that may be helpful for improving welfare.

Client questionnaires

Client questionnaires are a good way to gather as much information as possible about the animal's normal environment, husbandry, diet and behaviour, and this provides a vital insight into the pet's welfare at home. Much of this information can be gained with the use of client questionnaires, which can be completed either prior to visiting the veterinary practice or during the consultation. Figure 2.4 details the important information that should form the basis of the questionnaire and examples of client questionnaires can be found at the end of the chapter.

The information gathered by the client questionnaire can be useful if the animal needs to be admitted to the practice, as it will allow the veterinary team to replicate as closely as possible the patient's home environment and routine. This can help to alleviate any unnecessary stressors for the patient and prevent misinterpretation of preference-based aversions as clinical abnormalities. In addition, the questionnaire may indicate the cause of the underlying condition(s) for which the animal has been presented, as often poor husbandry and diet lead to medical problems. If poor animal welfare in the home environment is identified, this can be flagged and discussed with the owner when the animal is discharged.

Parameter	Example questions
General	• What are the client's details? • What are the animal's details? • Where was the animal sourced from? • Does the animal have a bonded companion? If yes, what species? • Does the animal regularly have human interaction? • Are there any specific handling requirements for the animal?
Housing	• What is the normal home environment of the animal (e.g. indoor *versus* outdoor housing)? • What type of enclosure is normally provided (e.g. size, substrate, toys, hides)? • Where does the animal usually sleep? • When does the animal usually sleep? • Is there a specific type of bedding that is provided or that the animal prefers? • Does the animal have a 'comfort item'?
Feeding	• What is the normal diet? • Is there a food item which is regarded as 'high reward'? • What is the normal frequency of feeding and at what times is the animal fed? • How is food usually presented (ceramic/metal feeding bowls, shallow or deep bowls, raised or at ground level, scatter/puzzle/slow feeder used)? • Does the animal have any specific feeding requirements? • Does the animal have any food allergies? Or strong dislikes?

2.4 Examples of the important questions that should form the basis of the client questionnaire. (continues) ▶

Parameter	Example questions
Drinking	• How is water usually provided (e.g. bowl, bottle, mister)? • Does the animal have any specific requirements for the provision of water?
Elimination	• Is the animal trained to urinate/defecate to a specific command? • Does the animal prefer a specific substrate for elimination? • Does the animal require assistance/stimulation to urinate or defecate? • Is the animal currently incontinent (urine or faeces) or constipated?
Grooming	• Does the animal require manual grooming? • Does the animal enjoy being groomed? • What grooming equipment is the animal used to?
Behaviour	• What is the animal's normal temperament? • Does the animal show any typical signs when they feel anxious or upset? • Are there any concerns about the animal's behaviour?
Exercise	• What is the animal's normal exercise routine? • Are there any concerns about the animal's motility?
Health and medication	• Are there any concerns about the animal's health? • Is the animal currently on any medication? If yes, what drug(s), dose, frequency and when was it last administered? • Is the animal currently receiving any prophylactic preventative treatments (e.g. vaccinations, treatment for fleas or worms)? If yes, what drug(s), dose, frequency and when was it last administered? • Does the animal pose a zoonotic risk to any other animals or staff within the veterinary practice?

2.4 (continued) Examples of the important questions that should form the basis of the client questionnaire.

Ethograms

An ethogram is a catalogue of different behaviours seen in a specific animal. This may include behaviours most commonly seen or a particular class of behaviours. It is important to understand the natural behaviour of the animal when creating an ethogram and to adapt the behaviour list so that it is specific to that individual.

Ethograms are a good way to start any behavioural investigation: the observer should monitor the individual or group of animals and make a note against the ethogram of how many times a particular behaviour is performed within a given timeframe (Figure 2.5). The best way to observe any animal is without their awareness of being watched; therefore, the use of cameras is ideal, although this option may not be available to everyone.

Ethograms can be used to identify behaviours associated with poor welfare. Changes can then be made to the environment or interactions with the animal and the ethogram repeated. This will provide a quantifiable way of determining whether there has been a reduction in behaviours associated with poor welfare.

Species-specific ethograms

The following figures show ethograms that have been developed for wolves (Figure 2.6), rabbits (Figure 2.7) and lizards (Figure 2.8). The large carnivore ethogram for wolves can be adapted for other large carnivores in a zoo environment by including behaviours such as pacing, deferred aggression, tail flicking, grooming, vocalization and digging. This ethogram can also be adapted for use with dogs and should include behaviours such as tail chasing, excessive licking of an area, scratching, nose rubbing and barking (K Atkinson, personal communication). For further information on animal behaviour, the reader is referred to Chapter 3.

Record no.: ....

Date: .... Time: ....

Weather: ....

Species: ....

Environment (wild/zoo/rescue/vet): ....

Time (mins)	Behaviour (examples)			Comments
	Grooming	Playing	Aggression	
30				
60				
90				

Descriptions
• Grooming: describe grooming behaviour for that species
• Playing: describe play behaviours for that species
• Aggression: describe aggressive behaviours for that species

2.5 General ethogram template.

Record no.: ....

Date: .... Time: ....

Weather: ....

Species: ....

Environment (wild/zoo/rescue/vet): ....

Time (mins)	Behaviours					Comments
	Search	Approach	Attack – group	Attack – individuals	Capture	
30						
60						
90						
120						
150						
180						
210						
240						
270						
300						

Descriptions
- Search: travelling without fixating on or moving towards prey
- Approach: travelling towards or fixating on prey
- Attack – group: running after a fleeing group or lunging at a standing group whilst glancing about at different group members
- Attack – individual: running at or lunging at a solitary or single member of a group whilst ignoring all other group members
- Capture: biting and restraining prey

2.6 Ethogram for wild wolves. Note that this example is based on a study of animals with access to live prey, which is illegal in the UK.
(MacNulty, 2007)

Record no.: ....

Date: .... Time: ....

Weather: ....

Breed: ....

Environment (wild/zoo/rescue/vet): ....

Time (mins)	Behaviours										Comments
	Binky	Grooming	Eating caecotrophs	Hiding	Vocalization	Thumping	Mating	Eating	Aggression	Playing	
30											
60											
90											
120											
150											
180											
210											
240											
270											
300											

Descriptions
- Binky: jumps into the air and twists its head and body in opposite directions before falling back to the ground
- Grooming: licking a companion or self-grooming
- Eating caecotrophs: bending over and eating caecotroph faeces directly from the anus
- Hiding: out of direct view from potential predators, either in tunnels or in a hide
- Vocalization: grunting/growling vocalizations
- Thumping: stomping the floor with either one or both back legs
- Mating: with a companion or object within the environment. This should include pre-mating chasing behaviour
- Eating: consuming any environmental vegetation and/or diet provided by the owner
- Aggression: lunging and darting towards or biting/boxing a companion
- Playing: direct and deliberate interaction with any toys or non-food objects that are within the enclosure

2.7 Ethogram for rabbits.

Record no.: ....

Date: .... Time: ....

Weather: ....

Species: ....

Environment (wild/zoo/rescue/vet): ....

Time (mins)	Behaviours										Comments
	Head bob	Tongue flick	Approach	Intimidating posture	Chase	Bite	Fight	Dorsum display	Tail wave	Retreat	
30											
60											
90											
120											
150											
180											
210											
240											
270											
300											

Descriptions
- Head bob: vertical wave of head and anterior part of the body. This motion is repeated several times at different amplitudes
- Tongue flick: tongue projection outside the mouth bringing it back quickly, touching the substrate, air or body of an opponent
- Approach: movement straight towards an opponent at a fast or slow speed
- Intimidating posture: rise of the anterior part of the body or the whole body, curving the head towards the ground, curving the dorsum. Sometimes inflation of the gular region
- Chase: quick move towards retreating opponent; bites may or may not occur
- Bite: biting an opponent, mainly in the neck and tail base regions, releasing it afterwards. The approach towards a bite is either lateral or dorsal
- Fight: both individuals attempt to bite or tail wave against each other. Usually lateral approach with their heads positioned in opposing directions
- Dorsum display: lift of the anterior part of the body, exposure of the gular region and lateral inclination of the upper body. Changes the angle of the scapular waist, expanding the thoracic region and showing the full dorsum towards an opponent
- Tail wave: the ventral part of the body is in contact with the substrate whilst waving only the final section of the tail laterally in rapid movements
- Retreat: move rapidly directly away from an opponent

2.8 Ethogram for lizards.

Welfare during hospitalization

Hospitalization can be very stressful for all species, but by making small changes it is possible to reduce the stress experienced by patients and to shorten recovery times. Mimicking a normal routine, including diet and exercise, can help provide the best welfare for hospitalized patients. Where possible, prey and predator species should be separated in order to reduce stress and better observe patient behaviour to assess pain and progress. Cameras can be used within the ward to observe the patient's behaviour, as many prey species will hide pain and clinical signs of disease as a self-preservation tactic.

Hospitalizing patient companions may also help reduce stress and recovery times (Figure 2.9); it is recommended that the animals are separated for a short time overnight in order to reliably track what the patient is eating, drinking and eliminating; using a wire cat carrier or clear separator screen still allows the patient to see, smell and interact with their companion whilst facilitating monitoring. In addition, some species carry out the majority of their activities at night or when it is quieter, so allocating sleep time and administering medications together (where possible) will allow rest and consequently better welfare for the more stressed patients.

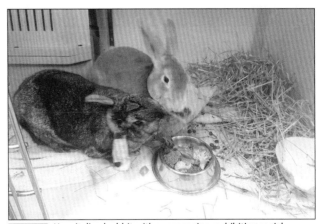

2.9 Hospitalized rabbit with a companion, exhibiting social behaviours and showing an interest in fresh food.

Hospitalization forms

The use of hospitalization forms (Figure 2.10), comparing physical parameters such as heart rate, respiratory rate, temperature and blood pressure, in conjunction with body condition scoring and pain scoring systems (see below) will facilitate a much more clinical view of the patient and

Surname:...

Patient no.: ....

Microchip no.: ....

Animal:..

A downloadable form is available for this manual from the BSAVA Library

Sex:.. Age: ....

Date:.. Day:...Tel: ....

Condition..Weight ....Admit weight...

Kennel...Vet ....

	0800	1000	1200	1400	1600	1800	2000	2200	0000	0400	0600
Vet/RVN initials											
Temperature											
Heart rate											
Respiration rate											
MM/CRT											
Demeanour											
Pain score											
Gut sounds (L) if applicable											
Gut sounds (R) if applicable											
Urine											
Faeces											
Drinking											
Food offered (weigh in grams)											
Food eaten (weigh out)											

Treatment / Frequency / Route	*	9	10	11	12	13	14	15	16	17	18	19	20	21	22	23	24	1	2	3	4	5	6	7	8
Fluid type/rate: Check/flush intravenous catheter																										

Special considerations (am) Initials:	Nursing/VCA comments	Vet comments/plan
Special considerations (pm) Initials:	Owner called: Y/N Notes on computer: Y/N	Summary

2.10 Example of a hospitalization form that should be completed for each patient. CRT = capillary refill time; MM = mucous membrane.

aid in interpreting results. They can also be a useful visual prompt for nursing interactions and interventions (e.g. administration of medications). Hospitalization forms can be adapted to reflect species-specific needs, such as temperature gradients for reptiles and reversed daytime for nocturnal species. In-house training should be carried out to ensure that the veterinary team understand the importance of adapting nursing care for different species.

Body and muscle condition

During hospitalization, accurate daily recording and comparison of bodyweight, as well as body and muscle condition scoring, will determine whether the current interventions are proving successful and help identify cases where further evaluation and/or alteration of nutritional management is required. Body and muscle condition scoring should also form part of the general care and maintenance of an individual or group of animals outside of a clinical setting. It is suggested that the body and muscle condition of animal collections be evaluated at least biannually, in order to prevent caregivers overlooking gradual changes that occur over a longer time period. Although published body and muscle condition scoring systems are not available for all species, Figures 2.11 to 2.15 demonstrate the type of resources available for dogs, cats and birds.

Pain

The International Association for the Study of Pain (IASP) defined pain as 'an unpleasant sensory and emotional experience associated with actual or potential tissue damage or described in terms of such damage' in 1979. As pain is associated with both physical and psychological mechanisms, the monitoring and recording of pain in non-verbal species is complex and has a huge scope for misinterpretation.

"Verbal description is only one of several behaviours to express pain; inability to communicate does not negate the possibility that a human or non-human animal experiences pain" (IASP, 2019). A pain stimulus is often categorized as somatic or visceral pain. Some commonly recognized conditions that are well documented to be painful are listed in Figure 2.16.

The negative effects of pain (Thomas and Lerche, 2011):

- Produce a catabolic state (energy release), which may lead to wasting
- Suppress the immune response, predisposing to infection or sepsis and increasing hospitalization time and cost
- Promote inflammation, which delays wound healing
- Cause patient suffering, which is also stressful for owners and caregivers.

Regular, repeatable and comparable assessments of the patient's perceived pain must be conducted throughout periods of hospitalization and whilst the animal is under veterinary care during 'normal' living conditions.

Scoring systems

The effective treatment of pain is crucial for animal welfare. In order to achieve this, an appreciation of how painful certain procedures and conditions are likely to be is required, along with the ability to recognize and quantify that pain. Thus, pain scoring should be part of the routine

ongoing assessment for each patient whilst they are in the hospital.

Veterinary pain scoring systems have been developed from human models. When assessing pain in non-verbal, non-human animals, the ability to recognize and assess changes in physiology and behaviour is paramount, as is identifying the presence of painful stimuli and the extrapolation of information. There are a multitude of pain scoring systems available for veterinary use, including:

- **Visual Analogue Systems (VAS)** – VAS use a plottable line to record results. The line is often 10 cm in length. The line starts and ends with two polar opposite outcomes (e.g. no pain at 0 cm on the left-hand side and extreme pain at 10 cm on the right-hand side). The line is marked at a point corresponding to the assessment of pain. The distance of the mark from 0 cm is then measured to give a numerical score. These systems are subjective and therefore open to a wide degree of variation between assessors
- **Numerical Rating Scales (NRS)** – NRS use numbers to grade pain (e.g. 0 indicates no pain and 10 indicates extreme pain). These systems are commonly used in human medicine by patients to assess their pain level
- **Simple Descriptive Scales (SDS)** – SDS are the least sensitive means of pain assessment. They often comprise a set of descriptions, which the assessor uses to grade the level of pain (e.g. no pain, mild pain, moderate pain, severe pain, extreme pain). Assessments undertaken using SDS are very subjective and do not take into consideration more subtle pain behaviours that may be exhibited
- **Tailored/composite objective scales** – These scales merge the three systems described above (i.e. VAS, NRS and SDS) into a more useable veterinary model for non-verbal patients. However, the vast differences in the way that different species respond to painful stimuli complicates the production of a single form and species-specific scales are required. Examples of species-specific pain scoring systems used in practice include:
  - Glasgow Composite Measure Pain Scale (Canine – Short Form) (Figure 2.17a)
  - Glasgow Composite Measure Pain Scale (Feline)
  - UNESP-Botucatu Multidimensional Composite Pain Scale (Short Form)
  - Colorado Canine Acute Pain Scale
  - Colorado Feline Acute Pain Scale (Figure 2.17b)
  - Rabbit Grimace Scale (Figure 2.17c)
  - Mouse Grimace Scale.

Each scoring system has its limitations, so the person performing the assessment must be aware of these when interpreting the results. All veterinary personnel responsible for carrying out pain assessments must be fully trained in the use of scoring systems and, most importantly, the subsequent actions should pain be detected in the patient.

Assessment and interpretation

Whichever pain scoring system is chosen, it should be dynamic and interactive. All assessments should start with observation from a distance so that the patient is not aware that they are being watched. This will allow evaluation of the patient in the absence of stimulation. The assessor should then move closer to the animal,

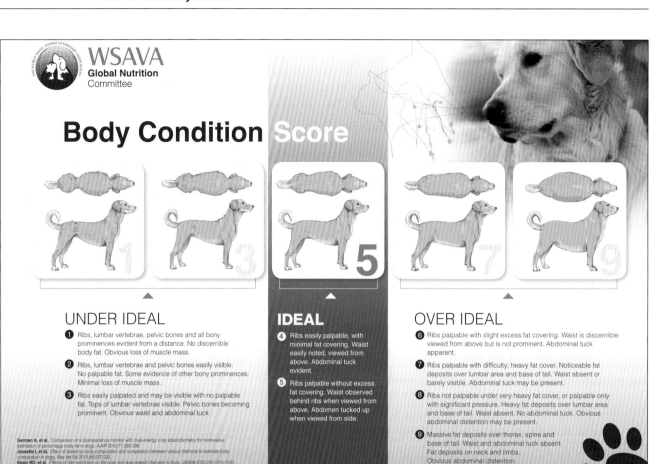

2.11 Body condition scoring chart for dogs.
(Provided courtesy of the World Small Animal Veterinary Association (WSAVA). Available at the WSAVA Global Nutrition Committee Nutritional Toolkit website: https://wsava.org/global-guidelines/global-nutrition-guidelines/. Accessed 14 July 2020. © WSAVA, 2013)

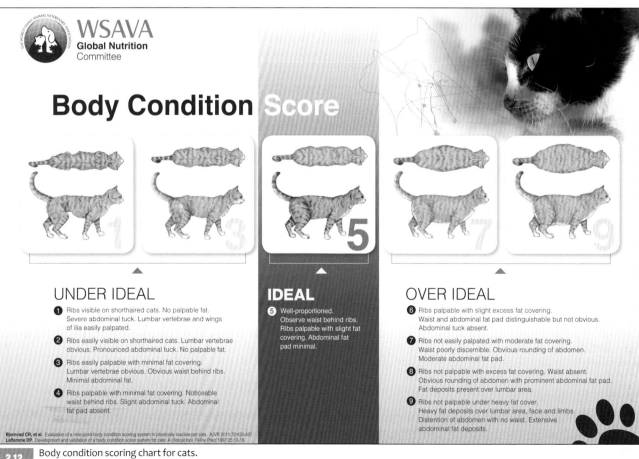

2.12 Body condition scoring chart for cats.
(Provided courtesy of the World Small Animal Veterinary Association (WSAVA). Available at the WSAVA Global Nutrition Committee Nutritional Toolkit website: https://wsava.org/global-guidelines/global-nutrition-guidelines/. Accessed 14 July 2020. © WSAVA, 2013)

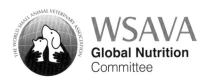

Muscle Condition Score

Muscle condition score is assessed by visualization and palpation of the spine, scapulae, skull, and wings of the ilia. Muscle loss is typically first noted in the epaxial muscles on each side of the spine; muscle loss at other sites can be more variable. Muscle condition score is graded as normal, mild loss, moderate loss, or severe loss. Note that animals can have significant muscle loss if they are overweight (body condition score > 5). Conversely, animals can have a low body condition score (< 4) but have minimal muscle loss. Therefore, assessing both body condition score and muscle condition score on every animal at every visit is important. Palpation is especially important when muscle loss is mild and in animals that are overweight. An example of each score is shown below.

Normal muscle mass	Mild muscle loss

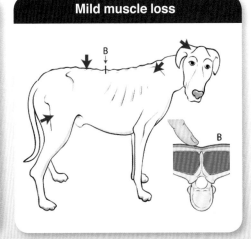

Moderate muscle loss	Severe muscle loss

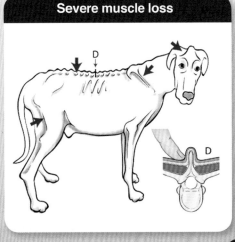

wsava.org

2.13 Muscle condition scoring chart for dogs.
(Provided courtesy of the World Small Animal Veterinary Association (WSAVA). Available at the WSAVA Global Nutrition Committee Nutritional Toolkit website: https://wsava.org/global-guidelines/global-nutrition-guidelines/. Accessed 14 July 2020. © Tufts University, 2013)

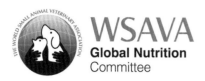

Muscle Condition Score

Muscle condition score is assessed by visualization and palpation of the spine, scapulae, skull, and wings of the ilia. Muscle loss is typically first noted in the epaxial muscles on each side of the spine; muscle loss at other sites can be more variable. Muscle condition score is graded as normal, mild loss, moderate loss, or severe loss. Note that animals can have significant muscle loss even if they are overweight (body condition score > 5/9). Conversely, animals can have a low body condition score (< 4/9) but have minimal muscle loss. Therefore, assessing both body condition score and muscle condition score on every animal at every visit is important. Palpation is especially important with mild muscle loss and in animals that are overweight. An example of each score is shown below.

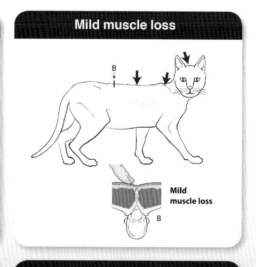

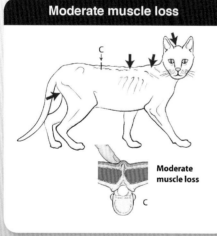

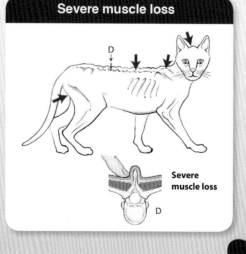

wsava.org

2.14 Muscle condition scoring chart for cats.
(Provided courtesy of the World Small Animal Veterinary Association (WSAVA). Available at the WSAVA Global Nutrition Committee Nutritional Toolkit website: https://wsava.org/global-guidelines/global-nutrition-guidelines/. Accessed 14 July 2020. © Tufts University, 2014)

Bird Size-O-Meter

 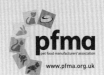
www.pfma.org.uk

Size-O-Meter Score: Characteristics:

viewed from above   skyline view of breast bone and muscle

1 Very Thin
- Breast bone is very sharp to the touch
- Loss of breast muscle and no fat cover

2 Thin
- Breast bone is easily felt and sharp
- Loss of breast muscle and little or no fat cover

3 Ideal
- Breast bone easily felt but not sharp
- Breast muscle rounded

4 Overweight
- Pressure is needed to feel the breast bone
- Well rounded breast muscle and some fat cover
- May see some fat below where breast bone ends

5 Obese
- Very hard or not possible to feel the breast bone
- Very rounded muscle and possible to feel or see fat moving under the skin.
- Fat also obvious below where the breast bone ends

Produced with assistance and advice from Anna Meredith MRCVS

☐ Your pet is a healthy weight
☐ Seek advice about your pet's weight
☐ Seek advice as your pet could be at risk

How to check your birds shape

- Getting hands on is key. Not all birds are used to being handled but it is difficult to judge if your bird is the right weight by sight. You will need to gently feel your bird, using restraint if necessary.
- Use bare hands and not gloves to handle birds as then you can judge the tightness of grip. If you need to protect yourself – use a cloth or towel.
- Small birds can be held in one hand with the neck between the first and second finger and the bird's back against the palm so that the wings and body are gently restrained in the closed hand.
- Larger parrots may take two people, one to hold the bird and the other to assess its body condition. A towel or cloth is used over the open hand to grasp the bird firmly behind its head and neck. The towel is then wrapped around the wings and body to prevent flapping. Gently stroking the top of the head and talking to the bird gently will help to calm it.
- Gently run your fingertips down the centre of the front of the bird in the midline over the breast area. You should be able to feel a bony ridge (known as the keel or breast bone). This should be easy to feel but not too prominent.
- Next, run your fingers at right angles to the keel across the breast muscles. If these feel shrunken so that the keel sticks out prominently your bird is too thin. If the breast muscles are just rounded but you can still feel the keel your bird is in good condition. If you cannot feel the keel and the muscles are very rounded or you can feel or see fat moving underneath the skin your bird is overweight.
- The breast muscle can also vary in size depending on how much exercise your bird gets – so if it flies a lot it will have larger firmer breast muscles than a bird who does not fly. However, the same criteria still apply in assessing body condition – prominence of the bony keel and presence of fat underneath the skin.

Bird Size-O-Meter

Results:

Feeding tips:

- Pet birds can get obese (fat) quickly if they are fed an improper diet, and especially in combination with lack of exercise.
- The most common cause of obesity in parrots is feeding a diet that is too high in seeds (e.g. sunflower seeds) – these are high in fat and cholesterol and low in many essential vitamins and minerals, and lead to many health problems.
- Although some smaller birds such as finches, canaries and budgerigars, will do well on a largely seed-based diet, larger parrots do not. Complete pelleted diets that are nutritionally balanced are widely available for most species of pet parrots and can be supplemented with a variety of fruits, vegetables and nuts. Different species will have differing nutritional requirements.
- Consult your vet for dietary advice for your bird.

Increasing Exercise:

- It is ideal to let your bird out of the cage at least twice a day to fly freely. Pet parrots can easily be trained and should never need to have their wings clipped. Flying is a key part of a bird's normal behaviour. Always make sure the area is secure. i.e. close all windows and doors, away from other pets that may harm them (e.g. cats and dogs).
- Where appropriate free flight in a large aviary outdoors is ideal. Exposure to natural sunlight is also very important for birds, as long as they do not get too cold. Indoors special UV lights for birds can be used.
- Parrots enjoy playing with toys and these should be used to provide mental stimulation as well as physical exercise.

Your Bird is score 1 Very Thin — A score of one suggests that your bird is very likely to be underweight. Your bird may have a naturally lean physique but we would recommend you speak to your local vet to rule out any underlying medical reasons such as kidney disease. If your pet is healthy, but otherwise underweight, your vet is likely to advise some dietary and lifestyle changes.

Your Bird is score 2 Thin — A score of two means your bird is thin and potentially underweight. Your bird may have a naturally lean physique but we recommend you speak to your local vet for a health check up. If your bird is healthy but otherwise underweight, your vet may advise some dietary and lifestyle changes.

Your Bird is score 3 Ideal — Congratulations your bird is in ideal body condition! This is great news, as being at ideal weight increases the chances of your bird living a long and healthy life. To keep your bird in tip top shape, monitor its weight and body condition on a regular basis (e.g. once a month) and be careful what you and everyone else in the family feeds it. Remember any changes in lifestyle (e.g. reduced exercise, extra treats or other factors such as stress) can result in weight-change. To help you keep on track – check out our feeding and exercise tips.

Your Bird is score 4 Overweight — A score of four means your pet is potentially overweight. Being overweight is unhealthy for birds as it can lead to a shortened life-span, atherosclerosis, heart and liver disease and other health complications. Please speak to your local vet for advice and a thorough health check-up. The vet will look for any underlying medical reasons as to why your bird may be too heavy. If there are no underlying health issues, a change of diet and lifestyle is likely to be suggested. Many vet practices run free weight management consultations led by the veterinary nurse, ask about these services when you ring to book an appointment.

Your Bird is score 5 Obese — A score of five means your bird is likely to be obese and this can have serious medical implications. Being overweight is unhealthy for pets as it can lead to a shortened life-span, shortened life-span, atherosclerosis, heart and liver disease and other health complications. Please speak to your local vet for advice and a thorough health check up. The vet will look for any underlying medical reasons as to why your pet may be too heavy. If there are no underlying health issues, a weight loss programme will probably be individually developed for your bird and should include diet and lifestyle changes.

For more information and details of how to perform the assessment and check your bird's shape please visit **www.pfma.org.uk**. In addition to providing useful tips on how to keep your pet healthy and happy, a team of veterinary nutrition experts are on hand to answer your pet nutrition questions in the 'Ask the Expert' section.

2.15 Body condition scoring chart for birds.
(© Pet Food Manufacturers' Association)

Type of pain	Associated organs	Common examples
Somatic	Pain that originates from damage to bones, joints, muscle or skin and is described in humans as localized, constant, sharp, aching and throbbing	Burns, trauma to tissues, arthritis, fractures
Visceral	Pain that arises from stretching, distension or inflammation of the viscera and is described in humans as deep cramping, aching or gnawing without good localization. The respiratory, digestive, urinary and reproductive systems are affected	Organ distension (colic, gastric dilatation–volvulus, urethral obstruction) Inflammation (pancreatitis, gastric ulcers)

2.16 Examples of conditions that are reported to result in somatic or visceral pain.
(Gaynor and Muir, 2014)

SHORT FORM OF THE GLASGOW COMPOSITE PAIN SCALE

Dog's name: ....

Hospital number: .... Date............/............./.............. Time:..

Surgery: Yes/No (delete as appropriate)

Procedure or condition: ....

....

....

In the sections below please circle the appropriate score in each list and sum these to give the total score

A. Look at dog in Kennel

Is the dog?

(i)

Quiet	0
Crying or whimpering	1
Groaning	2
Screaming	3

(ii)

Ignoring any wound or painful area	0
Looking at wound or painful area	1
Licking wound or painful area	2
Rubbing wound or painful area	3
Chewing wound or painful area	4

> In the case of spinal, pelvic or multiple limb fractures, or where assistance is required to aid locomotion do not carry out section **B** and proceed to **C**
> *Please tick if this is the case* ☐ then proceed to **C**.

B. Put lead on dog and lead out of the kennel.

When the dog rises/walks is it?

(iii)

Normal	0
Lame	1
Slow or reluctant	2
Stiff	3
It refuses to move	4

C. If it has a wound or painful area including abdomen, apply gentle pressure 2 inches round the site.

Does it?

(iv)

Do nothing	0
Look round	1
Flinch	2
Growl or guard area	3
Snap	4
Cry	5

D. Overall

Is the dog?

(v)

Happy and content or happy and bouncy	0
Quiet	1
Indifferent or non-responsive to surroundings	2
Nervous or anxious or fearful	3
Depressed or non-responsive to stimulation	4

Is the dog?

(vi)

Comfortable	0
Unsettled	1
Restless	2
Hunched or tense	3
Rigid	4

(a) © University of Glasgow

Total score (i + ii + iii + iv + v + vi) = _____

2.17 Examples of species-specific pain scales. (a) Glasgow Composite Measure Pain Scale (Canine – Short Form). Further examples are included in the *BSAVA Guide to Pain Management in Small Animal Practice* and the *BSAVA Textbook of Veterinary Nursing*. (continues)
(© University of Glasgow 2008; licensed to NewMetrica Ltd). ▶

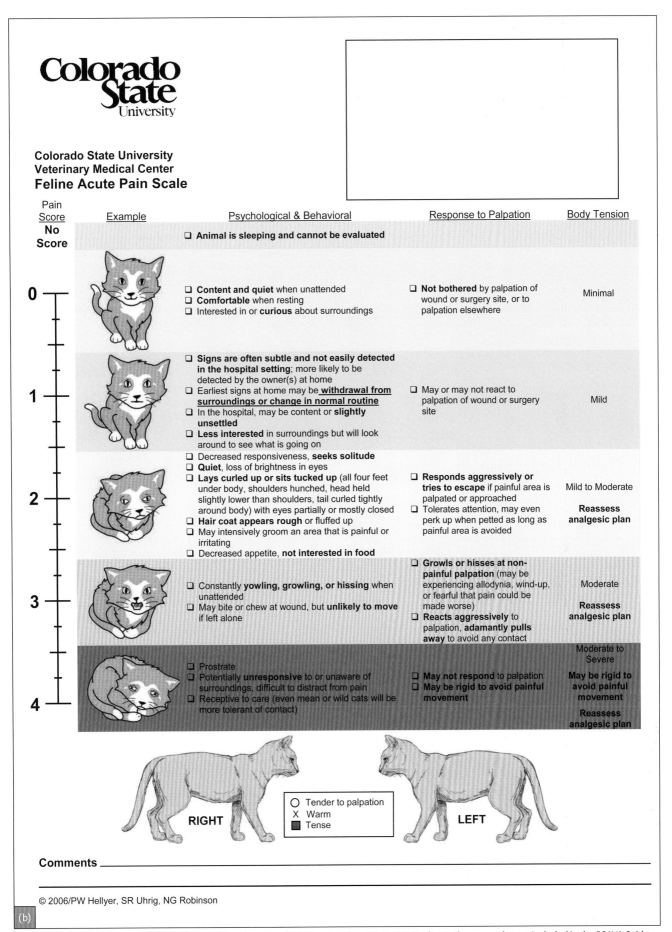

Colorado State University Veterinary Medical Center
Feline Acute Pain Scale

Pain Score	Example	Psychological & Behavioral	Response to Palpation	Body Tension
No Score		☐ **Animal is sleeping and cannot be evaluated**		
0		☐ **Content and quiet** when unattended ☐ **Comfortable** when resting ☐ Interested in or **curious** about surroundings	☐ **Not bothered** by palpation of wound or surgery site, or to palpation elsewhere	Minimal
1		☐ **Signs are often subtle and not easily detected in the hospital setting**; more likely to be detected by the owner(s) at home ☐ Earliest signs at home may be **withdrawal from surroundings or change in normal routine** ☐ In the hospital, may be content or **slightly unsettled** ☐ **Less interested** in surroundings but will look around to see what is going on	☐ May or may not react to palpation of wound or surgery site	Mild
2		☐ Decreased responsiveness, **seeks solitude** ☐ **Quiet**, loss of brightness in eyes ☐ **Lays curled up or sits tucked up** (all four feet under body, shoulders hunched, head held slightly lower than shoulders, tail curled tightly around body) with eyes partially or mostly closed ☐ **Hair coat appears rough** or fluffed up ☐ May intensively groom an area that is painful or irritating ☐ Decreased appetite, **not interested in food**	☐ **Responds aggressively or tries to escape** if painful area is palpated or approached ☐ Tolerates attention, may even perk up when petted as long as painful area is avoided	Mild to Moderate **Reassess analgesic plan**
3		☐ Constantly **yowling, growling, or hissing** when unattended ☐ May bite or chew at wound, but **unlikely to move** if left alone	☐ **Growls or hisses at non-painful palpation** (may be experiencing allodynia, wind-up, or fearful that pain could be made worse) ☐ **Reacts aggressively** to palpation, **adamantly pulls away** to avoid any contact	Moderate **Reassess analgesic plan**
4		☐ Prostrate ☐ Potentially **unresponsive** to or unaware of surroundings, difficult to distract from pain ☐ Receptive to care (even mean or wild cats will be more tolerant of contact)	☐ **May not respond** to palpation ☐ **May be rigid to avoid painful movement**	Moderate to Severe May be rigid to avoid painful movement **Reassess analgesic plan**

RIGHT   LEFT

○ Tender to palpation
X Warm
■ Tense

Comments _____

© 2006/PW Hellyer, SR Uhrig, NG Robinson

2.17 (continued) Examples of species-specific pain scales. (b) Colorado Feline Acute Pain Scale. Further examples are included in the *BSAVA Guide to Pain Management in Small Animal Practice* and the *BSAVA Textbook of Veterinary Nursing*. (continues)
(Reproduced with permission from Peter W. Hellyer, College of Veterinary Medicine and Biomedical Sciences, Colorado State University, USA)

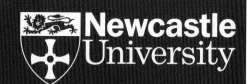

NC 3Rs
National Centre
for the Replacement
Refinement & Reduction
of Animals in Research

Newcastle University

The Rabbit Grimace Scale

Research has demonstrated that changes in facial expression provide a means of assessing pain in rabbits.

The specific facial action units shown below comprise the Rabbit Grimace Scale. These action units increase in intensity in response to post-procedural pain and can form part of a clinical assessment alongside other validated indices of pain.

The action units should only be used in awake animals. Each animal should be observed for a short period of time to avoid scoring brief changes in facial expression that are unrelated to the animal's welfare.

	Action units		
	Not present "0"	**Moderately present "1"**	**Obviously present "2"**
Orbital tightening • Closing of the eyelid (narrowing of orbital area) • A wrinkle may be visible around the eye			
Cheek flattening • Flattening of the cheeks. When 'obviously present', cheeks have a sunken look. • The face becomes more angular and less rounded			
Nostril shape • Nostrils (nares) are drawn vertically forming a 'V' rather than 'U' shape • Nose tip is moved down towards the chin			
Whisker shape and position • Whiskers are pushed away from the face to 'stand on end' • Whiskers stiffen and lose their natural, downward curve • Whiskers increasingly point in the same direction. When 'obviously present', whiskers move downwards			
Ear shape and position • Ears become more tightly folded / curled (more cylindrical) in shape • Ears rotate from facing towards the source of sound to facing towards the hindquarters • Ears may be held closer to the back or sides of the body			

2.17 (continued) Examples of species-specific pain scales. (c) Rabbit Grimace Scale. Further examples are included in the *BSAVA Guide to Pain Management in Small Animal Practice* and the *BSAVA Textbook of Veterinary Nursing*.

(Reproduced with permission of the NC3Rs; www.nc3rs.org.uk/grimacescales; Keating *et al.*, 2012; images provided by Dr Matthew Leach, Newcastle University).

incorporating verbal cues, before progressing to physical interaction and palpation of the areas of interest, where pain is likely to exist. "Pain signs may be obvious, such as increased heart rate and blood pressure, increased respiratory rate and vocalization. More subtle behavioural changes that occur such as general restlessness, decreased appetite, not sleeping, resenting handling and not assuming a normal position may be even more significant" (Goldberg and Shaffran, 2015).

Rabbits

Prey species, such as rabbits, often do not demonstrate outward signs of debilitation as a means of self-preservation, as to do so would make them targets for predation

Chelonians

Chelonians may only exhibit subtle changes in response to chronic illness and/or pain, which may be missed by an owner or caregiver, leading to dehydration and anorexia

Dysphoria is defined as a state of anxiety or restlessness, which is often accompanied by vocalization. Differentiating dysphoria from pain can be challenging, especially in traumatic or surgical cases. In addition, pain and dysphoria can occur simultaneously, which may complicate the clinical picture. However, the observant practitioner can discern clues to differentiate dysphoria from pain. Dysphoric animals are often difficult to distract or calm by interaction or handling (Hellyer et al., 2007).

In addition, having a full history of current medications that the patient is on which may affect the pain scoring assessment is useful to avoid misinterpreting side effects such as sedation or emesis as a pain response or clinical anomaly.

Analgesia

Analgesic medication selection is important as different species can have differences in the distribution and quantity of receptor sites, meaning that each drug chosen will have a species-specific pharmacokinetic effect. The presence of a renoportal or hepatoportal system also needs to be taken into consideration as this may alter the site of drug delivery and potentially the medication selection, depending on the species and underlying disease processes. Where there is a delayed onset of action, the half-life of the drug may be altered.

Environmental and behavioural considerations are not only important in terms of welfare, but also act as adjuncts to analgesia and can be extremely helpful in enhancing analgesic effects from pain medications. In addition, preemptive analgesia should be considered ahead of any planned investigation or surgical procedure.

Nursing care
Nursing process and models

The nursing process (Figure 2.18) provides a structure for nursing care that enables each individual animal's needs to be taken into consideration. By nursing in this manner, holistic care rather than care focused solely on the disease or injury present can be delivered. The nursing process can be divided into six steps:

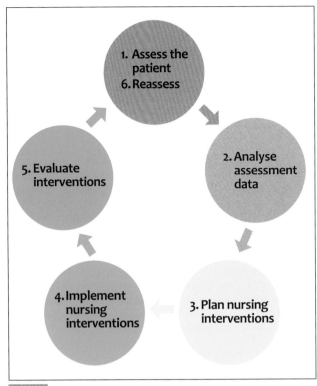

2.18 The nursing process (see text for further details).

1. **Assess the patient** – gather data based on the patient's physical status, diagnosis, life stage and ability to perform the 'activities of living' (see Figures 2.19 and 2.20).
2. **Analyse assessment data** – identify problems and potential problems and create a nursing diagnosis, taking into account the 'activities of living' and the ability of the patient to perform them unassisted. It is important to remember that these variables can change regularly, based on the response of the patient to treatment, and that destabilization can occur at any point (even if a patient seems well).
3. **Plan nursing interventions** – write a care plan to rectify/prevent the problems identified. Make sure that the plan is concise and that the goals of the plan are clearly stated. Ensure that all caregivers are aware of the goals and the appropriate techniques to implement the plan.
4. **Implement nursing interventions** – carry out the care plan, documenting all interventions and communicating them to the wider veterinary team. Ensure that all equipment and consumables are available for the required nursing interventions. Observe appropriate hygiene practices (e.g. handwashing, use of personal protective equipment) and ensure the safety of both the patient and staff carrying out the nursing interventions at all times.
5. **Evaluate nursing interventions** – collect objective data on whether the goals of the care plan have been met, as well as the efficacy of the interventions. The following questions should be posed: can we do something better? Are we doing too much? Do all primary caregivers agree with the observations?
6. **Reassess the patient** – reassess the patient following evaluation of the nursing interventions. It is at this stage that new problems, or limited capabilities if the patient is decompensating, may be identified. Review the current interventions and equipment with a view to improving practices. Communicate all findings to the veterinary team.

The nursing process offers a systematic approach to care but is limited in its function unless it is integrated into a model of nursing (see *BSAVA Textbook of Veterinary Nursing*). There are many nursing models that can be used to assist with the nursing process, including:

- The Roper, Logan and Tierney Model (Figures 2.19 and 2.20)
- Orem's Model
- The Ability Model.

These models often list a patient's needs and assess how well the patient can achieve those needs based on their underlying disease or condition. If a patient is limited in its ability to achieve one of the needs, then nursing intervention is required to assist the animal. These models can be adapted to concentrate on the animal and its welfare, focusing on what needs the animal has and the steps that can be taken to improve welfare. This assessment should be completed when the animal is admitted to the hospital to flag any concerns with the accommodation or treatment and should form the basis of the care plan. The assessment should be reviewed regularly as the animal's needs change with their life stage.

Care plans

Care plans translate the theory of nursing models into practice. They should include details of the patient's needs and the nursing assessment of whether the animal is able to achieve them, list any existing or potential problems, state the nursing goals and the interventions required to achieve them, and evaluate the care provided. Care plans should be clear and concise to ensure continuity of care.

Care bundles

A 'care bundle' is the term given to a group of documents that collectively help assess, monitor and record practices related to a particular condition or disease. Care bundles are widely used in human-centred nursing, eitheralongside or as an alternative to nursing care plans (Ballantyne, 2016), and their use is gaining traction in veterinary nursing.

Veterinary care bundles need to be carefully considered and tailored to the individual animal. They can be useful in a variety of situations, ranging from evaluation of general housing and wellbeing, to recognition and adaptation to the changes associated with life stage, through to requirements during hospitalization for procedures that involve intensive nursing care and the provision of end-of-life palliative care.

A care bundle is produced by identifying the type of care that will be required for a particular condition or disease and compiling the supporting documents. Documents that may be included in a veterinary care bundle include:

- Client questionnaires
- Ethograms
- Hospitalization forms
- Pain scoring systems
- Nursing care plans
- Fluid therapy plans

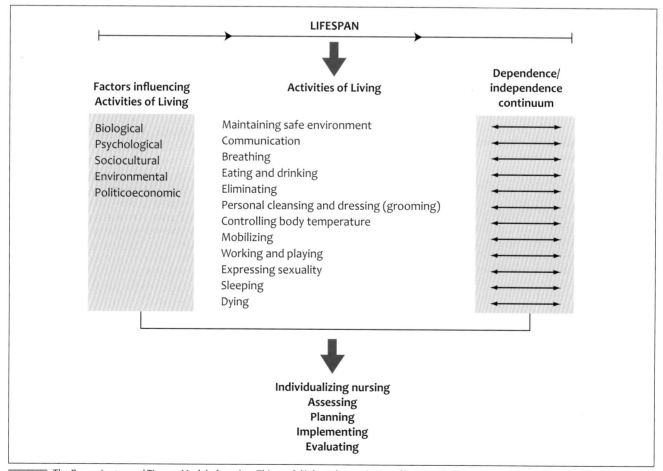

2.19 The Roper, Logan and Tierney Model of nursing. This model is based on activities of living and is often used to assess how the life of the patient has changed due to disease, injury or admission to the hospital.
(Roper et al., 1993) (Reproduced from the *BSAVA Textbook of Veterinary Nursing*, 6th edn)

Activity	Comments
Breathing, eliminating and maintaining body temperature	All animals share these needs but individuals may require different facilities to help support these needs. For example, a litter tray in the hospital if the patient is trained to use one or a heat and ultraviolet lamp for reptile patients
Sleeping	In human nursing, the emphasis for the sleeping activity is its restorative power. Many veterinary patients are crepuscular or nocturnal, so mimicking this will allow more natural behaviours. Rest time is important for animal patients and taking this into account when determining timing for the administration of medication will help reduce recovery time and stress
Mobilizing	The mobility of the patient is very important, especially for prey species that have a strong flight reaction when threatened. If mobility is limited, changes to the enclosure (e.g. provision of hides) will need to occur, as well as physical therapy
Cleaning and grooming	Many species never wash in water, so providing the correct cleaning environment is essential (e.g. sand baths for chinchillas). Smell is important to animals, so fragrant soaps should not be used. Clipping fur is often favoured to bathing as this can be very stressful. There is also the risk of hypothermia if the animal is not warmed and dried. Care should be taken when clipping certain areas of animals; for example, the pedal aspect of rabbits should never be fully clipped as the thick fur can protect them from developing pododermatitis (however, large knots should be brushed out as these can cause pressure points)
Communication	Gaining an owner's perspective of the individual's normal behaviours will better allow interpretation of communication. For example, if the animal is normally aggressive but is docile due to illness, aggression may occur when it is feeling better. This is an important distinction to aggression due to pain. Good, two-way communication will improve the welfare of the animal and safety of the veterinary personnel
Sexuality	Linking this to the relevant life stage of the animal to suggest neutering for optimum welfare will vary between species. For example, most female rabbits should be neutered before they are 6 months old (depending on breed) to reduce the risk of uterine adenocarcinoma, whereas neutering of ferrets is not recommended due to the link with hyperadrenocorticism
Working and playing	Companionship and enrichment are essential for the welfare of certain animals. If appropriate, a companion can be hospitalized alongside their sick partner to help reduce stress and recovery times. On the other hand, human interaction and companionship may be very stressful for the patient; understanding species-specific communication and withdrawing for the patient's best interests may be necessary
Eating, drinking and maintaining a safe environment	Almost all of these activities are controlled by the owner. Providing hides and access to high and low areas will help create a safe environment. It is also the responsibility of the owner to provide a secure enclosure away from predators. Provision of basic food and water alone is not adequate; a correct, species-specific and life stage appropriate diet should be provided to maximize welfare. A poor diet can result in secondary health problems, leading to compromised welfare (e.g. inadequate hay for small herbivores may cause dental and digestive problems)
Factors affecting activities of living	
Sociocultural	The cultural and religious beliefs of the owner may affect the activities of living (e.g. may limit some treatment options)
Politico-economic	Financial challenges will always be a factor limiting care; however, this does not mean that the owner should not be given the gold standard options (e.g. computed tomography (CT) scans are often not recommended because the veterinary surgeon has taken the view that the 'owner would not go for that' or that 'it is just a guinea pig'). The veterinary team should present all the available options and then work with the owner to decide what can and cannot be achieved
Environmental	The environment is very much within the control of the owner and they are responsible for providing a suitable environment based on their pet's requirements. Using the Five Freedoms to determine the type of environment that should be provided will help achieve good welfare
Psychological	This aspect is not always considered when it comes to animals, but is just as important as physical health. Addressing the animal's mental health and providing enrichment and stimulation will improve welfare and reduce many behavioural problems. This should be remembered during periods of hospitalization: providing safe toys or enrichment will help address mental health in hospital. A radio or television may be useful if the animal is used to this in the home environment. Some animals, such as African Grey parrots, may exhibit fearfulness with new enrichment, so toys from home may be beneficial

2.20 Examples of the activities of living that are central to the Roper, Logan and Tierney Model of nursing.

- Assisted feeding plans
- Physiotherapy plans
- Care sheets
- Diet plans
- Enrichment plans.

Care bundles should be structured and formalized, as well as adaptable to accommodate the wide range of species and veterinary working environments that the team will encounter. It is essential that all staff members are trained in the use of care bundles, including patient assessment and recording, monitoring and communicating changes identified.

Care sheets

Care sheets should be put together for all species seen in the practice. The care sheet should contain the relevant information to allow the patient's home or natural environment to be replicated and its basic needs to be met. Figure 2.21 details the factors that should be considered when putting together a care sheet. It should be remembered that for some of the less frequently encountered species, data may still be being gathered regarding feeding habits and preferences, so care sheets should be regularly reviewed and updated with the most current evidence-based research available.

Factor	Considerations
Species information	• Species • Life span • Life stage • Origin
Nutrition	• Carnivore/herbivore/omnivore (further specialist diets) • Feeding frequency and amounts • Food quantity
Environment	• Diurnal/nocturnal/crepuscular • Terrestrial/arboreal/fossorial/aquatic • Additional heating/lighting requirements (e.g. preferred optimum temperature range, ultraviolet light) • Perches/hides • Water requirements • Enrichment for both physical and mental stimulation
Special considerations	• Social species • Unusual feeding habits (e.g. 'feeding off the wing')
Potential zoonosis	• Personal protective equipment required/vaccinations • Handling/restraint requirements • Staff risks/cautions/biosecurity measures • Disease risk to other patients (e.g. rabbit haemorrhagic disease)

2.21 Factors that should be considered when designing a care sheet.

Care sheets can also be given out to owners to help improve welfare of the pet in the home environment. Nursing clinics are an ideal opportunity to discuss animal welfare with owners and to provide them with information. 'Pre-purchase' clinics can be set up to provide information to potential new owners about the species they are interested in; this will help ensure that the best possible set-up is available in the new home before the pet arrives.

Welfare charts

Welfare charts can be created to give a quantitative score based on the individual's circumstances (Figure 2.22). Changes can then be implemented and a revaluation carried out to determine whether the animal's welfare has improved.

Special considerations
Neonates

When treating neonates or adults with dependants, special considerations should be discussed by the veterinary team. Neonates will be almost completely dependent on basic nursing care for survival, from active warming to reduced starvation times and nutritional support, and perhaps even stimulation for elimination purposes. Consideration should be given to removing the infants from the parent in order to minimize stress on both sides. In the case of an adult with dependants, consideration should be given to the type of medication provided and whether passive transfer via the milk supply is likely to be a problem.

Welfare score	Behaviour	Body language	Comments
1	• Bright and responsive • Interacting with surroundings and environment • Behaving in a recognizable way for that individual • 'Binkying'/'flopping' frequently • Eating and defecating regularly	• Ears up and alert (if applicable, e.g. lop breeds are unable to raise ears) • Whiskers forward facing • Eyes open and clear • No teeth grinding • No zygomatic tension	• Welfare is good • Enclosure size should exceed minimum requirements • Access to a hide and shade • Access to *ad libitum* water and hay • Correct life stage diet offered
2	• Bright but may not have objects to interact with in the environment • Behaving in a recognizable way for that individual • Eating and defecating regularly	• Ears up and alert (if applicable, e.g. lop breeds are unable to raise ears) • Whiskers forward facing • Eyes open and clear • No teeth grinding • No zygomatic tension	• Welfare could be improved with more enrichment (i.e. objects to interact with) • Enclosure may not be big enough to allow full interaction or 'binkying' • Access to a hide and shade • Access to *ad libitum* water and hay
3	• Quiet and less responsive to environment • Not moving around much • Sitting in more of a hunched position than normal • Using hide more • Acting in a way that is unusual for the individual • Change in appetite	• Ears not in a normal position but not fully flat to the head at all times • Whiskers forward facing • Eyes open and clear • No teeth grinding • No zygomatic tension • Missing fur	• May not be showing any grimace behaviours, but welfare is seriously compromised • Enclosure is accessible to predators, leading to chronic stress (e.g. family dog, children or birds flying overhead) • Inappropriate diet • Variable access to water and hay • Changes to the environment are required and a veterinary health check should be undertaken to rule out illness and pain
4	• Quiet and less responsive to environment • Not moving around much • Using hide more • Acting in a way that is unusual for the individual • Reduced appetite • Faeces becoming smaller, harder and fewer in number	• Ears down • Whiskers flat • Eyes squinting or closed • Teeth grinding • Hunched position • Missing fur/wounds • Abdominal pressing • Inappetence • Zygomatic tension • Head tilt	• Welfare is a serious concern and veterinary attention should be sought immediately • Likely to be in pain and discomfort • Dental disease possible • Gut stasis likely • Enclosure is accessible to predators, leading to chronic stress • Inappropriate diet • Variable access to water and hay • Husbandry changes required

2.22 Welfare chart for rabbits. Photographs can be added for a visual representation.

Social species

Hospitalization of social species can be challenging as they can suffer from additional stress when removed from a bonded companion and isolated in a foreign environment. Where plausible and not contraindicated, hospitalizing pairs can help reduce stress levels. Social and/or herd species that require long periods of isolation for a treatment course may suffer unnecessarily and a pragmatic approach should be considered.

Hierarchical species, such as primates, require more tactical planning for procedures where individuals are removed from the group. A team would need to be available to monitor the possibly lengthy reintroduction of the individual to the group, and this is often not a straightforward procedure.

Nocturnal species

If long periods of hospitalization and medical intervention are required for nocturnal species, the implementation of reverse lighting systems may be beneficial, as they allow the vital rest period to commence during a quieter working period. In the shorter term, lighting can be used to help reduce the stress associated with handling; for example, with diurnal birds, dimming the lights will enable the practitioner to observe and catch patients quickly and effectively.

Dangerous animals

Animals that pose serious risks to the care staff, such as venomous species, predators or large animals, must be handled by competent and confident, trained professionals in order to ensure safety and maintain high welfare practices.

Reverse barrier nursing

Barrier nursing is a familiar concept in a veterinary environment when dealing with infectious and zoonotic diseases; however, it is often overlooked when dealing with 'at risk' patients. Reverse barrier nursing should be performed for young, unvaccinated or immunocompromised patients to prevent cross-contamination from other animals that have the potential to affect their health and welfare.

Non-ambulatory patients

Patients with a reduced ability to ambulate (that is likely to continue for more than a couple of hours) will require interventions from caregivers to ensure that the circulation and joint and muscle movements are maintained. Interventions can vary from simple passive range of movement exercises and gentle rotation to change recumbency, to a fully planned course of physiotherapy and/or hydrotherapy. It is essential that caregivers recognize periods of debilitation and ensure that appropriate interventions are instigated to prevent further complications from developing in the recovering patient.

Enrichment

Enrichment is the provision of something within the environment that allows an animal to act out its natural behaviours and is essential for good mental welfare (Figure 2.23). Enrichment should be varied and tailored to the normal behaviours of the species being kept; for example, scatter feeding to mimic foraging, placement of food rewards in a

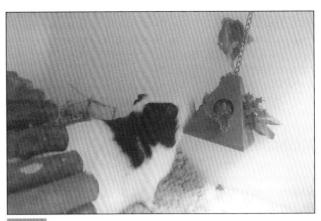

2.23 Enrichment for a guinea pig.

toy to encourage the animal to problem solve, or placement of enrichment items up high for arboreal species. Enrichment does not always have to be a food reward, but can be olfactory such as perfume, herbs or animal smell trails. It is vital to remember that enrichment should not be used as a remedy for substandard enclosures.

When selecting enrichment, ensure that nothing is toxic and in the case of destructive animals, such as ferrets and larger predators, that the materials used will not be a foreign body risk. Some species can be afraid of new toys (e.g. African Grey parrots), so the introduction of enrichment should be gradual and the complexity can be increased based on individual skill. Enrichment will reduce unwanted stereotypical behaviours, such as pacing and feather plucking, and should be provided for all animals.

See Chapter 4 for more information on enrichment.

Training

Training is viewed as enrichment as it is an example of mental stimulation, even though the animal is not strictly exhibiting a natural behaviour. Training can improve animal welfare hugely, particularly in zoo and captive environments. Poor welfare is often associated with a lack of control over interactions within the environment (Brando, 2012). Training reinforces empowerment given to the animal, as the repeatability of the behaviour is within the animal's control. Training behaviours such as presenting an arm for injection or conscious blood sampling has reduced the need for manual restraint and darting injectables in many zoological collections. Parrots, for example, can be trained to open their beak, open their wings and to step on to weighing scales; training to undertake these activities reduces the need for manual restraint and thereby reduces stress during veterinary examination. Many owners undertake basic training with their pets (e.g. teaching a dog to sit or give a paw) but owners are rarely encouraged to teach their pets techniques that can be helpful within a veterinary setting (e.g. getting dogs used to having their tails lifted and restrained over their backs so a rectal temperature can be obtained). It is worth considering creating an owner guide that explains which species-specific behaviours may be useful to teach their pet to help them feel more calm and relaxed within a veterinary setting. There are many online resources and forums that offer advice and guidance on species-specific animal training. For those working in a zoo environment, other zoological collections will often share resources and the training plans that have worked well with the same species in their collection.

See Chapter 6 for more information on welfare-focused animal training.

Welfare until the end

The quality of life (QOL) and welfare of patients receiving palliative care should be closely monitored and scored in order to identify when an animal is suffering and euthanasia should be recommended. Client questionnaires can be useful to help owners monitor the QOL of their pet and reach a decision regarding the timing of euthanasia (see Chapter 8).

Methods of euthanasia

Euthanasia means 'good death'. To achieve this outcome, techniques that induce an immediate loss of consciousness following, or in conjunction, with cardiac and respiratory arrest are required (Woods et al., 2010). When deciding upon the method of euthanasia, the following need to be considered:

* Animal welfare (minimal stress, pain and fear should be strived for)
* Patient restraint (chemical or physical)
* Safety of the veterinary team
* The need to preserve tissues (e.g. brain tissue) for post-mortem examination.

Figures 2.24 and 2.25 provide information on the methods of euthanasia for a number of different species. Although there are no official guidelines in the Royal College of Veterinary Surgeons (RCVS) Code of Professional Conduct regarding best practice for euthanasia, welfare should be the most important consideration. Chemical restraint or gaseous anaesthesia should be considered in small animals or if it is unlikely that intravenous access will be achieved in a stress- and pain-free manner. Intracardiac injections are preferred to an intraperitoneal technique, as the drugs can take up to 30 minutes to be effective when administered via this route, which can compromise welfare, especially if the animal is conscious. Each method of euthanasia requires a level of skill and training in order to be performed quickly and efficiently. It should be noted that cost may also affect the method of euthanasia in some cases (e.g. livestock where the cost of a lethal injection, which must be performed by a veterinary professional, and body disposal need to be taken into account). Further information on euthanasia techniques can be found on the American Veterinary Medical Association (AVMA) website (www.avma.org).

Species	Method	Comments
Dogs	• Intravenous via the cephalic or saphenous vein	
Cats	• Intravenous via the cephalic or saphenous vein • Intra-kidney can be used if vascular access unavailable	• Intra-kidney injection is extremely painful and should not be performed without heavy sedation or anaesthesia
Rabbits	• Intravenous via the lateral/marginal ear vein (Figure 2.25a), cephalic or saphenous vein	• Sedation (e.g. with midazolam) can be useful prior to anaesthesia • Cephalic vein access is difficult unless the animal is sedated or 'flat'
Guinea pigs Chinchillas	• Intravenous via the cephalic vein or cranial vena cava • Intracardiac	• The cranial vena cava is the route of choice, but injections must be performed under anaesthesia • Intravenous access to the cephalic vein is more successful with a 'cut down' technique as the skin over this area is very tough • Intracardiac injections should not be performed without heavy sedation or anaesthesia
Rats	• Intravenous via the cephalic or tail vein or cranial vena cava • Intracardiac	• Intravenous access is unlikely in a conscious or collapsed rat • Intracardiac or intravenous access via the cranial vena cava should only be performed under anaesthesia (Figure 2.25b)
Small rodents	• Intracardiac (Figure 2.25c)	• Intracardiac injection should only be performed under anaesthesia
Large animals	• Penetrative captive bolt • Shot gun	• Training and specific equipment required • Chemical restraint may be needed
Birds	• Intravenous via the jugular (Figure 2.25d), wing (Figure 2.25e) or medial metatarsal (Figure 2.25f) vein • Intracardiac (Figure 2.25g)	• Medial metatarsal intravenous placement can be achieved in conscious birds, particularly waterfowl and poultry • The right jugular vein is bigger in all birds • Anaesthesia should be used to gain access to other vessels or if unsure whether technique will be successful. Birds should not be placed in a gas chamber due to the risk of breaking their wings during excitation. If using gaseous anaesthesia, this should be delivered via a mask with the bird safely restrained • Intracardiac access is more difficult to achieve than intravenous due to the keel bone and should only be performed under anaesthesia
Tortoises Turtles	• Intravenous via the subcarapacial (Figure 2.25h) or jugular vein	• Helpful to warm up reptiles prior to euthanasia (if appropriate). Must be kept warm for several hours after euthanasia and the heart checked for over a minute to ensure it is not beating before pithing and placing in a freezer
Lizards Snakes	• Intravenous via tail vein (Figure 2.25i) • Intracardiac	• Helpful to warm up reptiles prior to euthanasia (if appropriate). Must be kept warm for several hours after euthanasia and the heart checked for over a minute to ensure it is not beating before pithing and placing in a freezer • Sedation or anaesthesia required for intracardiac injection
Amphibians	• MS222 anaesthetic overdose • Gaseous anaesthesia	• Water must be buffered with bicarbonate of soda if MS222 is used due to its acidity • If gaseous anaesthesia is to be used, the amphibian should be placed in a bag with water and the bag filled with gas
Fish	• MS222 anaesthetic overdose • Intravenous	• Water must be buffered with bicarbonate of soda if MS222 is used due to its acidity

2.24 Euthanasia techniques for various species. Note that this list is not exhaustive.

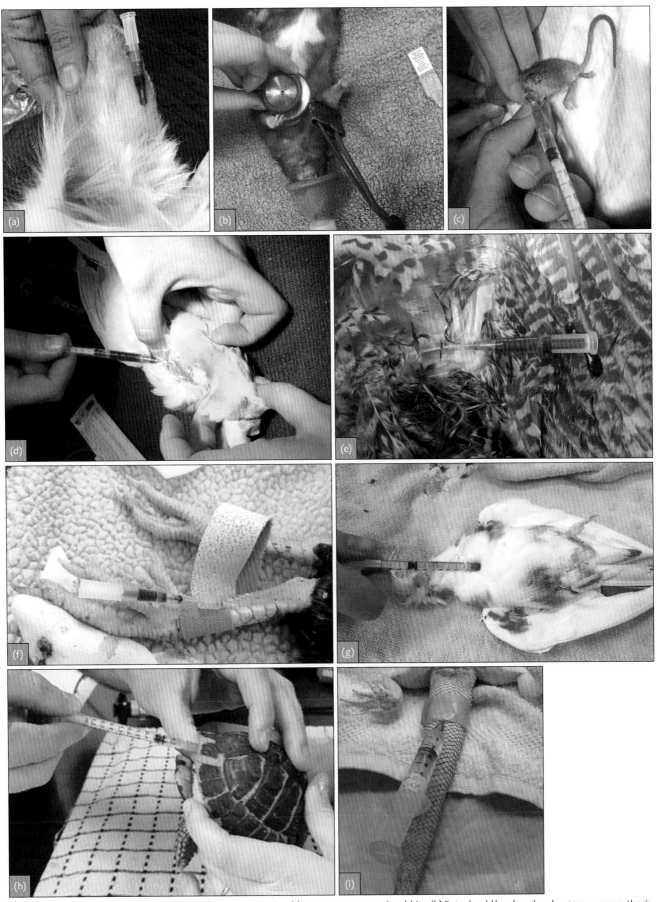

2.25 Examples of euthanasia techniques for various species. (a) Intravenous access in rabbits. (b) Rats should be placed under gaseous anaesthesia prior to obtaining intracardiac or intravenous access. (c) Intracardiac access in a small rodent (under anaesthesia). Intravenous access in birds via the (d) jugular, (e) wing and (f) medial metatarsal vein. (g) Intracardiac access in a bird (under anaesthesia). (h) Subcarapacial access in a chelonian. (i) Intravenous access via the tail vein in a lizard.
(c, i, courtesy of Vicki Baldrey; h, courtesy of Abigail Edis)

Case example 2: Fish

In 2017 it was estimated that 44% of UK households owned pets. Of these, indoor and outdoor fish were found to be present in 8% and 5% of homes, respectively (Pet Food Manufacturers' Association, 2017), and yet their welfare is often overlooked. Due to their seemingly low maintenance needs, fish are a popular choice of pet and can be easily purchased without any policing regarding suitable ownership or husbandry knowledge. Thus, owners should be educated to provide the best possible care and welfare for their aquatic pets.

Welfare considerations

Fish are ectothermic, meaning that they rely on water temperature for enzyme activity, metabolism and other bodily functions. Fish have an optimum water temperature range, which can vary between species. Some species are capable of surviving in a wide range of temperatures (eurythermic), whereas others are restricted to a narrow temperature range (stenothermic).

Owners should be advised to follow the recommendations below in order to maintain good animal welfare:

* Provide as large a tank as possible (spherical tanks should be avoided)
* Place the tank where minimal noise and banging will occur
* Determine and provide the optimum water temperature range for the species of fish being kept
* Monitor the water temperature and avoid rapid changes
* Perform routine water quality checks (kits can be purchased and the instructions provided explain results and how to make changes, or a sample of the tank water can be taken to a veterinary surgeon for testing)
* Only one-third of the water in the tank should be changed when cleaning. This is essential to maintain commensal bacterial colonies
* Provide a cleaning filter and change filters when needed
* Provide low level ultraviolet lighting and mimic daylight hours (this can be achieved manually or with an automatic timer)
* Provide heating (if applicable)
* Provide safe plant life for hiding, oxygenation and food
* Provide hides
* Provide appropriate diet (pelleted food, if possible, to avoid selective feeding)
* Provide suitable companions (determine which species will thrive together).

Routine monitoring of the water quality of a tank is advised, as poor water quality often precedes disease. Temperature, pH, nitrate concentrations and nitrite concentrations should be monitored weekly and a full water quality check performed monthly. Unfortunately, it is more common for water quality checks to be performed and problems identified once the fish start exhibiting clinical signs.

Stress

Stress is a vital factor in fish health. The most basic response to stressors, such as handling, vibrations or, in captivity, the owner attempting to catch the fish for either transfer or examination, is to escape from the perceived danger. Preparing the body for escape involves the release of hormones. This has detrimental long-term effects on the fish. For example, the release of adrenaline disturbs osmoregulation and cortisol affects lymphocytes, reducing the effectiveness of the immune system. A fish that undergoes this type of response, as a result of stress applied even for a short period of time, can take several hours or even days to recover its equilibrium. If fish are frequently moved between collections, then positive reinforcement training should be considered to reduce the negative effects of stress and improve welfare.

Pain

Although protected under the Animal Welfare Act 2006, which protects all animals from unnecessary suffering, fish have less legal protection than other animals as it was thought that they do not have a complex enough nervous system to feel pain in the same way as other animals. However, a study by Sneddon (2019) demonstrated that many fish that have undergone painful experiences (e.g. being caught with a hook or shocked) will refuse to eat, rub the affected area, avoid the location where the event occurred and hyperventilate. Extreme heat was also seen to have a negative effect on zebrafish and goldfish, which was alleviated with pain relief drugs. This would suggest that fish do feel pain and that when undergoing procedures pain relief should be provided.

Veterinary consultations

Due to their low cost, many owners do not see the value of seeking veterinary advice for fish, when a replacement animal can be purchased for less than a consultation fee. However, owners should be made aware that the animal may be suffering and encouraged to bring them into the practice when they start exhibiting clinical signs, even if it is for humane euthanasia, rather than for treatment. The cost of a veterinary consultation *versus* the cost of the animal will always be a struggling point; however, taking on a pet is a commitment, no matter the price or the species, and the owner has a responsibility to protect that animal from unnecessary suffering.

Examples of client questionnaires

Admissions questionnaires

Small mammal admission questionnaire

Date: ....Time: ....

Name(s) of recorder: ....
....
....
....
....

A downloadable form is available for this manual from the BSAVA Library

Patient details

Name: .... Patient no.: ....

Owner's name: ....

Microchip no.: .... Microchip location: ....

Ring no.: .... Ring location: ....

Insured?　　[ ] Yes　　　[ ] No　　　Company ....

Species: .... Breed/colour: .... Age: ....

Sex: .... Reason for admission: ....

History

Where was the animal sourced from?　[ ] Breeder　　[ ] Pet shop　　[ ] Rescue　　[ ] Other ....

How long has the animal been in the owner's possession? ....

How is the animal housed?　　　[ ] Indoor cage　[ ] Outdoor cage　[ ] Indoor hutch　[ ] Outdoor hutch　[ ] Tank

[ ] Shed　　　　[ ] Aviary　　　　[ ] Other

Substrate(s) used ....

Is the animal housed alone or in a pair/group? ....

Type of food offered ....

Amount offered .... Amount eaten ....

How is drinking water offered?　　[ ] Bowl　　　[ ] Bottle

Has there been an increase in thirst?　　[ ] Yes　　[ ] No

What, if any, vitamin/mineral supplements are used? ....

Clinical signs

How long has the animal been ill for? ....
....
....

What clinical signs have you noticed? ....
....
....

List any disease history of this pet ....
....
....

List any disease history of any in-contact pet ....
....
....

What treatments have already been tried? ....
....
....

Reptile admission questionnaire

Date: .... Time:..

Name(s) of recorder: ....
....
....
....

A downloadable form is available for this manual from the BSAVA Library

Patient details

Name: .... Patient no.:..

Owner's name:..

Microchip no.: .... Microchip location: ....

Ring no.: .... Ring location: ....

Insured? [ ] Yes   [ ] No   Company ....

Species: .... Breed/colour:............................ Age:...........................

Sex:... Reason for admission:...

Source

Where was the animal sourced from?   [ ] Breeder   [ ] Pet shop   [ ] Rescue   [ ] Other................................

How long has the animal been in the owner's possession? ....

What is the animal's natural habitat?   [ ] Aboreal – vertically arranged environment   [ ] Terrestrial – horizontally arranged environment

  [ ] Desert – dry environment   [ ] Rainforest – high humidity   [ ] Aquatic

Specifications for enclosure

Size of enclosure: Length ....Depth...Width................................

Substrate(s) used..

Lighting provided including UV ....

Temperature: Daytime range .... Night-time range .... Day length ....

Humidity: Daytime .... Night-time ....

Exposure to other reptiles

Have there been any other reptiles sharing the vivarium in the last 6 months?.....................................

Have any been sick or died? Details..

Diet

Type of food offered..

Amount offered .... Amount eaten .... Frequency..........................

How is drinking water offered?   [ ] Bowl   [ ] Spray   [ ] Other

What, if any, vitamin/mineral supplements are offered and how?...

Progression and type of clinical signs

How long has the animal been ill? ....
....

What clinical signs have you noticed?..
....
....

List any disease history for this animal..
....
....

List any disease history of any in-contact reptile..
....
....

What treatments have already been tried? ....
....

Bird admission questionnaire

Date: .... Time: ....

Name(s) of recorder: ....
....
....
....

A downloadable form is available for this manual from the BSAVA Library

Patient details

Name: .... Patient no.: ....

Owner's name: ....

Microchip no.: .... Microchip location: ....

Ring?   [ ] Yes   [ ] No   Ring no.: ....

Insured?   [ ] Yes   [ ] No   Company: ....

Species: .... Breed/colour: .... Age: ....

Sex: .... Reason for admission: ....

Source

Origin of the bird   [ ] Captive bred   [ ] Wild bred*   [ ] Unknown

*Note, the following wild bred species can be legally held in captivity: ....

Where was the bird sourced from?   [ ] Breeder   [ ] Pet shop   [ ] Importer   [ ] Rescue

[ ] Other..

How long has the bird been in the owner's possession? ....

How is the bird kept?   [ ] Cage   [ ] Aviary   [ ] Free indoors   [ ] Outdoors   [ ] Other..........................

Exposure to other birds

Are there any other birds in the house? ....

Are the birds sick? Have any died? ....

Diet

Type of food offered...

How is drinking water offered? ....

What, if any, vitamin/mineral supplements are offered? ....

Have there been any recent dietary changes?...

Progression and type of clinical signs

How long has the bird been ill? ....
....
....

What clinical signs have you noticed?..
....
....

List any disease history for this bird ....
....
....

List any disease history of any in-contact bird...
....
....

What treatments have already been tried? ....
....
....

Bird of prey admission questionnaire

Date: .... Time:..

Name(s) of recorder: ....

....

....

....

A downloadable form is available for this manual from the BSAVA Library

Patient details

Name: .... Patient no.: ....

Owner's name:..

Licence/registration no.:..

Microchip no.: .... Microchip location: ....

Ring?   [ ] Yes   [ ] No   Ring no.: ....

Insured?   [ ] Yes   [ ] No   Company: ....

Species: .... Breed/colour: .... Age:................

Sex:... Reason for admission: ....

Source

Origin of the bird   [ ] Captive bred   [ ] Wild bred*   [ ] Unknown

*Note, the following wild bred species can be legally held in captivity: ....

Where was the bird sourced from?   [ ] Breeder   [ ] Private owner   [ ] Rescue

     [ ] Other...

How long has the bird been in the owner's possession? ....

How is the bird kept?   [ ] Cage   [ ] Aviary   [ ] Free indoors   [ ] Outdoors   [ ] Other.............................

Exposure to other birds

Are any other birds kept?..

Are the birds sick? Have any died? ....

Diet

Type of food offered .... How much is given ....

Source of food: wild quarry (shot or caught) or farmed? ....

Is casting fed?..

When did the bird last cast? Was it normal? ....

What, if any, vitamin/mineral supplements are offered? ....

Weight

Normal flying weight? .... Normal moulting weight? ....

Weight normal for level of feeding? ....

Flying

Is the bird keen to fly? .... Is it tiring easily? ....

Progression and type of clinical signs

How long has the bird been ill? ....

....

What clinical signs have you noticed?...

....

List any disease history for this bird ....

....

List any disease history of any in-contact bird...

....

What treatments have already been tried? ....

....

Behaviour questionnaires

Canine behaviour questionnaire

Date: ....

A downloadable form is available for this manual from the BSAVA Library

Owner details

(Mr/Mrs/Miss/Ms) Surname/Family name: ....

First name or Initials: ....

Address: ....

....

....Postcode:...............................

Phone (day)...(evening)...............................

(mobile) ....Email...............................

Are you covered by a pet insurance policy? If so, please give details:...............................

Please include as much information as possible. The more detail available, the more accurate our assessment of the case can be. Please use additional sheets where necessary.

Have you owned a dog before?   [ ] Yes   [ ] No
Have you owned this breed of dog before?   [ ] Yes   [ ] No
Have you owned other pets previously?   [ ] Yes   [ ] No

Please list other current household pets

Type and breed	Name	Age	Spayed/neutered?	Relationship with dog (e.g. avoids, plays, fights)

Please list the names, ages and occupations of other family members who live at home

Name	Age	Occupation

Patient details

Name .... Breed ....

Sex   [ ] Male   [ ] Female   [ ] Male neutered   [ ] Female spayed

Date of birth...Age when obtained (if known) ....

Microchip no..Microchip location...............................

Date first acquired ....Source ....

▶

Canine behaviour questionnaire *continued*

Reason(s) for obtaining this dog

....

....

....

Has the dog ever been used for breeding?   [ ] Yes   [ ] No   If yes, at what age?...

How would you describe your dog's personality?

....

Do you consider your dog to be:

[ ] Aggressive? (growling, snarling, snapping, nipping or biting in any circumstances)

[ ] Destructive?   [ ] Hyperactive/restless?   [ ] Disobedient?   [ ] Housetrained?

[ ] Nervous?   [ ] Excitable?   [ ] Noisy/excessive vocalization?

[ ] Depressed?   [ ] Demanding attention?   [ ] Playful?

Medical history

1. Please give a brief medical history, especially recurrent problems and treatment. Use an extra sheet if necessary.............................

    ....

    ....

2. Vaccination status ....

3. Date last wormed ....

4. Is your dog currently on any regular medications (such as allergy medication, heartworm treatment, herbal or homeopathic remedies)?

Drug/remedy	Dose

5. Has your dog been on medication for their behaviour in the past?

Drug/remedy	Dose

6. Is your dog on any medication for their behaviour now?
    If yes, please list name and dosage (include herbals and homeopathics)

Drug/remedy	Dose

Early history

1. Please give details of the dog's early life, if known, including litter size, age of weaning, age when obtained, whether raised outside or indoors, if orphan or stray, whether hand-reared, etc.

    ....

    ....

    ....

▶

Canine behaviour questionnaire *continued*

2. How much interaction did the puppy have with people in the first year of its life?...

3. What method of housetraining was used?..

4. How did you react to any mistakes during housetraining?...

5. Did your puppy attend puppy 'parties' or classes? If so, please give details ....

Training and obedience

1. Has your dog ever attended training classes?   [   ] Yes   [   ] No

2. If Yes, please give details (when, where, age of dog, who took it to the class)..

3. What types of training techniques were used in the class?...

4. What training methods have you used?...

5. How well did your dog do in the class?   [   ] Very well   [   ] Average   [   ] Poor   [   ] Was asked to leave

    If asked to leave, please say why..

6. Do you think your dog is Good, Average or Poor at learning?   [   ] Good   [   ] Average   [   ] Poor

7. What tasks will the dog reliably perform for you on command?

    [   ] Sit   [   ] Stay   [   ] Down   [   ] Fetch   [   ] Other...

8. Does your dog do 'tricks' (such as shake, rollover)?..

9. Does your dog pull when on the lead?   [   ] Yes   [   ] No

10. Is your dog more obedient in some places than in others?   [   ] Yes   [   ] No

    If Yes, please give details...

11. Is your dog more obedient with some people than with others?   [   ] Yes   [   ] No

    If Yes, please give details...

12. How do you correct your dog when they misbehave?...

Diet and feeding

1. What types of food (and brands) do you give your dog?..

2. How much does your dog eat a day?...

3. When and where is the dog fed? (how often and at what time) ....

4. If there is more than one dog in the home, how many food bowls are provided?......................................

    Where are the food bowls situated?..

5. Who feeds the dog?..

6. Is the dog protective (stiffening, growling, snapping or biting) around the food?   [   ] Yes   [   ] No

    If Yes, please give details..

7. Is their appetite Good or Poor?   [   ] Good   [   ] Poor

8. Does your dog eat Quickly or Slowly?   [   ] Quickly   [   ] Slowly

9. What are their favourite foods?..

10. Do you have to be present for them to eat?   [   ] Yes   [   ] No

11. How much does your dog drink each day (in pints or litres)?...

12. Do you add supplements or titbits to the diet?   [   ] Yes   [   ] No

    If yes, what and why?...

13. Is your dog given bones or chews?...

    Are they possessive with these?..

14. Do you consider your dog to be at the correct weight?   [   ] Yes   [   ] No

    Please fill in your dog's weight ....

▶

Canine behaviour questionnaire *continued*

Daily activities

Sleeping and waking

1. Where does your dog sleep? ....

2. If your dog sleeps on the bed, who invites them up? ....

3. When does the dog get up in the morning? ....

4. Does your dog ever wake you at night?   [   ] Yes   [   ] No
   If yes, how often and why? ....

Going outside

5. When does your dog go outside and for how long? ....

6. How does your dog ask to go outside? ....

7. Do they roam free in a garden or yard? ....

8. What type of fencing is used to restrain the dog? ....

9. Is your dog keen to explore when on its own? ....

Toileting

10. Where does your dog tend to go to the toilet? ....

11. Does your dog spot mark with small amounts of urine?   [   ] Yes   [   ] No
    If so, where? ....

12. How often does your dog empty their bladder in a day? ....

13. How frequently do they empty their bowels? ....

Exercise

14. What sort of exercise (e.g. walking on/off lead, running off lead, agility training) does your dog receive and how much?

Type	Purpose	Amount	Frequency

15. Who takes the dog for exercise? ....

Play/training

16. Is there any specific time devoted to play and/or training on a daily basis?   [   ] Yes   [   ] No

17. Does your dog play games with you or other family members?   [   ] Yes   [   ] No
    If Yes, please give details ....

18 Who initiates play: people or the pet? ....

19 What types of toys does your dog play with? ....

'Home alone'

20. Is your dog left home alone in the house? ....

21. Where does the dog stay during the day when no one is home? ....

22. What do they do as you prepare to depart? ....

23. Does your dog ever bark or whine when you leave?   [   ] Yes   [   ] No

24. Does your dog ever [   ] vocalize, [   ] toilet, or [   ] engage in destructive behaviour while you are gone?

25. Typically, how long is your dog alone without people on any given day? ....

26. What arrangements are made for your dog when you go on holiday? ....

▶

Canine behaviour questionnaire *continued*

Family routine

27. What does your dog do during family meals?..

28. Has there been a change in your household routine (e.g. new work hours, new baby, moving, new roommate or visitors, boarding, diet change)?   [   ] Yes   [   ] No

   If Yes, please give details...

Favourite things

Please list 5 things your dog enjoys most; these may be foods, toys or activities

....

....

....

....

....

Interaction with family members

The home environment

1. What type of home do you have (e.g. flat/apartment, house)?..

2. What areas of the house does your dog have access to?...

3. Where does your dog sleep at night? ....

4. Do they have their own bed? ....

Reaction to handling by family members

5. Is there aggression in the following circumstances? This can include growling, snarling (showing teeth), lunging, nipping, snapping or biting. Please fill in the chart: (Y=Yes, N=No, N/A=does not apply).
   If biting has occurred in any of these circumstances, please describe the wound (tear, puncture, bruising)

	Adult owner (female)	Adult owner (male)	Children	Any specific individual
Handling/grooming				
Petting or hugging				
Disturbed when resting				
Disciplining				
Walking on the lead				
Taking food away				
Taking other objects				

Interaction with others

Reaction to visitors

1. How does your dog behave when visitors come to the house (e.g. barking, door charging)? ....
   ....

2. Is the behaviour different toward familiar and unfamiliar people?   [   ] Yes   [   ] No

   If yes, describe...

3. Is the behaviour different toward people outside the house and people inside the house?   [   ] Yes   [   ] No

   If yes, describe...

4. Does your dog display aggression (growling, snarling, snapping or biting) to visitors to your home?   [   ] Yes   [   ] No

   If yes, describe...

5. Has your dog ever bitten or attacked anyone?   [   ] Yes   [   ] No

▶

Canine behaviour questionnaire *continued*

6. Please fill in details of any regular visitors to the home

Name (if known)	Purpose	Time and days	Dog's reaction

7. What is the dog's response to other visitors?

Frequent visitors	Occasional visitors	Rare visitors

Reactions to other people

8. Please describe your dog's reaction to each of the following:

	In the home	Out of the home
Familiar men		
Familiar women		
Familiar children		
Unknown men		
Unknown women		
Unknown children		
Familiar dogs		
Unknown dogs		
Other animals		
Crowds/busy areas		

Reactions to other animals

9. What is the reaction to other dogs when out at exercise?

On a lead ....

Free exercise ....

10. What is the reaction to other animals, e.g. squirrels, unfamiliar cats? ....

....

Other behaviours

1. Does your dog ever show inappropriate mounting or other sexual activity?   [   ] Yes   [   ] No

   If so, to whom or what? ....

2. Is your dog ever protective over parts of their body (especially ears and feet)?   [   ] Yes   [   ] No

   If yes, which regions? ....

3. Does your dog lick or chew on themselves more than you would expect?   [   ] Yes   [   ] No

The current problem

1. What current problem(s) are you having with your dog? Please give a brief description ....

....

....

....

▶

Canine behaviour questionnaire *continued*

2.   When did it begin?...

3.   How long has it been present?..

4.   How old was the dog when it began?..

5.   Where does the problem occur?..

6.   With whom?...

7.   How often?...

8.   Other details..

....

....

Aggression

Please answer the questions below if the problem is aggression:

1.   Describe the most recent incident and the setting it occurred in (try to be very precise):

a)   Where was the dog?..

b)   Where was everyone in relation to the dog?..

c)   What was everyone doing before the incident?..

d)   What did the dog do? ....

e)   What was the dog's body posture? Describe the position of ears, tail, face, hair on back, or draw a picture if necessary ....

....

....

2.   What was your reaction to the behaviour?...

3.   How did the dog react to your reaction?..

4.   Was there any punishment? ....

5.   If there was a bite wound was it a puncture wound or a tear?...

6.   Going back in time, describe the 3 most recent incidents of the behaviour. Please use additional pages for this

....

....

....

7.   How frequently does the problem occur?   [   ] Times per day   [   ] Times per week

                                                                                     [   ] Times per month   [   ] Times per year

8.   When does the problem occur?

When left alone?   [   ] Always   [   ] Usually

                                                              [   ] Rarely   [   ] Never

When family members are present?   [   ] Always   [   ] Usually

                                                              [   ] Rarely   [   ] Never

9.   What has been done to correct the problem?..

10. Is the problem getting: [   ] Better?   [   ] Worse?   [   ] No change?

11. Do you suspect any cause?..

House soiling

If the problem is house soiling, does it take place:

When you are not present?   [   ] Yes   [   ] No

When someone is home?   [   ] Yes   [   ] No

▶

Canine behaviour questionnaire *continued*

Destruction

If the problem is destruction, does it take place:

When you are not present?   [   ] Yes   [   ] No

When you are home?   [   ] Yes   [   ] No

Other problems

What other behaviours does your dog engage in that are objectionable to you?..
....
....

Does your dog's behaviour cause arguments at home?...
....
....

You and your dog

1.   How would you describe your relationship with this dog?

     Adult owners (female)..

     Adult owners (male)..

     Children ....

2.   What are your feelings about the dog's present behaviour?

     Adult owners (female)..

     Adult owners (male)..

     Children ....

3.   How would you ideally like your dog to be?..

4.   Under what circumstances would you consider euthanasia?...

5.   What is your expectation for change?...

6.   Is there anything else you would like to add about your dog and its behaviour?..............................
     ....
     ....
     ....
     ....
     ....
     ....

Please give any other information you think is relevant to the case...
....
....
....
....
....
....
....

Questionnaire completed by (print)...

Signature ....Date...

Feline behaviour questionnaire

Date: ....

Owner details

(Mr/Mrs/Miss/Ms) Surname/Family name: ....

First name or Initials: ....

Address: ....

....

....Postcode:...

Phone (day)...(evening)..

(mobile) ....Email ....

Are you covered by a pet insurance policy? If so, please give details:.....................................

A downloadable form is available for this manual from the BSAVA Library

Please include as much information as possible. The more detail available, the more accurate our assessment of the case can be. Please use additional sheets where necessary.

Have you owned a cat before?   [   ] Yes   [   ] No
Have you owned this breed of cat before?   [   ] Yes   [   ] No
Have you owned other pets previously?   [   ] Yes   [   ] No

Please list other current household pets

Type and breed	Name	Age	Spayed/neutered?	Relationship with cat (e.g. avoids, plays, fights)

Please list the names, ages and occupations of other family members who live at home

Name	Age	Occupation

Patient details

Name .... Breed ....

Sex   [   ] Male   [   ] Female   [   ] Male neutered   [   ] Female spayed

Date of birth...Age when obtained (if known) ....

Microchip no..Microchip location.................................

Date first acquired ....Source ....

▶

Feline behaviour questionnaire *continued*

Reason(s) for obtaining this cat

....

....

....

Has the cat ever been used for breeding?   [ ] Yes   [ ] No   If yes, at what age?.............................

How would you describe your cat's personality?

....

Do you consider your cat to be:

[   ] Aggressive? (growling, hissing, scratching, nipping or biting in any circumstances)

[   ] Destructive?   [   ] Hyperactive/restless?   [   ] Disobedient?   [   ] Litter trained?

[   ] Nervous?   [   ] Excitable?   [   ] Noisy/excessive vocalization?

[   ] Depressed?   [   ] Demanding attention?   [   ] Playful?

Medical history

1. Please give a brief medical history, especially recurrent problems (such as fur balls and fight injuries) and treatment. Use an extra sheet if necessary..

    ....

    ....

2. Vaccination status..

3. Date last wormed..

4. Is your cat currently on any regular medications (such as allergy medication, herbal or homeopathic remedies)?

Drug/remedy	Dose

5. Has your cat been on medication for their behaviour in the past? If yes, please list name and dosage (include herbals and homeopathics)

Drug/remedy	Dose

6. Is your cat on any medication for their behaviour now? If yes, please list name and dosage (include herbals and homeopathics)

Drug/remedy	Dose

Early history

1. Please give details of the cat's early life, if known, including litter size, age of weaning, age when obtained, whether raised outside or indoors, if orphan or stray, whether hand-reared, etc.

    ....

    ....

    ....

▶

Feline behaviour questionnaire *continued*

2. How much interaction did the kitten have with people (frequency, number of people) in the first year of its life?.....................

3. What method of litter training was used?.....................

4. How did you react to any mistakes during litter training?.....................

5. Did your kitten attend kitten 'parties' or classes? If so, please give details.....................

Diet and feeding

1. What types of food (and brands) do you give your cat?.....................

2. How much does your cat eat a day? Please state actual weight if known.....................

3. When and where is the cat fed?.....................

4. Who feeds the cat?.....................

5. How many food bowls are provided?.....................

6. Where are the food bowls placed?.....................

7. Is their appetite Good or Poor?   [ ] Good   [ ] Poor

8. Does your cat eat Quickly or Slowly?   [ ] Quickly   [ ] Slowly

9. What are their favourite foods?.....................

10. How much water does your cat drink each day (in pints or litres)?.....................

10. How much milk does your cat drink each day (in pints or litres)?.....................

12. Do you add supplements or titbits to the diet?   [ ] Yes   [ ] No

    If yes, what and why?.....................

Daily activities

Sleeping and waking and resting

1. Where does your cat sleep at night?.....................

2. Where do they sleep during the day?.....................

3. Is your cat very active at night?   [ ] Yes   [ ] No

4. When do they get up in the morning?.....................

5. Does your cat tend to seek out high places to rest?   [ ] Yes   [ ] No

6. Where can the cat normally be found during the day?.....................

Toileting

7. Do you provide a litterbox?   [ ] Yes   [ ] No

    If Yes, how many are there?.....................

8. Where is/are the box/boxes located?.....................

9. Does the cat use a litterbox on a regular basis?   [ ] Yes   [ ] No

10. How often is/are the box/boxes cleared of waste material (scooped out)?.....................

11. Does your cat ever eliminate outside the litterbox inside the house?   [ ] Yes   [ ] No

    If yes, please complete section **'Elimination and marking problems'** below.

Going outside

12. Does your cat have access to a garden or yard?   [ ] Yes   [ ] No

13. Is access controlled or free through a cat door?.....................

14. How often do you see other cats in your garden?   [ ] Daily   [ ] Several times a week

                                                      [ ] Once a week   [ ] Rarely

15. How much time is spent outdoors by your cat each day?   In summer.....................

                                                              In winter.....................

▶

Feline behaviour questionnaire *continued*

Roaming

16. What area is available to the cat to roam?..

17. How far do they roam on average? [ ] Stays in the garden [ ] May go to next door or two
             [ ] Further ranging

18. Does your cat stay away from home for several days at a time? [ ] Yes [ ] No

Territory

19. Does the cat defend territory against other cats? [ ] Yes [ ] No

  If yes, describe your cat's reaction ....

Hunting

20. Does your cat catch prey and bring it into the house? [ ] Occasionally [ ] Regularly [ ] No

21. If so, what type of prey do they catch?...

'Home alone'

22. How long is your cat alone without people on any given day?...

23. What arrangements are made for the cat if you are away from home for a while, e.g. on holiday?......................................

Play

24. Is your cat playful? [ ] Yes [ ] No

25. Is there any specific time devoted to play on a daily basis? [ ] Yes [ ] No
  If so, how much?...

26. Who initiates play: People or the Cat?   [ ] People [ ] Cat

27. What types of toys does your cat play with?...

28. Does your cat come home when called or do any 'tricks'? [ ] Yes [ ] No

Scratching

29. Do you have a scratching post? [ ] Yes [ ] No
  If yes, please describe it...
  How many are available in the home?..
  Where are they placed?...

30. Does your cat use the scratching post? [ ] Yes [ ] Sometimes [ ] Never

Family routine

31. Has there been a change in your household routine (e.g. new work hours, new baby, moving, new roommate or visitors, boarding, diet change)? [ ] Yes [ ] No

  If Yes, please give details...

The home environment

1. What type of home do you have (e.g. flat/apartment – ground floor/upper floor, house)?...

2. How would you describe your home? [ ] Quiet [ ] Lively   [ ] Chaotic

3. What areas of the house does your cat have access to?..

4. Please draw on a separate sheet of paper a map of the layout of your home with the cat's key areas (e.g. feeding, litterbox, favourite rest areas) indicated. Please indicate any windows through which the cat can see the outside.

5. Is your can keen to explore? [ ] Yes [ ] No

6. If you have more than one cat, when do you see them all in the same room?..

7. Do some cats spend most of their time in only certain locations? [ ] Yes [ ] No
  If yes, which cats and where do they stay?...

Interaction with others

1. How does cat behave when visitors come to the house (e.g. hides, acts interested, interacts with them)?...........................

2. Is the behaviour different toward familiar and unfamiliar people? [ ] Yes [ ] No

  If yes, describe...

▶

Feline behaviour questionnaire *continued*

3. Is your cat quick to approach new people?   [   ] Yes   [   ] No

4. Has your cat ever bitten anyone?   [   ] Yes   [   ] No

    If yes and this is NOT the primary complaint, please give brief details of circumstances..

    If yes and this IS the primary complaint, please complete section **'Aggression'**

5. Please fill in details of any regular visitors to the home

Name (if known)	Purpose	Time and days	Cat's reaction

6. What is the cat's response to other visitors?

Frequent visitors	Occasional visitors	Rare visitors

7. Please describe your cat's reaction to each of the following:

	In the home	Out of the home
Familiar men		
Familiar women		
Familiar children		
Unknown men		
Unknown women		
Unknown children		
Familiar dogs		
Unknown dogs		
Familiar cats		
Unknown cats		

Other behaviours

1. When does your cat miaow?..

2. When does your cat growl?..

3. When does your cat purr?..

4. Is your cat aggressive when denied something they want?   [   ] Yes   [   ] No

5. Does your cat ever show inappropriate mounting or other sexual activity?   [   ] Yes   [   ] No

    If so, to whom or what?..

6. Does your cat Tolerate, Enjoy or Resist: Handling   [   ] Tolerate   [   ] Enjoy   [   ] Resist

                                                 Grooming   [   ] Tolerate   [   ] Enjoy   [   ] Resist

7. Does your cat lick or chew on themselves more than you would expect?   [   ] Yes   [   ] No

8. How do you correct your cat when they misbehave?..

    ....

    ....

    ....

▶

Feline behaviour questionnaire *continued*

The current problem
Please also refer to specific sections below

1. What is the current problem you are having with your cat? Please describe it briefly ....
    ....
    ....

2. When did it begin? ....

3. How long has it been present? ....

4. How old was the cat when it began? ....

5. Did the onset of the problem coincide with any event, or action, you can identify? ....
    ....

6. Where does the problem occur? ....

7. With whom? ....

8. How often? ....

9. Other details ....
    ....
    ....

10. What has been tried to correct or change the problem? ....

11. Is the problem getting: [   ] Better   [   ] Worse   [   ] No change?

12. Do you suspect any cause? ....

13. Describe the 3 most recent incidents of the behaviour. Use separate pages as required.
    ....
    ....
    ....

Elimination and marking problems (house soiling)
Please answer the questions below if the problem is elimination or marking (house soiling)

Elimination behaviour

1. Does the cat use a litterbox?   [   ] Yes   [   ] No   How often? ....

2. Does the cat use the litterbox for: [   ] Urine only   [   ] Faeces only   [   ] Neither

3. Does the cat bury their urine?   [   ] Yes   [   ] No

4. Does your cat bury their faeces?   [   ] Always   [   ] Usually   [   ] Occasionally
                                               [   ] Rarely   [   ] Never   [   ] Do not know

5. Is there much digging and scratching in and around the litterbox?   [   ] Yes   [   ] No

6. Does your cat ever eliminate outside the litterbox inside the house?   [   ] Yes   [   ] No

Litterbox

7. How many litterboxes are there? ....

8. What type (e.g. covered, uncovered)? ....

9. What shape and size? ....

10. Where is/are it/they located? ....

Litter

11. What type of litter material do you use? ....

12. Do you always use the same brand?   [   ] Yes   [   ] No

13. Are there odour control granules added? [   ] Yes   [   ] No

Litterbox cleaning

14. How often is the litterbox cleared of waste material (scooped out)? ....

15. How often is it completely cleared out and washed? ....

16. What do you use to clean the litterbox? .... ▶

Feline behaviour questionnaire *continued*

17. Have you recently changed the litter material or cleaning solution used?   [   ] Yes   [   ] No

18. How often do you provide a completely new box?...

Problem details

19. Is the cat leaving faeces, urine or both outside the litterbox?   [   ] Faeces   [   ] Urine   [   ] Both

20. How often does this occur?   [   ] Once a week   [   ] Once a month

                                                  [   ] Once a day   [   ] Always

21. What time of day do you usually find the urine or faeces outside the litterbox (a.m., p.m., before work, overnight, etc)?.................

    ....

22. How big is the spot of urine?..

23. How many times a day does your cat defecate?...

24. Do you recall the first time you found urine or faeces outside of the litterbox? [   ] Yes   [   ] No

    If yes, please provide the details surrounding the incident?...

25. Where is the cat depositing urine/faeces outside the litterbox? Please list the room/rooms and all the locations in the room/rooms. Also specify if the deposits are found near windows, doors, plants, furniture, etc. How many spots/deposits are there in a given room?

Room	Locations	Number of spots/deposits

26. Please draw a floor plan of the house, noting litterbox location and sites of urination and/or defecation outside the litterbox. Please also include resting places in cases of conflict between cats and indicate any specific locations of such conflict

27. Has there been a change in litterbox location?   [   ] Yes   [   ] No

    If yes, how recent was this?...

    From where to where? ....

28. Has there been a change in litter type?   [   ] Yes   [   ] No

    If yes, how recent was this?...

    From what to what?...

29. Has there been a change in litterbox cleaning routine?   [   ] Yes   [   ] No

    Is the box cleaned Less or More often?   [   ] Less often   [   ] More often

30. When the problem first began, can you recall any unusual incident or anything that might have upset the cat? (For example, moving house, new roommates, unusual noises, new work hours, addition of another pet, a new baby, food changes)..

    ....

31. Have there been any recent changes in your personal routine? ....

32. Have there been any recent changes in living arrangements?..

33. Have you ever caught the cat depositing urine or faeces outside the litterbox?   [   ] Yes   [   ] No

    What was your response?...

    What was the cat's response? ....

34. What posture does the cat assume when urinating or spraying outside the box?   [   ] Standing [   ] Squatting

35. Where is the urine located?   [   ] On the floor   [   ] On the walls about 6 to 8 inches up from the floor?

36. Is this Spraying or Urination?   [   ] Spraying   [   ] Urination?

37. Are there many cats outdoors in the immediate vicinity of your cat?   [   ] Yes   [   ] No

38. Is your cat agitated by the presence of other cats?   [   ] Yes   [   ] No

39. Are you the cat's first owner?   [   ] Yes   [   ] No

    If no, were there similar problems in a previous home?   [   ] Yes   [   ] No

40. If you have more than one cat, are there additional litterboxes? [   ] Yes   [   ] No

    How many?...

    Where are they? ....

▶

Feline behaviour questionnaire *continued*

41. Does this cat interact with the other cats in the home?   [   ] Yes   [   ] No

42. Does this cat fight with or avoid any of the other cats in the home?   [   ] Yes   [   ] No

    If yes, which cats do they fight with or avoid? ....

    Which cats do they associate with? ....

43. Does this cat have a previous history of urinary tract infections?   [   ] Yes   [   ] No

44. When was the last time a urine sample was examined? ....

45. What have you done in the past to try and change the behaviour? ....

    ....

Aggression

Please answer the questions below if the problem is aggression:

1. Describe the most recent incident and the setting it occurred in (try to be very precise, as if you were drawing a picture):

    a)   Where was the cat? ....

    b)   Where was everyone in relation to the cat? ....

    c)   What was everyone doing before the incident? ....

    d)   What did the cat do? ....

    e)   What was the cat's body posture? Describe the position of ears, tail, face, hair on back, or draw a picture if necessary ....

        ....

        ....

2. What was your reaction to the behaviour? ....

3. How did the cat react to your reaction? ....

4. Was there any punishment? ....

5. If there was a bite wound was it a puncture wound or a tear? ....

6. How frequently does the problem occur?   [   ] Times per day   [   ] Times per week

                                                   [   ] Times per month   [   ] Times per year

7. When does the problem occur?

    When left alone?   [   ] Always   [   ] Usually   [   ] Rarely   [   ] Never

    When family members are present?   [   ] Always   [   ] Usually   [   ] Rarely   [   ] Never

Other problems

Does your cat have any other behavioural problems (e.g. scratching, excessive miaowing, plant eating)? ....

....

....

....

....

You and your cat

1. How would you describe your relationship with this cat?

    Adult owners (female) ....

    Adult owners (male) ....

    Children ....

2. What are your feelings about the cat's present behaviour?

    Adult owners (female) ....

    Adult owners (male) ....

    Children ....

Feline behaviour questionnaire *continued*

3. How would you ideally like your cat to be?...

4. Under what circumstances would you consider euthanasia?...

5. What is your expectation for change?..

6. Is there anything else you would like to add about your cat and its behaviour?...

....

....

....

....

....

....

Please give any other information you think is relevant to the case..

....

....

....

....

....

....

....

Questionnaire completed by (print)..

Signature ....Date..

Rabbit behaviour questionnaire

Date: ....

A downloadable form is available for this manual from the BSAVA Library

Owner details

(Mr/Mrs/Miss/Ms) Surname/Family name: ....

First name or Initials: ....

Address: ....

....

Postcode: ....

Phone (day).. (evening)..

(mobile).. Email..

Are you covered by a pet insurance policy? If so, please give details: ....

Please include as much information as possible. The more detail available, the more accurate our assessment of the case can be. Please use additional sheets where necessary.

Referring veterinary surgeon

Address:..

....

....

Tel: ....

Patient details

Name: .... Breed:...

Age (if known) ....

Sex   [ ] Male   [ ] Female   [ ] Male neutered   [ ] Female spayed

If your rabbit is neutered when was it done? ....

Microchip no..Microchip location..............................

Has this rabbit ever been used for breeding?...

How much does your rabbit weigh? ....

How long is your rabbit from nose to tail when lying down on their side?.........................

Early history:

How old was your rabbit when you obtained them?..

Where did your rabbit come from? Did they, for example, come from a breeder, rescue centre or pet shop?.........................

....

....

Medical history

Does your rabbit have any current medical problems to your knowledge? ....

Do you know of any previous medical problems? ....

Is your rabbit on any current medication?...

Has your rabbit had any teeth problems?..

Does your rabbit have to have regular dental procedures? If so, how often?.......................

Do you clip your rabbit's nails or do you take them to the vet?....................................

How often are the nails clipped?...

Please ask your veterinary surgeon to provide your rabbit's complete veterinary records. ▶

Rabbit behaviour questionnaire *continued*

Interactions with family members

Please describe other members of your household.

Person's name	Person's age

Who interacts with the rabbit? ....

Does the rabbit have a favourite person or people? If so, who?...

Who is responsible for the following tasks:

Cleaning the rabbit's cage/hutch?..

Cleaning the rabbit's run? ....

Grooming the rabbit?...

Clipping the rabbit's nails?..

Interactions with other animals

Please provide details of any rabbits that share a hutch or other area with the patient

Rabbit name	Breed/type	Age	Sex	Spayed/neutered (yes/no)	How long lived with rabbit patient?

Do you ever see these rabbits lying next to each other? Please give details of who lies with whom ....
....

Do you ever see these rabbits licking/grooming each other? Please give details ....
....

Do you ever see these rabbits mounting (attempting to mate) each other? Please give details..........................
....

Do you ever see these rabbits chasing each other? Please give details..
....

Do you ever see these rabbits pulling fur from each other? Please give details..
....

Do you have any other rabbits, besides those described above?

Rabbit name	Breed/type	Age	Sex	Spayed/neutered (yes/no)

▶

Rabbit behaviour questionnaire *continued*

Other pets

Do you have any other animals?

Type and breed	Name	Age	Sex	Relationship with the rabbit patient (e.g. avoids/no interaction, stalks, stares, grooms, plays)

Cats in the neighbourhood

Do cats come into your garden?...

Have you ever seen them staring at/stalking your rabbit?...

Your rabbit's home:

Please provide diagrams of your rabbit's enclosure/hutch/cage/run with dimensions including height.

Please indicate where litter trays, water bowls/bottles, food bowls and hay racks are location.

Please indicate where other items such as pipes and boxes are located.

Please give as much detail as possible about where your rabbit lives.

What sort of bedding do you give your rabbit?   [ ] Hay   [ ] Straw   [ ] Sawdust/woodshavings
Please tick all that apply   [ ] Blanket/towel/Vetbed   [ ] Other ....

Outside-living rabbits

If your rabbit lives outside, does it live: [ ] In a converted shed enclosure?   [ ] In an aviary enclosure?   [ ] In a cage/hutch?
                [ ] In a cage/hutch with an attached run?   [ ] In a cage/hutch with a separate run to which you carry your rabbit?

If the run is attached, does your rabbit have access to the run: [ ] Always   [ ] Daytime only   [ ] Dry days only

Other (please describe)..

If the run is separate, when do you put your rabbit in the run: [ ] Every day   [ ] Dry days only

                                                       [ ] Summer only   [ ] Weekends only

Other (please describe)..

How long on average does your rabbit have access to the run per week?...

Whether attached or separate, is the run: [ ] On concrete?   [ ] On decking?   [ ] On tiles?   [ ] On grass?

Do you move the run to fresh patches of grass? If so, how often?...

Do you move your rabbit into a shed/garage in the winter? If so, please describe any difference in its accommodation in summer and winter.........

....

....

....

House rabbits

If your rabbit lives in your home, do they have access to all areas of the house?   [ ] Yes   [ ] No

Please state which rooms your rabbit has access to?...

Does your rabbit have an enclosure/hutch/cage in the house?...

Is your rabbit confined to the enclosure/hutch/cage at night?..

Is the rabbit confined to the enclosure/hutch/cage during the day? If so, for how long?...

Does the rabbit ever go outside? If so, please describe when and where...

Outdoor run for house rabbits

If your rabbit spends any time in an outdoor run please answer the following:

Is the rabbit's outside run: [ ] On concrete?   [ ] On decking?   [ ] On tiles?   [ ] On grass?

Do you move the enclosure/run to fresh patches of grass? If so, how often?...

▶

Rabbit behaviour questionnaire *continued*

Toileting

Does the rabbit use a litter tray? If so, what kind of litter do you use?..

How many litter trays do you have in the areas the rabbit lives in?   [   ] Enclosure   [   ] Cage/hutch

                                                                             [   ] Run   [   ] Your house

How often do you clean the litter trays?...

How often do you clean the rest of the cage/hutch?...

How often do you clean the rest of the run?...

Have you noticed your rabbit spraying inside or outside?   [   ] Yes   [   ] No
(Spraying is when the rabbit runs past and twists their hindquarters, letting loose a jet of urine.)

If so, on what items/people does your rabbit spray?..

Describe your rabbit's droppings...

Chewing

Does your rabbit chew their enclosure/hutch/cage or run?..

Do they chew the wooden parts?...

Do they chew plastic parts?...

Do they chew metal parts, e.g. wire or bars?...

If indoors in your home, does your rabbit chew:

Furniture? If so, are there any items in particular?...

Carpets? ....Other?..

Diet

What do you feed your rabbit and how often? (Please list all that apply)

Food	Brand/type	Fed daily	Fed weekly	Fed occasionally
Commercial compressed rabbit pellets				
Commercial rabbit mix (muesli style mix)				
Commercial extruded pellets				
Hay				
Plants/forage				
Fresh grass/herbs				
Fruit (please specify)				
Household greens (please specify e.g. carrot, turnip, broccoli)				
Other (treats)				

Do you give any supplements, e.g. salt block?...

Does your rabbit enjoy their food or would you say they are fussy?...

Do you give any titbits? If so, what and how often? ....

Do you give any commercial rabbit treats? If so, please give details ....

Where does your rabbit have access to water? Please tick all that apply

In its cage/hutch: [   ] In a bowl   [   ] In a water bottle

How often do you change the water?...

In its run: [   ] In a bowl   [   ] In a water bottle

How often do you change the water?...

▶

Rabbit behaviour questionnaire *continued*

Please state how many of each item are in the cage/hutch and in the run.

Item	Cage/hutch	Run
Food bowls		
Hay racks		
Water bottles		
Water bowls		

Human interaction

Does the rabbit have any toys? Please describe...

....

Do you play with the rabbit? Please describe the games and approximately how long each day you play with the rabbit......................................

....

....

Have you clicker, target or voice trained your rabbit?...

Does your rabbit know any tricks? If so, please give details...

....

....

....

The problem

Describe the problems you are having with your rabit in as much detail as possible. (Please use additional sheets as necessary)

....

....

....

....

As rabbit communication is very subtle and difficult to describe, it would be EXTREMELY helpful if you could send a video showing the problem you are having with your rabbit. It this is not possible, please describe your rabbit's behaviour in as much detail as possible, e.g. are its ears flat or upright, is it making a noise, struggling, kicking, biting? Please do try, however, to provide a video. Thank you.

What happens immediately before your rabbit displays these behaviours? Try to think both what you/others and your rabbit are doing when the problem occurs..

....

....

What happens immediately after? Again, think about what you/others and the rabbit do..

....

....

When did the problem begin? Can you remember the first time it happened?...

When does the problem occur? Is it in any particular circumstances?..

....

How frequently, on average, does the problem occur? Do you think it is becoming more frequent, less frequent, or staying about the same?

....

....

Where does the problem occur? Is it, for example, always in the same place?..

Who is usually present at the time, if anybody?...

When was the last incident, and can you describe this? ....

....

▶

Rabbit behaviour questionnaire *continued*

Have there been previous attempts to cure this problem? (if so, please describe)...
....
....
....

Other problems:

Does your rabbit have any other problems? For example, is it nervous of:

[ ] Children?   [ ] Strangers?   [ ] Any family members?   [ ] Dogs?   [ ] Other?   [ ] All of these?

Does your rabbit struggle/bite/kick when you   [ ] Groom them?   [ ] Stroke them?   [ ] Pick them up?

If so, please give details..
....
....
....

What sort of brush do you use to groom your rabbit? ....

Are there any other problems with the rabbit that you would like to discuss at the consultation? ....
....
....
....

Rehabilitation

How much time do you feel able to commit to working with your rabbit to solve these problems?..........................
....

What would you envisage happening if the behaviour problem persists? ....
....

Finally, to help us understand more, it is helpful if you can give us information about rabbits that you have owned before.

Breed	Age of rabbit when obtained (if known)	How long was the rabbit owned for	Were there any behaviour problems encountered? If so, please describe	What was the outcome? (e.g. behaviour improved, someone else in family looked after rabbit (I was a child at the time), rabbit was rehomed/given to a rescue charity, rabbit was euthanased)

Thank you very much for your cooperation in filling in this questionnaire. If you have any queries, please do not hesitate to contact me.

I look forward to meeting you and your rabbit or speaking to you on the telephone.

References and further reading

Ballantyne H (2016) Beyond the nursing care plan: an introduction to care bundles. *Veterinary Nursing Journal* **31(2)**, 43–46

Ballantyne H (2017) *Veterinary Nursing Care Plans: Theory and Practice.* CRC Press, London

Brando SI (2012) Animal learning and training: implications for animal welfare. *Veterinary Clinics of North America: Exotic Animal Practice* **15(3)**, 387–398

Coelho FEA, Bruinjé AC and Costa GC (2018) Ethogram with the description of a new behavioural display for the Striped Lava Lizard, *Tropidurus semitaeniatus. South American Journal of Herpetology* **13(1)**, 96–101

Cooper B, Mullineaux E and Turner L (2020) *BSAVA Textbook of Veterinary Nursing, 6th edn.* BSAVA Publications, Gloucester

Gaynor JS and Muir WW (2014) *The Handbook of Veterinary Pain Management, 3rd edn.* Elsevier, Philadelphia

Goldberg ME and Shaffran N (2015) *Pain Management for Veterinary Technicians and Nurses.* Wiley Blackwell, Oxford

Hellyer P, Rodan I, Brunt J, Downing R, Hagedorn JE and Robertson SA (2007) AAHA/AAFP pain management guidelines for dogs and cats. *Journal of the American Animal Hospital Association* **43(5)**, 235–248

Horwitz DF and Mills DS (2009) *BSAVA Manual of Canine and Feline Behavioural Medicine, 2nd edn.* BSAVA Publications, Gloucester

International Association for the Study of Pain (2019) IASP's proposed new definition of pain. Available from: www.iasp-pain.org

Kagan R and Veasey J (2010) Challenges of zoo animal welfare. In: *Wild Mammals in Captivity: Principles and Techniques for Zoo Management, 2nd edn,* ed. DG Kleinman *et al.,* pp. 11–21. The University of Chicago Press, London

Keeling LJ, Rushen J and Duncan IJ (2011) Understanding aninal welfare. In: *Animal Welfare, 2nd edn,* ed. MC Appleby *et al.,* pp. 13–14. CABI Publishing, Oxford

MacNulty DR (2007) A proposed ethogram of large carnivore predatory behaviour, exemplified by the wolf. *Journal of Mammalogy* **88(3)**, 595–605

Malik A (2018) Pain in reptiles: a review for veterinary nurses. *Veterinary Nursing Journal* **33(7)**, 201–211

Malik A and Valentine A (2017) Pain in birds: a review for veterinary nurses. *Veterinary Nursing Journal* **33(1)**, 11–25

Mellor DJ (2016) Updating animal welfare thinking: moving beyond the 'Five Freedoms' towards 'A Life Worth Living'. *Animals* **6**, 21

Mellor DJ (2017) Operational details of the five domains model and its key applications to the assessment and management of animal welfare. *Animals* **7(8)**, 60

Pet Food Manufacturers' Association (2017) Pet Population 2017. Available from: www.pfma.org.uk/pet-population-2017

Rollin BE (2006) *An Introduction to Medical Veterinary Ethics: Theory and Cases, 2nd edn.* Blackwell Publishing, Oxford

Roper N, Logan W and Tierney A (1993) *The Elements of Nursing: A Model for Nursing Based on a Model for Living.* Churchill Livingstone, Edinburgh

Schwaller F and Fitzgerald M (2014) The consequences of pain in early life: injury-induced plasticity in developing pain pathways. *European Journal of Neuroscience* **39(3)**, 344–352

Self I (2019) *BSAVA Guide to Pain Management in Small Animal Practice.* BSAVA Publications, Gloucester

Sneddon LU (2015) Pain in aquatic animals. *Journal of Experimental Biology* **218**, 967–976

Sneddon LU (2019) Evolution of nociception and pain: evidence from fish models. *Philosophical Transactions of the Royal Society B* **374**, 20190290

Thomas J and Lerche P (2011) *Anesthesia and Analgesia for Veterinary Technicians, 4th edn.* Elsevier, Philadelphia

Wildgoose W (2001) *BSAVA Manual of Ornamental Fish, 2nd edn.* BSAVA Publishing, Gloucester

Woods J, Shearer JK and Hill J (2010) Recommended on-farm euthanasia practices. In: *Improving Animal Welfare,* ed. T Grandin, pp. 186–200. CABI Publishing, Oxford

Useful websites

American Veterinary Medical Association (AVMA)
www.avma.org

Rabbit Welfare Association and Fund
rabbitwelfare.co.uk

The People's Dispensary for Sick Animals (PDSA) Which Pet? toolkit
www.pdsa.org.uk/which-pet

Online extras

- This chapter includes forms that are available to download and print from the BSAVA Library.
- Each form is marked in the text with a download symbol.

Access via QR code or: bsavalibrary.com/welfareforms_2

Chapter 3

Animal behaviour

Anne McBride and Jo Hinde-Megarity

Introduction

"Behaviour is the internally coordinated responses (actions or inactions) of whole living organisms (individuals or groups) to internal and/or external stimuli, excluding responses more easily understood as developmental changes" (Levitis *et al.*, 2009).

Behaviour comprises those activities (or inactivity) that we can see and measure. All behaviours are coordinated by the processing of sensory information and actions of the endocrine system or neurotransmitters in response to changes in the external or internal environment. Body temperature is one example of an internal stimulus; if it is elevated, the behavioural response of moving to a shady spot may be observed. Responses to external stimuli include solving puzzles to access food, for example, a crow using sticks to catch insect larvae (Troscianko and Rutz, 2015) or a squirrel finding a safe route to a bird feeder and discovering how to get seeds out.

Behaviour is crucial to survival. What the animal will do next depends on the information it receives in response to its current behaviour. This information is gained through both external and internal sensory processors and enables the animal to learn which behaviours are worth repeating (i.e. are successful). Did they get the food? Did it make them feel sick? Did they avoid being chased by the dog in the garden or do they have to try something different?

Behaviour also incorporates communication of how an individual is feeling and its intention in social interactions. This is important for establishing friendly relationships, as seen in play behaviour and mutual grooming. It is also integral to defending oneself or important resources, and in escaping or defusing a social threat. For example, a dog who is anxious and feeling threatened by being in a new place (e.g. the veterinary clinic) with an unfamiliar person (e.g. the veterinary surgeon (veterinarian)) will put back its ears, turn its head away and lick its lips to deter any approach. The dog will relax a little if the threat (the veterinary surgeon) retreats – the behaviour was successful. If the veterinary surgeon responds by touching the dog, then clearly the behaviour was unsuccessful, and the dog may decide to escalate its defensive signalling by growling and snapping. Regrettably, this can also happen when others do not recognize and respond to signals appropriately, as with young children (Figure 3.1).

Understanding animal behaviour is imperative if we are going to manage and interact with animals to the benefit of their welfare and our own. You may wonder just how much

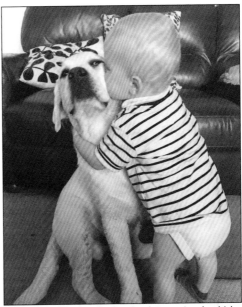

3.1 A dog showing low-level stress signals which are not being recognized and attended to.

you need to know. After all, you probably consider yourself a pet owner, animal carer or veterinary professional, not an academic, like the author [AM], who is interested in some esoteric aspect of animal behaviour or cognition.

You would not be alone in thinking that all you really need to know are the animal's signals of friendliness, frustration and fear, and how to respond appropriately. Some, especially those working with dogs, horses or elephants, may also think it important to know how these animals learn, so they can be trained to perform desired behaviours when asked to do so. Yet, regardless of species or the reasons why we are interacting with them, both these knowledge areas are essential as alone they are not sufficient to ensure welfare-friendly interactions.

To be able to maintain even good, let alone the highest, standards of animal welfare so the animal can have a life worth living (Mellor, 2016), we need to understand the factors that influence behaviour at a species, breed and individual level. Broadly speaking, these influences are the individual's genetic make-up, the environment and any gene–environment interaction. Gene–environment interaction is fundamental to the evolution of a species and its behaviour through natural selection.

Natural selection is considered the main process of evolution by which a species alters over time in response to changes in the physical and social environment. Species that do not change effectively become extinct. Natural selection works at an individual level, although its effects are seen at a population level. Those individual organisms whose phenotype (body and behaviour) is better adapted to the current environmental conditions tend to survive and produce more offspring, thus more of their genotype is present in the population. Natural selection has led to the bewildering and fascinating variety of adaptions seen across the different species that are the Earth's fauna and flora.

Major selection pressures can be summarized under three broad headings, which the authors refer to as the 'Three Rules of Life' (see below). These are: get enough to eat, avoid being killed and reproduce successfully. This chapter will introduce some basic concepts relevant to these life rules and how they relate to domesticated species and wild species in captivity. It will provide some underpinning knowledge that complements the more applied focus of later chapters.

Further reading

The authors would like to highlight that this chapter provides a surface level introduction to these topics. The reader is exhorted to read further around all aspects of animal behaviour. A truncated set of references is provided here. The complete reference and further reading list for this chapter is available from the BSAVA Library (see 'Extra references' at the end of the chapter).

Nature and nurture

As mentioned above, an animal's behaviour at any moment in time is the result of its individual genetics, current environment and experiences with past environments. The study of these interactions is known as behavioural genetics. Behavioural genetics aims to estimate the relative extent to which differences in the behaviour of individuals are due to genetically imprinted information and the experiences of the individual during development (e.g. pre- and post-natal nutrition, pre-natal exposure to maternal stress hormones, parental care, physical and social environmental conditions, learning). Behavioural genetics is part of the study into individual differences in one mammal species relevant to all readers – Homo sapiens. It is also of increasing interest to those studying individuality in non-human species. To quote Wynne and Udell (2013):

"...many researchers in this field have embraced "temperament" as a term for the biological (genetic) predispositions of an animal, and "personality" as a generally consistent but moderately adaptable product of the interactions between an animal's behavioural predispositions and its environment."

These authors go on to remind us that the study of temperament and personality is intended to compare individuals of the same species and it may not even be applicable to extend such comparisons across breeds (strains), saying:

"If an entire strain or species contrasts with another on a trait, this may not be due to personality at all."

We are interested in assessing the behaviour of individual animals for various reasons, not least to judge the state of their welfare. Common first indications of compromised physiological or psychological welfare are behavioural. We also assess behaviour when determining an individual's potential usefulness in a given setting (e.g. farm, laboratory, zoo, home). This could be for breeding, as an assistance animal, to ride or carry/pull loads, to find items (e.g. people, landmines) or to function as a social and emotional companion (pet). We can, and should, assess the individual human so that both working and/or companion human–animal relationships have the best chance of success. This is an area that would benefit from further consideration and application. Ongoing behaviour assessment is also crucial to the success of training an animal, in identifying the aetiology of problematic behaviour and developing an appropriate behaviour modification programme. All behavioural assessments entail an application of behavioural genetics, albeit in a somewhat rudimentary form.

Genetic influences need to be considered at three levels: species, breed/strain and the individual's family line.

Species

Species have evolved to be physically and behaviourally adapted to particular ecosystems (Alcock, 2013). It is imperative that we understand as much as possible about species' normal, natural behaviour (Olsson et al., 2003). It may seem obvious that we should not assume that a cat is a small dog, but we may be more inclined to take shortcuts when considering less familiar species. It would be a mistake, for example, to assume that a dwarf hamster, guinea pig, degu and gerbil are the same simply because they all happen to be small, social rodents (Yeates, 2019).

Breed

Differences in behaviour are also due to the breed or strain of the species. For thousands of years, humans have meddled with animals through artificially selecting (breeding) for specific phenotypes (i.e. physical and behavioural characteristics). Originally, humans selected predominately for tameness and physical features relevant to how we wanted to use the animal or its products. For example, selective breeding of horses and other livestock prioritized features such as size, speed, strength, type of wool and fattiness of meat (marbled meat was more highly prized in the past; now we select for leanness). Likewise, dogs were selected for size, speed and strength, but also for character traits such as independence and tenacity in vermin catchers (terriers) or responsiveness and biddability in herding dogs. Up until the mid-20th century, companion animals were mainly selected to be both physically and behaviourally capable, and thus physically and behaviourally healthy. Physical health and welfare have been lesser concerns in livestock breeding, as seen in selection for an ever-increasing milk yield in cows (Oltenacu and Broom, 2010) and in selection for the expression of specific genes in laboratory animals.

In the 21st century, this widening disconnect between human desires and animal welfare is increasingly seen in the companion animal world, across all species. The results can be disastrous for the individual animals concerned and serve no other purpose than to satisfy human pleasure and whim. Inbreeding with disregard for welfare is comparable to that of livestock and produces equally, if not more, exaggerated features that we say we find 'attractive and appealing'. This includes, but is not limited to, breeding for dwarfism, gigantism, exaggerated fur length, elongated necks, sloping backs, curled tails, unnatural gaits, lop-ears and brachycephaly. We do not restrict our genetic sieving to a single species, for example, we select for brachycephaly in dogs, rabbits, cats and the show strains of the Arabian horse (Figure 3.2).

As chromosomes and genes do not work in isolation, artificial selection for one characteristic affects more than one aspect of the individual's genome and unintended consequences can occur, such as differences in 'normal' vision (McGreevy et al., 2004). Additionally, selection for one set of traits can increase predisposition to disease (Universities Federation for Animal Welfare, 2018), be that a wide range of systemic disorders (Summers et al., 2010); sensory losses, such as deafness and degenerative eye disorders (Strain, 2011; Mellersh, 2014); or behavioural issues, as in the neurologically linked 'wobble' of the 'spider' colour morph Ball Pythons, which diminishes both mobility and feeding ability (Rose and Williams, 2014), predisposition to nervousness (Jones and Gosling, 2005), and aggression associated with colour morphs in some breeds of dog (Amat et al., 2009). Deliberately or accidentally selected conformation and colour distortions can detrimentally affect behaviour in any species. Reducing the animal's ability to clearly communicate its emotional state and behavioural intention increases general levels of anxiety and interferes with learning, which in turn can lead to further exposure to stress and development of problem behaviours.

The similarity of phenotype that results from inbreeding is the main attraction of, and source of the higher value allocated to, 'pure-bred' or pedigree animals. There is a higher probability that such an individual will breed true to type, and thus we can make reasonable estimates about an offspring's physique and behavioural characteristics. In contrast, outbreeding using different strains/breeds leads to hybrid vigour – the more genetic variation the greater the vigour. In this respect, the mongrel is better off than the crossbreed or even the 'designer' crossbreed, which is bred from only two pure-breeds. The breeding population of mongrels has a greater range of genotype. This reduces the chance of any individual inheriting undesirable genes that would predispose it to welfare-compromising conditions. However, it also reduces the ability to predict adult physique and behavioural characteristics. As this more complex mixed genotype will breed true, in that it continues across generations, one might relabel these as 'pedigree mongrels'. Labels are very powerful influencers of human behaviour (Rahim, 2010; Wilkins et al., 2015).

Thus, simply relabelling the 'pedigree mongrel' (of any species) may raise their standing in the public's eye to the improvement of the overall welfare of that species.

Increasing hybrid vigour by outbreeding within a species is an established concept. However, true hybridization where two or more different species are interbred may have a very different outcome. The effects on physical and behavioural characteristics are more difficult to judge. This is particularly so where hybrids are from allopatric species (i.e. those that have evolved for different habitats). In nature these species would never interbreed, and they are genetically dissimilar in many subtle ways. The first hybridization experiment produced the mule, the result of crossing a horse and a donkey. The horse has 64 chromosomes and the donkey 62: the offspring mule has 63, inheriting an extra 'loose' chromosome from its horse parent. The lack of similarity in the chromosomes means that the mule is sterile as its cells cannot undergo meiosis, so it produces no sperm or eggs. Fortunately for the mule, the extra chromosome does not carry with it any obvious predisposition to welfare-compromising conditions (but this is indeed due to luck, not planning!).

Over the last few decades, we have seen an increase in this crossbreeding of species, the deliberate concocting of mutant animals for the pet market, especially in reptiles and cats (Figure 3.3). Examples include the Bengal Cat (domestic cat x Asian leopard cat (Prionailurus bengalensis)) and Savannah Cat (domestic cat (including Bengal) x serval (Leptailurus serval)). There are issues relating to infertility in these hybrids. In addition, although breeders tend to deny any, whether there are other deleterious genetic effects on the physical or behavioural welfare of these animals awaits further research. Just as with inbreeding the pedigree for specific (often mutant) characteristics, the driver for cross-species hybridization is simply human desire with little or no regard for ethical or welfare concerns.

Individual

Finally, genetic influence must be considered at individual level, that is the specific chromosomes an animal has inherited from its parents. What one inherits from one's family line has implications for one's physical and behavioural phenotype. As we have seen, this is a more complicated matter for the species hybrid.

Familial genetic inheritance is influential in establishing temperament. In human research, studies of identical and non-identical twins, and natural and adoptive families, have clearly indicated genetic determinants predisposing to a range of behaviours, including those related to anxiety and addiction. Comparable work in non-human

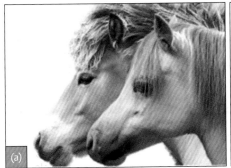 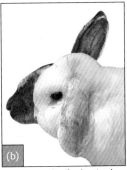 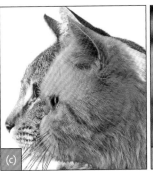 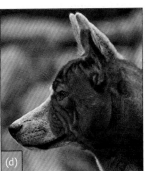

3.2 (a–d) Examples of brachycephalic distortions as a result of selective breeding.
(Reproduced with permission from vetsagainstbrachycephalism.com; b, © Dyrlaegehuset Farum and Rabbit Welfare Association & Fund; c, © International Cat Care; d, © Campaign for the Responsible Use of Flat-Faced Animals)

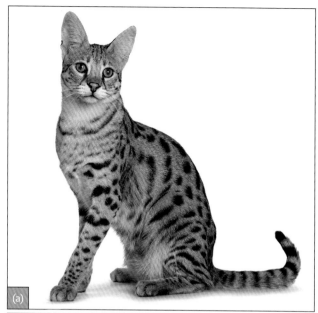

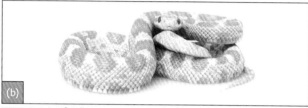

3.3 Artificially concocted animals. (a) Savannah Cat: an example of cross-species hybridization. (b) A cross-species hybrid between a corn snake and a Great Plains rat snake.
(a, Shutterstock.com/Nynke van Holten; b, Shutterstock.com/fivespots)

animals includes controlled breeding studies, but these are few (Hradecká *et al.*, 2015). Key examples include the 40+ year study of silver foxes (Kukekova *et al.*, 2008), Scott and Fuller's (1974) seminal work on the domestic dog in the 1960s and McCune's (1995) robust study of genetic and maternal behaviour effects on boldness (confidence) in the domestic cat. McCune found that boldness was influenced by the genetic contribution of the kitten's sire. Given 50% of genetic inheritance is from the male, it is curious that we rarely ask breeders about the sire's character. However, genes are not the whole story. As Hradecká *et al.* (2015) summarize in their meta-analysis of research on predicting suitability of puppies and adolescents as working dogs, differences in the breeding environment make the study of heritability elusive.

Whilst genes predispose, environmental factors throughout development determine how the genotype is expressed in the animal's physical phenotype and personality. The roles of nature (genes) and nurture (environment) are not separate. Environmental effects on behavioural resilience and cognition range from the perhaps more obvious influences of appropriate nutrition and exercise post weaning to stress experienced almost from conception to adulthood.

Pre-natal or pre-hatch stress can have long-term effects on emotional regulation (e.g. depression, anxiety, aggression), cognitive ability (e.g. attention deficits) and overall development in both humans and animals (Weinstock, 2008; Løtvedt and Jensen, 2014), and these effects can be passed on to the next generation. What may be of surprise is that stress does not have to be major or chronic to affect humans (O'Donnell *et al.*, 2009) or non-humans (Weinstock, 2008), and this is seen in both pre-cocial (highly developed at birth) and altricial (fetus-like at

birth and fully dependent on adult care) species. Animal studies have used non-social and social stressors. For example, the short-term housing of pregnant pigs with two familiar and three unfamiliar females (which usually results in a degree of aggression) for two separate 7-day periods (12% of the 115-day gestation) had long-term effects on the (precocial) piglets (Rutherford *et al.*, 2014). These piglets were more anxious and female offspring showed impaired maternal behaviour toward their own young. A similar effect occurs in rats, an altricial species, if a pregnant individual is placed in the cage of an unfamiliar lactating female for just 10 minutes across 5 consecutive days (0.2% of the 21-day gestation) (Brunton and Russell, 2010; Grundwald and Brunton, 2015). Whilst we may consider the length of exposure to be quite minor in respect of the whole pregnancy, clearly these 'short' stressors are significant to the female. Moreover, they are enough for her physiological reactions to affect the brain development of the fetus to a 'pro-anxiety phenotype', with effects on later resilience to stress, learning and memory ability, and how female offspring care for their own young. Many pregnant animals are exposed to man-made stressors including fireworks, travel, visits to the veterinary clinic, hospitalization and, for many farm animals, relocation to a different home pen and thus different social neighbour. Likewise, we may separate the female from the male, or from all her companions, even when their ethology shows that other females and/or the sire are directly or indirectly involved in the care of the dam and the young (Gubernick and Klopfer, 1981; Braun and Champagne, 2014). More research is needed on how stress can be reduced for breeding females. That notwithstanding, the evidence to date calls for a far more cautionary approach to be taken by breeders of any species and all others involved in the care of pregnant animals and neonates, including veterinary professionals.

Developmental stages

Lack of or inappropriate experiences at important developmental stages will have lasting effects on behaviour. These stages can be divided into the neonatal/infant period (naturally ended by weaning), juvenile period (between weaning and sexual maturity), adolescence (sexual maturity) and finally adulthood (social maturity). Throughout these periods, individuals change both physically and in their emotional and cognitive abilities. We need to remember that the developmental period is from conception to full *social* maturity. Adulthood is reached in humans at around 25 years of age (10+ years after adolescence begins), horses and some parrot species at around 5 years and dogs at around 24 months. Of course, further developmental changes occur throughout adulthood and old age. How the individual copes with these later changes will be determined by the foundations laid prior to reaching adulthood.

Neonatal/infant: Maternal behaviour post birth/hatch can affect individual offspring. At a gross level, we sometimes take this into consideration – think of the advice to see the bitch before buying a puppy to check whether she is friendly to them and unfamiliar people. This is important indeed, but does not provide the whole story. Care of the infant (be that maternal, paternal or by another member of the social group) comprises far more subtle and significant components (Braun and Champagne, 2014). For example, in dogs and rodents, care quality extends even to the amount of licking of the neonate – too much or too little can affect its confidence and ability to cope with potentially stressful environments in adulthood (Czerwinski *et al.*, 2016; Lezama-Garcia *et al.*, 2019). This should not be of surprise. We already know the importance of various subtle behaviours of the primary caregiver for human infants, especially during the first 12 months. Care quality influences the development of secure or insecure infant attachment styles and has onward repercussions for adult mental and behavioural health, resilience to social and non-social stressors, relationships with others and own future caregiving style (Mikulincer and Shaver, 2012).

Mammalian weaning, or the avian equivalent, is characterized by the parent no longer being the sole provider of food and protection. The parent's behaviour is less tolerant and food is no longer available on demand, making this a stressful time for the offspring (and parent). Weaning marks the end of infancy and the start of a new, more independent, phase of life – the juvenile stage. For most species, weaning is not the end of the relationship with the dam, which may continue for many months or even years and gradually lessen in intensity. However, for the vast majority of captive animals weaning is a highly traumatic process, performed at a time decreed by humans and usually during, not at the end of, infancy, and too often during early infancy. Further, it involves an unnatural total and abrupt separation of mother and offspring. This loss of support is itself potentially damaging to the long-term welfare of the offspring. In addition, it is frequently accompanied by other extremely stressful experiences. These include sudden exposure to human handling (from familiar and unfamiliar people) and being transported to new accommodation where both the physical and social environment is unfamiliar, (Dybkjaer, 1992; Ahola *et al.*, 2017; McMillan, 2017). Research from all species studied, including cattle, pigs, rats and horses, shows that early weaning predisposes to stress ulcers, other physical conditions and behaviour abnormalities, such as wind sucking, pica and enteric and respiratory conditions (Fraser, 1978; Nicol and Badnell-Waters, 2005; Waters *et al.*, 2010; Ahola *et al.*, 2017; McMillan, 2017). For these animals, the start of the juvenile stage of development may be substantially compromised.

Juvenile: The juvenile stage may be weeks, months or years in length, depending on when the species becomes sexually mature. It is a very important period in which animals continue to be close to and learn from their parents, other adults and peers about finding food, avoiding danger and how to interact with their own kind. This socializing and general widening of experience is crucial to the development of the confident and capable adult and should continue throughout adolescence (see 'Socialization', below). In summer, the author [AM] enjoys watching garden birds, such as juvenile robins, goldcrest and blue tits, learning these lessons. The juvenile stage is the period between infancy and pubescence/adolescence. Pubescence and adolescence are terms that are often used interchangeably, the former referring more to the physiological changes relating to sexual maturity and reproductive capacity, and the latter to the psychosocial developments that occur in this period. In much the same way as the sweet, if cheeky, juvenile human child of 8–9 years changes to the rather less obliging 13-year-old, the juvenile 14-week-old puppy changes as it morphs into an adolescent 24-week-old.

Adolescence: Adolescence is a period of psychological change in the individual that triggers changes in their social environment – others behave differently towards this changeling that is neither child nor adult. In humans, it covers the second decade of life and in rats (a cardinal species used in adolescence research) it covers weeks four to seven (Sturman and Moghaddam, 2011). During adolescence, some genes switch off and others switch on, resulting in hormonal and neurotransmitter changes. These changes drive alterations in physique and the appearance of secondary sexual characteristics, such as the red breast of the robin, the adult coat of the dog and the facial hair of the human. It is "a time of dramatic structural and functional neurodevelopment" (Sturman and Moghaddam, 2011) which results in changes in cognition, social and non-social behaviour. Methodological advances in the study of electrophysiological brain activity in laboratory animals and humans have expanded our knowledge of how changes in the 'social brain' (Blakemore, 2008) influence social behaviour and the behavioural vulnerabilities that can lead to problem behaviour and mental illnesses that manifest during adolescence.

As with earlier developmental periods, adolescence is one of continuing change across its course. However, adolescence seems to be more complex, with various aspects of change starting and ending at different times (Sturman and Moghaddam, 2011). Resultant behaviour changes are characteristic across all species studied and include:

- Development of new interests
- Increased social behaviour, particularly with peers
- Emotional instability (moodiness)
- Increased interest in novel scenarios and sensations
- Increased risk taking and impulsivity
- Increased conflict with others and reduced compliance with requests. This is seen in humans, and in adolescent animal interactions with their human caretakers (Asher *et al.*, 2020), a point not only for pet owners to note, but also veterinary professionals, farmers and others.

From an evolutionary perspective, adolescence is an important time when the individual is learning how to make their own way in the world with their peers. If it does so successfully, it will likely reproduce and pass on its genes to the next generation. Adolescence is a time of great discovery and lots of uncertainty and thus anxiety, a time of change. Novelty seeking and exploration are important parts of this process for discovering both new environments and new physical and mental activities. For our animals, this means we need to continue to expand their opportunities for enrichment activities and mental stimulation. This should be done in a gentle and gradual way so that exploration is pleasant and not overpowering or fear provoking.

Regrettably for many animals, adolescence is a time when pet owners find their expectations are no longer being met – the behaviour of the changeling is just too much to deal with. Similar to some teenagers whose home life is socially disrupted and who find themselves homeless, both physically and emotionally abandoned, so an animal may be abandoned by their owner on the roadside or in the countryside to fend for themselves. However, most will be put up for rehoming or be euthanased. Evidence strongly suggests that this period of transition from juvenile to adult is an extremely risky time for our pets in this regard (O'Neill *et al.*, 2013; Hazel *et al.*, 2018). Veterinary professionals have an essential role in ensuring owners of young animals are prepared for these changes and are directed to appropriate advice on how to guide their pet through this period.

One main cause of owner stress is the increased impulsivity associated with adolescence. Impulsivity is basically a lack of patience and a tendency to act before thinking. One way this is assessed is by testing the individual's preference for smaller rewards that occur sooner, rather than larger rewards that require waiting, indicating the 'I want it, and I want it now' effect. This is a natural part of adolescence, along with increased independence and emotional instability. Knowing this makes it easier to understand, and thus explain to owners (and parents), the outbursts of frustration seen in adolescent humans and other animals when asked to comply with requests not in line with their own immediate desires. Forcing the issue for compliance is unlikely to be of help and will only increase stress and aggressive behaviour on both sides. A better tactic is for the adult/owner to remain calm and change the situation, and thus the mood of the adolescent, before trying again. Keeping frustration and anxiety to a minimum is imperative for welfare throughout life, and especially during development. This is achieved through clear communication, positive reinforcement and consistently applied rules (see 'Learning and cognition'). Remember, there is light at the end of the turbulent teens. Whilst no parent/caretaker is perfect, with understanding and planning, adolescence can be negotiated successfully. After all, we are all evidence of successful developmental journeys we undertook together with our caretakers.

Learning and cognition

This section introduces some fundamental basics of how we and other animals learn. It is not intended to give sufficient grounding for training animals or dealing with behaviour issues. Rather, the aim is to give a flavour of this fascinating area and of its core importance to welfare. The reader is encouraged to explore further and there are many good, accessible chapters that cover learning and associated areas in psychology textbooks such as Haselgrove (2019), as well as books focused solely on the science of learning (Domjan, 2015, 2017) or its application to training (Burch and Bailey, 1999; McGreevy and Boakes, 2011). Welfare-focused animal training is covered in Chapter 6.

Humans are anthropocentric; we consider ourselves unique and superior to other species. Indeed, we are unique, as is every species. In some ways we are also superior to non-humans, notably our greater range of tool use – thanks to the evolutionary accident of the fully opposable thumb (Ambrose, 2001; Young, 2003). For 20,000 years or more, we have been aware of our skills deficits and have domesticated animals not only for their body products (meat, milk, eggs, fur and feathers), but to complement these deficits for our profit by, for example, carrying loads and finding food. We train a range of animals, such as dogs, raptors, water buffalo, camelids, donkeys, horses and truffle-hunting pigs. More recently, rats have been trained to detect landmines and illnesses, such as tuberculosis (Mahony *et al.*, 2014; Reither *et al.*, 2015; Figure 3.4).

To maintain our view of humanity and condone how we use animals, we have consistently underestimated and disregarded their capabilities to learn, think and feel. In the modern era this was reinforced by Descartes' conclusion that animals cannot reason nor feel pain and are basically unthinking machines. Only since the 1950s has there been a slow but noticeable shift in this view

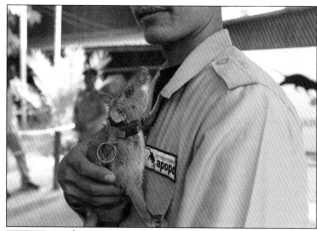

| 3.4 | An African giant pouched rat that has been trained for landmine detection. |

(Shutterstock.com/Adi Haririe)

accompanied by the growth of the scientific field of animal welfare (Ristau, 1991; McBride and Baugh, 2022). Since then, research has exposed such views for the comfortable and comforting misperceptions that they are (Herzog, 2010). The interest in this area continues and, seemingly weekly, papers are published that provide further evidence of the abilities of animals to learn, their cognitive skills and the complexity of their emotional lives.

Learning involves the mental processes of thinking, knowing, remembering and problem solving, which are essential to survival and meeting the 'Three Rules of Life' (see below). Science has already revealed much about animal minds and cognition. We have evidence of their long-term memory, use of tools, innovation, concepts of amount, number, time and place, capacity for self-recognition and use of symbols to communicate with humans, and ability to abstract information as in categorizing objects, to be sensitive to the actions of others, to show empathy and altruism, and to cooperate (Heyes, 2012; Wynne and Udell, 2013). We may almost expect to discover such abilities in chimpanzees, elephants, dogs, dolphins or parrots – animals we perceive as of a 'higher' order. Yet, most people are likely both unaware and would be quite amazed to know that rats, mice, cows, pigs, horses, chickens, pigeons, crows, various fish, reptiles and amphibia, cephalopods, and other invertebrates, insects and worms have been shown to have various of these abilities (Wynne and Udell, 2013; Reader *et al.*, 2016; McBride, 2017).

Creative use of technology is enabling better ways of asking questions of animals, with fascinating results. For example, Toda and Wantanabe (2008) showed that laboratory pigeons can recognize themselves in a video, even after a delay of 5 seconds before playback. This means pigeons do better than 3-year-old humans, who can only do this task if the delay is less than 2 seconds (Wynne and Udell, 2013). Likewise, the development of 'UV television' (Powell *et al.*, 2021) and various eye-tracking technologies, as used on dogs (Somppi *et al.*, 2012) and rats (Wallace *et al.*, 2013), has enabled us to better understand their perspective of the world. For the advancement of animal welfare, the study of animal cognition is an exciting and extremely important research area that is furthering our understanding of what animals can learn and how.

Learning is core to survival. Animals learn to avoid events they find aversive (unpleasant, noxious) and learn what predicts success in obtaining objects or experiences they find appetitive (pleasant). This requires the individual to be aware of how it feels, be able to remember associations between events, including its own behaviour, and being able to reason and plan. There are differences in the extent to which species and individuals do this, but evidence indicates the similarities may well outweigh these differences, further underscoring our responsibility to consider animal welfare more holistically (McBride and Baugh, 2022).

Modern interest in how human and non-human animals learn started with the work of Pavlov (1849–1936), Thorndike (1874–1949), Watson (1878–1958) and Skinner (1904–1990). The work of these and subsequent researchers has contributed greatly to animal and human welfare through changing attitudes on how best to teach others to behave in acceptable ways. Individuals learn continuously throughout their lives and use that learning to refine their behaviours, to become more efficient in finding and keeping the good things in life and avoiding/escaping the bad. Training (or teaching) is when one individual deliberately directs the learning of another. The principles underlying learning and training are the same. However, if these are not understood then they can easily be misapplied, potentially severely compromising the welfare of trainee and trainer (McBride and Montgomery, 2018).

Whilst the principles of learning theory apply across taxa, trainers need to be aware of biological factors, at species and individual level, that can influence learning and the animal's ability to respond in the way the trainer desires (Timberlake and Silva, 1994). It is a truism to say you cannot teach a pig to fly – it has no wings. Likewise, the trainer of a dog who has chronic low-level pain due to inherited conformation defects, or has compromised hearing/vision (at birth or later), should consider the behaviours they wish to train (e.g. substituting stand for sit) and/or their method of communication (Hayward, 2015).

Senses and learning

Learning relies on the animal obtaining information from its environment. This occurs through various organs, including whiskers (vibrissae) (McBride, 2017). Sensory differences between species means that stimuli that are obvious to a human may not be obvious to an animal and *vice versa*. For example, take a dog, a green tennis ball and green grass. Dogs have very good night vision, as they have more rods than we do, meaning they are accurate and acute detectors of motion. However, they are quite short-sighted and have dichromatic colour vision, seeing only blues and yellows. Reds and greens may appear more like different shades of grey (Figure 3.5). This is why, when the tennis ball stops on the grass, your dog changes from using its eyes to relying more on its nose to find it. In contrast, that slight body movement that you (unknowingly) repeatedly make when training may be more salient to the animal as a visual cue than an auditory word cue (Gibsone *et al.*, 2021).

Perceptual abilities are also central to the important topic of sensitization. Like us, in order to learn, animals need to be motivated (aroused) and at the same time relaxed and calm. If they are too mentally or physically aroused, then they are 'sensitized'. Sensitization puts the animal in a heightened state of alertness, especially to potentially threatening or dangerous stimuli. This is an important aspect of survival but can be counterproductive during training.

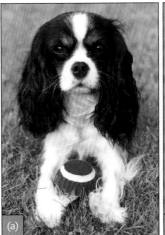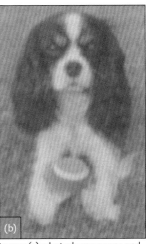

3.5 Colour vision differences between (a) what a human sees and (b) what a dog sees.
(Created using dog vision image processing tool: dog-vision.andraspeter.com)

Case example 1: Clever Hans

The classic study demonstrating accidental training is that of Otto Pfungst and Clever Hans the horse (Samhita and Gross, 2013). Clever Hans could allegedly calculate complicated sums, providing the answer by pawing the ground. In fact, Hans had learned that if he stopped pawing when a human gave a certain signal, he was rewarded. The signals (cues) he learned were unconscious and very subtle normal parts of human social behaviour, such as the flicker of a raised eyebrow used to indicate turn-taking in conversation.

Sensitization

Sensitization is essentially physiological arousal – what we call stress. Stress can be pleasant (eustress) or unpleasant (distress). Stress is caused by a wide range of internal and external factors, including being tired, hungry or thirsty, and being excited, anxious, frightened or frustrated (including being bored). We may not realize that under-stimulation can be as stressful (sensitizing) as over-stimulation, hence the necessity for appropriate enrichment to be provided throughout an animal's life (McBride, 2019; see Chapter 4). In terms of sensory perception, sensitization can be caused by an environment that is physically uncomfortable – for example, too hard, too soft, too hot, too cold, too noisy (including ultrasonic noise), too smelly, too bright or too busy.

What is comfortable for a human may not be so for an animal: a point we, intentionally or unintentionally, frequently ignore. Think of dogs being taken for a walk on a hot day – on hot pavements that their shoe-wearing owners are protected from – or horses and dogs being rugged or coated at temperatures that their owners may consider cold but they may not (Mejdell *et al.*, 2019). Few of us may be aware of potential sensitizing factors when we train or handle animals; for example, the potentially painful effects of normal office light levels on crepuscular and nocturnal rodents (McBride, 2017), the intense (and likely unpleasant) smell of anti-perspirant, perfume, the soap we have just used to wash our hands or disinfectant spray on the table (Nielsen, 2017), or the effects of anxiety pheromones left by an animal previously in the room.

Stimuli that sensitize can compound each other, causing a greater effect. Think of when you are tired or hungry or hot: little things that you can normally ignore become annoying. You are more likely to misinterpret and be irritated, or even feel anxious, at a passing comment meant as a bit of a joke. This serves to make you even more aroused. You may finally snap at something apparently trivial – 'the straw that broke the camel's back'. Trainers and behaviourists colloquially call this increased sensitization due to sequential or co-occurring arousing stimuli 'trigger stacking'. It is essential to be aware of this and aim to calm anxious animals, people or yourself down.

Learning requires motivation, but too much motivation leads to being too aroused and sensitized. This interferes detrimentally with the ability to learn new things and the ability to perform behaviours the individual has already learned. We experience this too: think of when you are excited because you are going on a dream date or anxious before an important interview. You may find you simply cannot tie your shoelaces or put on your mascara, and do stupid things like put your keys in the fridge! This is the basis of the Yerkes–Dodson law (Yerkes and Dodson, 1908).

The Yerkes–Dodson law states that, regardless of the source of arousal, after a certain optimum level of arousal is reached, arousal and performance are negatively correlated (i.e. the greater the arousal, the worse the performance) (Figure 3.6). Arousal levels should be kept low throughout training until the animal is consistently and reliably providing the right behaviour, and that behaviour is reliably on cue. Only then should the behaviour be strengthened by practice in circumstances that gradually increase the animal's arousal levels. It should also be remembered that less arousal is required for optimal learning and performance of a more difficult task. We may need to play music when doing a low motivating or less challenging task, such as housework, but need peace and quiet for difficult tasks, such as writing a book chapter or learning a new physical skill (Figure 3.7). An animal in a new or previously anxiety-provoking situation, such as when the veterinary surgeon is present, is already aroused. This may be further compounded because it is ill or in pain. Keeping the animal and

the veterinary team as calm as possible is essential for its welfare and will enable it to perform any behaviours it has learned that facilitate examination and treatment.

One of the most sensitizing factors is anxiety, and we often forget this when we are interacting with animals. Maslow's hierarchy of needs (see below) illustrates how the first two levels must be met if the animal (or human) is to be able to learn (Maslow, 1987). These are physiological and safety needs. Novelty is an immediate trigger for anxiety – this makes evolutionary sense, as anything new may be dangerous. So, we need to try and reduce the novelty of places, people and procedures that animals are exposed to. Ideally, owners should plan for possible future events. We can use trained cues to help make a new environment more familiar. We can also purposely use the process of habituation learning.

Maslow's hierarchy of needs

The behaviour of humans and animals is motivated by needs. Maslow (1987) developed the theory of the hierarchy of needs. These are illustrated in Figure 3.8 and can be grouped as basic needs (physiological, safety), psychological needs (belonging, cognitive) and self-fulfilment needs. The basic and psychological needs are known as deficit needs, and self-fulfilment as growth needs. Deficit needs motivate behaviour and do so more strongly the longer they are denied. At a general level, and in terms of learning and sensitization, being physiologically comfortable and feeling safe are needs that must be met before learning can occur in any efficient manner. This relates to arousal and the Yerkes–Dodson law. In terms of learning, and meeting the esteem and cognitive needs, it is clear that the animal must find the learning (training methods) pleasurable, otherwise the need for safety, and consequent increased arousal and sensitization, is likely to overwhelm the process.

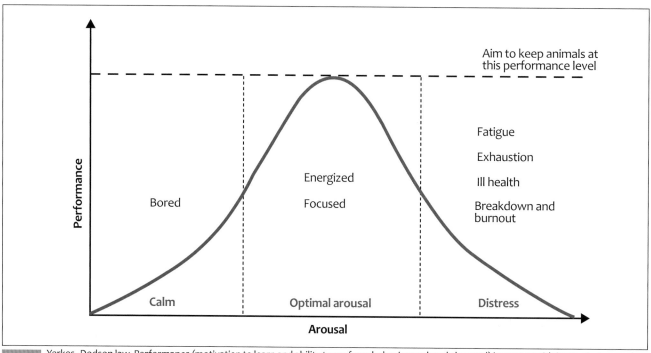

3.6 Yerkes–Dodson law. Performance (motivation to learn and ability to perform behaviours already learned) increases with increasing arousal up to an optimum level of arousal (indicated by the dashed line). Further increases in arousal result in decreased performance.

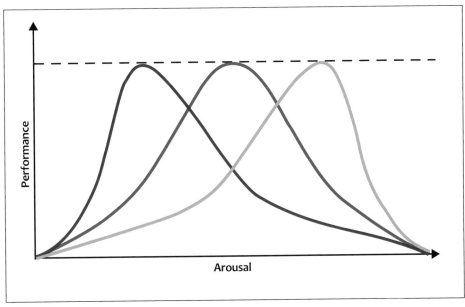

3.7 This graph shows how the difficulty of a task interacts with the Yerkes–Dodson law (blue line; see Figure 3.6). The red line represents a difficult task; the green line represents an easy task. External and internal sources of arousal need to be minimized during the learning phase of all tasks, when performing learned tasks that are more difficult or any task when the animal is already sensitized.

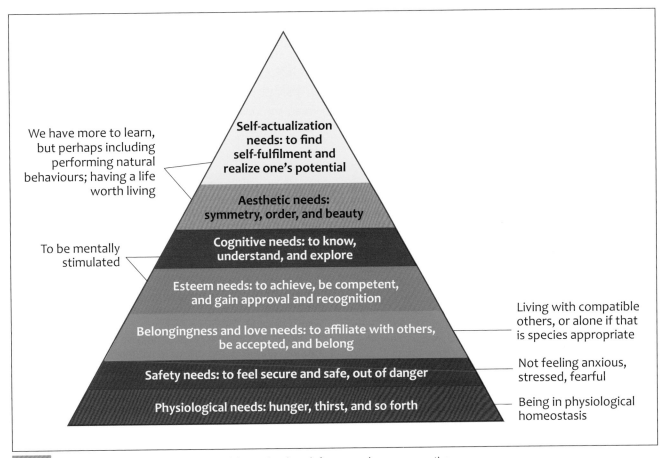

3.8 The author's [AM] adaptation of Maslow's hierarchy of needs from a non-human perspective.

Habituation

Habituation is the opposite of sensitization in that it is decremental – it decreases the tendency to respond. This reduction is due not to sensory adaptation or fatigue, or to motor fatigue, but to learning (Rankin *et al.*, 2009). Habituation is the simplest and weakest form of learning. The animal learns that *if* event A occurs, *then nothing* of interest follows. The animal is not learning a new behaviour but a reduction in a reflex response. It is evolutionarily very important and is seen across taxa, from single-celled organisms to humans (Haselgrove, 2019). Habituation allows conscious thought to be reserved for more complicated things like finding food, writing notes, interacting with others, or performing a clinical examination or surgical procedure. It acts as a filter for sameness and irrelevance in the environment and alerts the individual to change. In essence, it is our radar system (Rankin *et al.*, 2009).

Case example 2: Habituation to your environment

You can test your own habituation. Take a moment now to stop reading and notice things around you: the feel of the chair you are sitting on, the floor beneath your feet, the light and temperature level in the room, the gentle whirr of the computer fan, the sound of the birds outside, or the scent and breathing of your dog or cat next to you. Whilst your senses have perceived all this continuously, your brain has monitored 'no change' and has filtered out the information from your consciousness (Daleswartzentruber, 2007a). Should there be a change – a flicker of the light, a change in the pitch of the fan's whirr – or another extraneous stimulus, you would dishabituate and become alert, aroused and sensitized, and only rehabituate once you had decided that nothing exciting or threatening had occurred (Daleswartzentruber, 2007b). If you were to leave the room and come back minutes later or the next day, you would need to rehabituate to these things again upon your return. Your response to the stimuli would have spontaneously recovered (Daleswartzentruber, 2007c).

As illustrated in the case example, habituation is easily interrupted and dishabituation occurs. Depending on various factors, including the degree of sensitization, rehabituation may happen quickly or more slowly. It is this continual need to relearn that all is the same that makes habituation a very weak form of learning. To refine the initial description: in habituation the animal learns that *if* event A happens, *then nothing* of interest follows *in this place, at this time*. In technical terms, habituation learning is context and stimulus specific.

This does not mean that habituation is not useful. Used carefully, habituation training can help build resilience by letting an animal become accustomed to stimuli, reducing the probability of an aversive association with them later. Known as 'long-term habituation', this has been shown experimentally in various species and its effects can last for hours, days or even weeks (Rankin et al., 2009). For example, we may wish to habituate an animal to a confined area by enabling it to freely walk around or through it, or to a syringe by first granting the opportunity to investigate it, then very gently and repeatedly touching the skin with the blunt syringe. Allowing a horse to repeatedly investigate a saddle, or a dog a muzzle, before taking it on and off and gradually increasing the time spent wearing it is a use of habituation. But it is weak learning, and it is better to use non-context-specific classical learning (see below).

It is important to understand and remember that habituation is only part of the 'radar' analogy. Both habituation and sensitization processes are activated when an animal notices a stimulus, and its response is the summation of both. This is known as the dual-process theory (Groves and Thompson, 1970). If already aroused, then the individual will show an enhanced response. We may perceive this as 'over'-excited or 'over'-anxious or 'unnecessarily' irritable behaviour. When this occurs in children, friends or colleagues, we may think of an explanation (the sensitizing factors); for example, 'sugar rush', 'too tired', 'low blood sugar', 'too much coffee', 'not well' or that there is some form of stress or anxiety going on in their lives.

Hopefully, we do this even when we do not know the person well (e.g. when speaking with a client) and do not simply assume they have some form of temperament or personality flaw and are just difficult, rude or aggressive people. Yet, all too frequently, we assume precisely that when it comes to animals. This increases our own arousal, we become sensitized and may respond by jerking the leash or reins, yelling at the animal or gripping them more tightly. Whilst this may alter the animal's immediate behaviour, it will only serve to increase their arousal and the possibility of regrettable behavioural consequences in the future, as classical learning is also occurring. A better strategy would be to think, 'How can I change the balance of habituation to sensitization, that is, how can I reduce this animal's arousal state?'

> Remember: keep yourself calm, keep the animal calm, keep the owner calm, and carry on!

The animal's state of arousal, its level of sensitization, affects how well, and what, the animal learns. Thus, it is an especially pertinent consideration when a young animal is learning about its world through the process of socialization.

Socialization: experiencing the social and physical world

When we consider an animal's sensory abilities, it is clear that the human world is quite alien to that for which they are adapted. Stimuli we find tolerable or pleasant in terms of touch, smells, sounds, going to new places, meeting new people, heat, cold, etc. may to them be mildly or extremely distressing. Accounting for this is particularly pertinent during development. The type and quantity of social and environmental experiences can be too much, too aversive and can sensitize the animal. Likewise, a lack of appropriate experiences means that there is more of the world that is 'unfamiliar', 'novel' or 'scary', which is also sensitizing. The experiences that an animal has during its development, from pre-birth/pre-hatch to adulthood, will have long-term effects on its behaviour, confidence, resilience to stress and thus its welfare (McCune et al., 1995).

Numerous papers and books on dogs, horses, cats, rabbits and rodents provide evidence of the potential benefits of early and maintained socialization to humans through the gentle, gradual introduction of handling and other experiences, such as exposure to different objects and scents. This process should be introduced prior to weaning, so the infant has the emotional support of its mother and siblings. The terms 'gentle' and 'gradual' are important here and should be considered from the animal's perspective. Over exposure can also have detrimental effects (McCune et al., 1995). Some questionable practices have been suggested and the reader is urged to critically consider any new suggestions before applying them. Some may be more obviously inappropriate, such as the binding practices of traditional elephant training that involved forced interaction and restraint of the young infant (Locke, 2006). This is no longer deemed acceptable practice in UK zoos (Fagen et al., 2014). Yet, regrettably, many have applied, and no doubt many still do apply, a very similar process to horses. This is Miller's (1991) 'imprint training' of the neonatal horse, undertaken in the first few hours after birth.

Case example 3: Miller's imprint training of the neonatal horse

This method involves physical restraint (which itself mimics predation) and the very invasive, unnatural experiences of having an object (human finger) probing the ears, inserted up the nose and inserted in the anus (albeit gloved and lubricated). The process takes no account of the species and the world in which it has evolved. Horses are a prey species and this neonatal period is a time of great, if not the greatest, vulnerability in the wild. Being precocial, the neonate has well developed senses, but it is still unsteady on its feet and unable to move swiftly to try and escape threat. Such fear-provoking experiences have huge stress implications for both the foal and dam. In the wild, the dam would not leave the foal's side, but in captivity they are likely to be removed or tethered during this 'imprinting' procedure. Of course, even if not present, the dam would still be aware of stress pheromones on return to her foal.

Not surprisingly, the probings of this method were later found to be ineffective socializers (Simpson, 2002). The perceived outcome of a calm animal in later life is most likely a passive anxiety response, known as learned helplessness, instilled in the recipient by this traumatic and inescapable event.

Regardless of species, throughout development 'gentle' and 'gradual' are the watchwords, and methods should not involve the animal becoming stressed. The young of both precocial and altricial species (once the latter become mobile) should be encouraged, in a hands-off manner, to approach people and objects and to explore the environment. For example, if the animal needs to be on a lead, then this should remain loose. It is the animal not the human that dictates when it is feeling confident and secure enough to take the next step in discovery. Confident behaviour should be reinforced as appropriate for the individual given its species, age and observed preferences (e.g. parts of the body where it enjoys being stroked, particular food treats, play). Incidentally, this is the best way to introduce new things to human children and adults: gently, gradually and supportively. For useful guides on applying the principles to introducing young (and not so young) animals to different people, other animals (socialization) and environments, see Bailey (2008), Bradshaw and Ellis (2017), Atkinson (2018) and Rogers (2018).

The adage says: 'softly, softly catch'ee monkey'. This should be the underlying policy and mantra when introducing an individual animal to any new experience whatever its age – young, mature or aged. It is especially important during development. Using the dog as an example, owners are encouraged to attend good puppy parties and puppy training classes and are advised to socialize their puppy, especially for the first 14 weeks of life. All this is good, essential even, but it is not sufficient. To prepare for a confident, resilient adulthood, appropriate experiences must extend through the whole of development to social maturity. To be able to assess and compare methods to accomplish this requires understanding of behaviour. At a minimum, one should know about the basics of how animals learn, what they may learn that one

did not intend and how their emotional experience underlies this. Only then is one able to direct clients to the right sort of professional for the right sort of advice.

Classical and operant conditioning

As indicated above, animals can learn by different processes simultaneously. Whilst an individual is habituating to some stimuli in the environment, they are learning to associate others with outcomes. There are two types of associative learning: classical (Pavlovian) and operant (Skinnerian).

This section provides a brief introduction to some basic rules that apply to both classical and operant conditioning. The word conditioning simply means learning and both are used interchangeably. The animal may learn through its own experience or by proxy (i.e. by observing how others behave).

In classical conditioning, the animal learns that *if* stimulus A occurs, *then* stimulus B will follow (regardless of what behaviour I am doing) *and I will feel like... (and respond with a reflex behaviour)*. The animal learns to associate event A with event B.

In operant conditioning, the animal learns that *if* stimulus A occurs, *and I do* something, *then* stimulus B will follow *and I will feel like...* Here the animal is learning two sets of association: firstly between its behaviour and event B (the outcome), and secondly that this association only holds if event A (the cue) has occurred. It is called operant learning because the animal learns the outcome will only occur if it performs a specific behaviour – it 'operates' on the environment.

There are three important factors that enable classical and operant learning to occur. These are:

* Salience
* Contingency
* Contiguity.

Salience

Salience is the degree to which an item or event stands out from other stimuli. If too low, the animal's attention will not be captured and this will impede learning. For a stimulus to be salient, the animal must know it is there and must be able to detect and distinguish it from other stimuli also present. If it cannot, how can it learn about it? It should be remembered that sensory differences mean that what may be obvious (salient) to us may not be so for the animal, and what we find pleasant may not be so for them.

Contingency

Contingency refers to how contingent the second event is on the first. In other words, how reliably the first event predicts the second. The strength of this will depend on how frequently the two occur together and how recently the animal has experienced them. If the first event is not a reliable predictor, then the association will not occur. For example, if we repeatedly use a dog's name in general conversation the dog quickly learns that the word means nothing – no owner attention, no treat, nothing. It should, therefore, be no surprise that the dog does not respond immediately when you say its name and are wanting its attention. There is a simple solution to this: use the dog's name when you are talking to it and want its attention, and use a different 'code name' when you are talking about it. Then event A (the dog's name being spoken) remains a reliable predictor of event B (your attention).

Contiguity

Contiguity refers to how close in time events A and B occur. For best learning, they should not be separated by more than a few seconds, otherwise other events, thoughts and actions will have occurred in between, which makes it harder to learn that it was event A that reliably preceded event B. There is one notable exception to this, which is taste aversion (see 'Avoiding being killed', below).

Classical conditioning

Classical conditioning takes its alternative name, Pavlovian conditioning, from the well-known work of Ivan Pavlov. Originally a physiologist, Pavlov researched the digestive system, including saliva production. This reflex behaviour occurs in the presence of the sight, smell or taste of food. It requires no learning. It is an unlearned (unconditioned) response to an unlearned (unconditioned) stimulus (food). Pavlov realized that saliva production did not require the presence of food if an event reliably predicted that food was coming – such as a dog being put in the experimental harness it wore during research sessions (Figure 3.9). Whilst probably not the first to notice this phenomenon, Pavlov was the first to investigate it.

Initially, the harness had no connection with saliva production – it was a neutral stimulus. However, the dog learned that it was a reliable predictor of food, resulting in saliva being produced as soon as the harness was put on. The harness had become a conditioned (learned) stimulus. Further study showed that any stimulus the animal noticed could become a conditioned stimulus. These previously neutral stimuli could be olfactory, auditory, visual or tactile. Additionally, animals have been shown to 'generalize' their learning, displaying a conditioned response when presented with a neutral stimulus similar enough to a conditioned one. When the new stimulus is too different from the original, the animal will not respond to it – it will 'discriminate' between them. The conditioned stimulus can even be something we do reliably, for example, that particular sigh you only make just before you get off the sofa to take the dog out – this gives rise to situations where 'he seems to be able to read my mind!', but it is simply the result of classical conditioning.

Much of human behaviour is classically conditioned. For instance, a banknote is a neutral stimulus until we learn that it can predict the access to unconditioned stimuli such as food. The sound of an ice cream van or a picture of chocolate can make you salivate. A particular tune, or a variation of it, may make you feel happy or sad

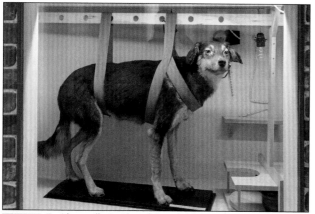

3.9 Taxidermy Illustration of the experimental set-up used by Pavlov.

(Shutterstock.com/Gilmanshin)

depending on associations you have made. This also occurs with names: if you think of the name of someone special to you and then you meet someone with the same name, you will have a slight positive bias in your behaviour towards them due to your learned pleasant classical associations with that name. Conversely, when first meeting someone who has the same name as a person who was nasty to you (a school bully, a bad colleague), then your behaviour will be more restrained, even slightly antagonistic. Classical learning is very powerful; it is not context specific and, once learned, the same stimulus evokes the same emotional response wherever it occurs.

For a classical association to be made, both the neutral and unconditioned stimuli must be salient and the former a reliable predictor of the latter. We can use this to our advantage, for example, giving pets many very pleasant associations with potentially scary events, such as stimuli associated with the veterinary practice – being handled, having someone stare into their face, being put on a table or, for cats, that the cat carrier means a trip to the veterinary surgery! Owners can help their pets learn pleasant classical associations: if the cat carrier is always out, has a comfortable bed and is where special titbits are given, the cat will learn to like it; if lifting and looking into the ear is always followed by a favourite treat, the animal will learn to accept handling; likewise with wearing a muzzle. It is well worth encouraging owners to practise these associations and even to bring their dog for frequent trips to the practice, for a game on the floor and a treat when placed on the clinic table, and then go home.

If this pleasant relationship no longer holds true because we do not bother to put treats in the cat basket every so often, the trips to the veterinary practice become less frequent or we forget the play and treats part, then the response will weaken and may seem to disappear – a process known as extinction.

Extinction is not a process of forgetting, simply a process of learning that 'for now that association is not relevant'. This is important to note if 'clicker' training methods are used. The click is a classically conditioned stimulus associated with food or other unconditioned stimuli. If this pleasant outcome does not reliably follow the click, the association will wane and eventually extinguish.

Case example 4: The round pound coin

Recently, UK residents have extinguished their response to a coin (a conditioned stimulus). In 2017, the round-edged £1 coin was replaced by a new 12-sided version. When the old coin lost its legal tender, it no longer predicted the acquisition of nice things (unconditioned stimuli) and the classical response to it was extinguished. However, if it were to come back into circulation with purchasing power, the previous response would recover very quickly.

We can see from the 'bully name' example that unpleasant classical associations can be made. Just as a neutral stimulus can predict something nice, so it can predict something aversive. The 'clicker' can be made to be scary just by pairing it with something the animal finds aversive. Indeed, all anxiety and fear associations are classical. It is important to realize that a fear association is learned very quickly: if an experience is very scary or painful, then one exposure to the association is enough, and this can override previously learned pleasant associations. This makes good biological sense. If we do not learn that lesson the first time we encounter a dangerous stimulus, we may not survive the second time.

Furthermore, if we are already sensitized, then an aversive experience does not have to be as scary for a fear association to form as it would if we were calm and relaxed. This is an example of trigger stacking. This underscores the need to facilitate resilience in the animals we care for so that they are less likely to make fear associations. With expert help, fear associations may be managed (made to go extinct) through a gradual process called desensitization and counter-conditioning, where the animal's arousal level is *carefully* monitored to keep it calm as it learns a new pleasant association. This new pleasant association is then *gradually* generalized to related salient stimuli that formed part of the whole jigsaw of conditioned stimuli that predicted the original fear-provoking stimulus. However, it is crucial to understand that fears are not forgotten, can never be cured and may resurface in the future.

Classical conditioning is a fundamental part of how we learn about the world, and understanding the process allows us to systematically use it in guiding that learning (training).

Operant conditioning

As with classical learning, research into operant learning continues to reveal the complex nuances of what might appear to be quite simple, especially as there is always reference to Thorndike (1874–1949) and Skinner (1904–1990), who were the founders of this fascinating area. The following section only touches the surface of this field of enquiry, and the reader is encouraged to read further – see 'References and further reading'.

Understanding operant learning means we can teach animals appropriate behaviours in a manner that promotes their confidence, willingness and cooperation. How to train is too broad a subject to cover here; it requires a deeper understanding of operant and classical learning, as well as of the training sequence. The latter includes deciding exactly what the behaviour is that the animal needs to learn and the cue to be used. For example, to fetch a ball an animal needs to learn that the ball, their mouth and their owner's hand have to be in the same place; and for 'leave', the animal must only learn to move its nose away from the object and look at the handler. That is, one needs to know the actual behaviour the animal must learn that leads to a desired outcome – a reinforcer. The starting point is explaining this clearly to the animal – a process that includes shaping, knowing when to raise criteria (e.g. moving the ball further from your hand), when to put in a cue, how to 'proof' the cue (discriminate it from other stimuli), how to strengthen the response using schedules of reinforcement and making the response robust even when the animal is aroused (sensitized), such as in distracting situations of excitement (e.g. in the park) and anxiety (e.g. at the veterinary practice). Underlying all of this is the concept that, to quote Skinner, 'The consequences of an act affect the probability of its occurring again.' – this is the foundation of the concepts of reinforcement and punishment. See Chapter 6 for a more detailed discussion of welfare-focused animal training.

Confusion, misunderstanding and emotional connotations about the concept of 'punishment' have led to the word being ostracized by those who care about animals. This is extremely regrettable as not talking about it, and not understanding it, means that (punishing) mistakes are made even by those who care. Additionally, lack of understanding means an inability to critically assess the latest training aid on the market and the language used to promote it. This too can lead to animal welfare concerns.

Punishment is part of life and learning cannot occur without it. We learn which of our behaviours are more successful than others through 'trial and error': those that are less successful are 'punished', and the probability of repeating that behaviour is reduced. Those behaviours that are more successful are more likely to be repeated. In other words, the probability of them occurring is 'reinforced' (increased, strengthened). People often muddle these terms; a useful mnemonic is to think 'reinforced' concrete is stronger than ordinary concrete.

Punishers and reinforcers

- Where the outcome following a behaviour serves to reduce the probability of the behaviour occurring again, the outcome is a punisher.
- Where the outcome following a behaviour serves to increase (strengthen) the probability of the behaviour occurring again, the outcome is a reinforcer.

As with classical conditioning, for learning to occur the general rules of predictability, contiguity and salience must be adhered to. With respect to salience, it should be remembered that the salience of both reinforcers and punishers is not an absolute but will vary between individuals and depend on their physical and emotional state and previous experience.

It is important to understand the *type* of reinforcement or punishment that is used. There are positive and negative reinforcers and positive and negative punishers (Figure 3.10). Positive and negative in learning theory do not relate to good or bad, but to the scientific meaning of adding and taking away. To remember this, think of a battery. The positive end is identified by the plus (+) symbol. The negative end of the battery is identified by the minus (–) symbol.

Reinforcement and punishment always work in tandem (Figure 3.11), both during the shaping of a behaviour and when it is on cue. For example, if the author [AM] is teaching a dog to sit, they will positively reinforce behaviours approximating to its bottom going on the ground (e.g. praise, treat) whilst negatively punishing all other behaviours (withhold the praise, treat). Likewise, if the dog has already learned the cue and the author [AM] asks it to sit, they will positively reinforce bottom-on-ground behaviour and negatively punish all other behaviours.

This so called 'reward-based' pairing engenders *pleasure* when the appetitive stimulus, the positive reinforcer, is attained and *frustration* when it is not. This frustration is the result of the animal's expectations (hopes) being thwarted. Basically, the relationship between behaviour and expected outcome is disrupted and extinction occurs. In the short-term, this leads to an 'extinction burst' where the animal's frustration leads it to try a bit harder and try other behaviours. Engendering this mild frustration is how trainers shape behaviours to the one they want, and frustration is how animals learn independently through trial and error. If the behaviour repeatedly fails (is negatively punished), then it will decline in frequency and extinguish. So even with positive reinforcement (reward-based) training, punishment, namely negative punishment (not getting the reward), is integral to the process.

Sometimes, undesirable behaviours are unwittingly taught through positive reinforcement. For example, not all

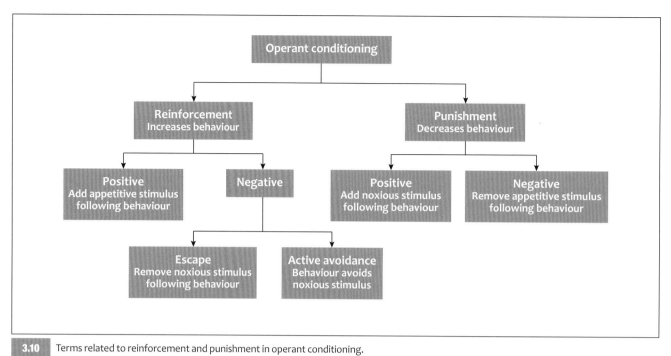

3.10 Terms related to reinforcement and punishment in operant conditioning.

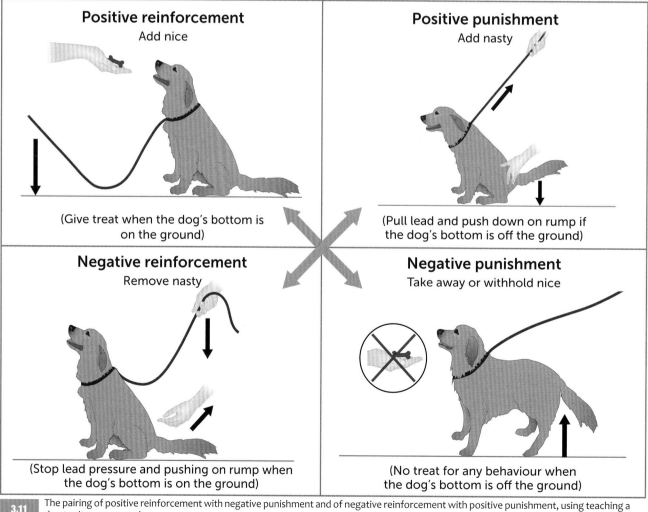

3.11 The pairing of positive reinforcement with negative punishment and of negative reinforcement with positive punishment, using teaching a dog to sit as an example.

repetitive behaviour is stereotypical. Imagine a dog who has a sore patch on its foot: it starts to lick and the owners try to stop the behaviour by touching the dog, saying 'don't do that' and possibly even distracting it with a treat. By giving the dog attention and food, they may simply have taught that licking behaviour is rewarded (positively reinforced), so it may continue even after the original medical cause has been resolved.

Knowing exactly the behaviour you want and the salience, timing and consistency of delivering the positive reinforcer are important. An example of what can go wrong otherwise is learned 'attention-seeking' behaviour, as seen in dogs who learn to bark at the TV or whine when their owner is on the phone because the owners then talk to them (even if the owners think they are telling them off). Yet, when it is lying quietly in the room the dog is ignored – lying quietly goes on to extinction. A timely 'good boy' or occasional treat will reinforce and strengthen the behaviour of lying quietly. Vague understanding by the owner of the desired behaviour can also lead to problems, as is the case with a dog who learns that the word 'come' means run to owner, get a treat, run away. It would perhaps be better to make 'come' mean 'stand in front of me, I then hold your collar' and to make that the behaviour that is rewarded.

Lack of clarity and of timing and consistency, even when using reward-based training, can lead to behaviours that are annoying or, far worse, can be injurious. The dog may pay with its life or have substantial restrictions placed on it. Under section 3 of the UK Dangerous Dogs Act (1991) this is the case for any dog if it causes injury (scratches, knocks someone over, nips or bites) or if a person has 'reasonable apprehension' that they may be injured. You may think this harsh for just a scratch. But scratches can lead to complications, for example, for those who are immunocompromised, even if from a small dog. This law applies to any dog, at home or away, and is regardless of the dog's motivation, which may have been to engage in friendly interaction. The owner may be fined or subjected to a community or prison sentence.

It is surprisingly easy to instil behaviours that can lead to such a situation. Take the example of the dog that jumps up to people in greeting. We sometimes respond positively to early more subtle requests for interaction, such as the animal trying to make eye contact, or gently making body contact (e.g. a nose nudge) and alternating its gaze between us and a ball. However, when we do not respond, the animal gets frustrated and an extinction burst happens. It will try different behaviours: pawing, harder nudges, barking, jumping up or even nipping. If we respond to these, then we have differentially reinforced them over the more subtle behaviours, which now go on to extinction. We have put the animal on a 'cycle of escalation' with positive reinforcement where early unrewarded signals are less likely to occur, and these escalated signals become its normal way of communicating (Figure 3.12).

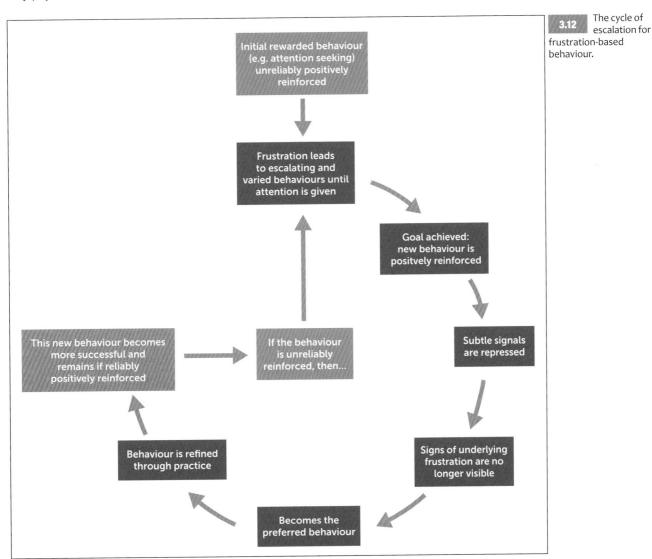

3.12 The cycle of escalation for frustration-based behaviour.

Preventing this problem requires owner awareness of the dog's communication, and consistent teaching, starting when it is a puppy, that attention (touch, eye contact and being spoken to) is contingent on all four feet being on the ground – the cues (commands) 'stand', 'sit' and 'lie down' can help. Of course, this must be consistently applied by the entire household and also requires getting all those people in the park who want to stroke or treat the dog to wait until it has obeyed this rule. It is far easier to teach what you want from the outset, rather than try to extinguish and replace unwanted behaviours. The principle holds for all other species: horses should be taught to keep their noses away from people's bodies to get their attention (and mints) and humans who always seem to be shouting can be ignored and rewarded for quiet communication.

To recap, positive reinforcement (reward-based) training is advocated for the teaching of new behaviours and their maintenance. This method engenders willingness, engagement (motivation) and appetitive (pleasant) emotions. Strengthening the behaviour in more arousing circumstances can be achieved through increasing the salience of the positive reinforcer, as we do when we give a gift, tip or bonus pay for hard and effective work. This could be a preferred treat or play with a preferred toy, for example. Negative punishment is part and parcel of reward-based, positive reinforcement-based training. Being aware of this means we can use it appropriately in shaping, and to avoid the cycle of escalation.

Problems with aversive methods

The alternative to reward-based training is the pairing of positive punishment and negative reinforcement (see Figure 3.11). This approach leads to far more significant problems. Here the desired behaviour is strengthened by negative reinforcement. That is the animal must learn which response will enable it to avoid an aversive event (the active avoidance behaviour, see Figure 3.10). Initially, the animal does not know what that behaviour is and can only learn through trial and error. Shaping is not an option in this form of training.

For a stimulus to be aversive, it must cause the animal anxiety, be that through being potentially threatening (e.g. sudden noise, strong smell) or causing pain. If the stimulus is too salient (strong or important), then the animal will become sensitized and that will interfere with its ability to learn. For example, imagine your computer goes blank, and you get really anxious at the possibility of losing all the work you have done. Somewhat frantically, you press lots of key combinations and all is restored… would you remember the combination of button presses (your behaviour) that allowed you to escape this very aversive stimulus? Probably not!

If the aversive event is too frightening, then all the animal may learn is that the situation is scary and form classical fear associations with contextual stimuli, including the trainer. Even if it later learns how to avoid the positive punisher, these fear associations will remain, as shown in studies using electronic training (shock) collars (Schilder and Van der Borg, 2004; Schalke et al., 2007). Whilst the debate regarding the use of such collars is ongoing (China et al., 2020; Cooper et al., 2021; Sargisson and McLean, 2021), this is not the only positive punishment training method used for dogs: leash jerks, spray collars, ultrasonic or sonic 'anti-bark' collars, invisible fencing and even kicks to the groin area, as have been promoted by certain celebrity trainers, are all forms of positive punishment.

Likewise, for equids, behavioural control is obtained through positive punishment: physical pressure via bits, stirrups, whips and nosebands and its release (negative reinforcement) when the desired behaviour is performed (McLean and McGreevy, 2010; Doherty et al., 2017). The aversive effect of these methods is rarely considered by trainers, owners or riders (Roberts, 1997; Ijichi et al., 2018). One reason for this is that the animal learns to comply, so from our perspective the training is a success. We simply do not look more closely at the signals that indicate the animal's distressed emotional state (Ziv, 2017; Squibb et al., 2018). We can consider these points in relation to other species as well: nose rings on livestock, pig boards and pig sticks are some examples.

Despite the aversion used in positive punishment–negative reinforcement training, the animal complies. One might wonder why the animal does not resist. Where the punishment is applied properly, that is, it is not too salient and when the animal performs the desired behaviour, it is immediately and reliably (negatively) reinforced by stopping the punisher, then the animal can learn that this is the active avoidance behaviour it needs to do when the cue is applied. The horse can learn to avoid the stirrup by moving forward to the cue 'walk on' or the pig can learn to move away from the pig board – they have learned how to control this aspect of their environment. However, if the punisher is too salient and/or the application and removal is inconsistent or badly timed, then the animal will suffer learned helplessness.

Learned helplessness: Learned helplessness is basically a state of resigned depression. Learned helplessness occurs when an animal has been repeatedly exposed to aversive stressors over which it has no control; there is a lack of contingency. It cannot discover the appropriate avoidance behaviour and learns that it lacks control over the situation. The punisher does not have to be extreme for this to happen. Learned helplessness was first described by Seligman and Maier (1967) in dogs who were exposed to unavoidable and unpredictable shocks. Learned helplessness results in decreased motivation (the animal is far less responsive and may even fail to respond when challenged with further aversive events), a reduced ability to learn subsequent avoidance behaviours and an emotional deficit inasmuch as that the animal is *behaviourally* less reactive to painful events; although, physiological measures reveal that animals experiencing learned helplessness are highly stressed. This reduced behavioural response is also the reason people think flooding (inescapable exposure to a scary stimulus) is an effective treatment for fear problems – it is not.

Learned helplessness is seen in humans, dogs, rats, other mammals and birds, and has even been observed in cockroaches, slugs and flies (Yang et al., 2013). Learned helplessness can emerge from, as well as exacerbate, states of anxiety, depression and post-traumatic stress disorder. Where aversive events are particularly pervasive through many or all aspects of the animal's environment, as in intensive farming, or are highly traumatic, physical issues can develop, such as ulcers, a reduced immune response, increased or decreased hunger and thirst, and intransigent repetitive behaviours (true stereotypies) (Broom and Fraser, 2015).

Positive punishment:
The problem of salience: The salience of an aversive stimulus presented as an outcome influences the predictability of the association between behaviour and outcome. When

positive punishment is used to train a behaviour, it is difficult to gauge the salience of aversive stimulus required to form an association. Too salient a punisher will elicit a fear response, which will seriously impair learning. Conversely, if the aversive stimulus is too mild, the animal will habituate to the punisher and it will lose any effectiveness (Azrin and Holz, 1966; Sargisson and McLean, 2021). The trainer may then increase the punisher, which will lead to either further habituation or a fear response.

The problem of timing and consistency: For an animal to learn an association with its behaviour, a punisher must be delivered as soon as the unwanted behaviour starts and must occur every time the behaviour occurs.

Case example 5: Timing as a pitfall of punishment

Azrin and Holz (1966) placed dogs in three groups:
A. Consistently punished for approaching a bowl of food – the start of eating behaviour
B. Punished as they started to eat
C. Punished after they had finished eating.

When tested with a bowl of food and no human present, only dogs in group A did not approach it. Those in group B still approached the food, albeit a bit hesitantly, and dogs in group C approached, ate and then become anxious – expecting punishment.

Outside of strictly controlled laboratory conditions, it is nigh on impossible to meet these requirements of timing and consistency. With mistiming, the punishment is not connected to the behaviour, so the animal cannot learn what to do to avoid the punishment. Learned helplessness is a likely outcome. Animals can easily generalize across similar stimuli and discriminate between those that are clearly different. However, where the application of punishment is inconsistent, in that sometimes the behaviour is punished and sometimes it is not, this becomes an impossible task. The animal has no way to discriminate

between the context cues that indicate it is 'safe' to do the behaviour and those that indicate it is not. This can lead to 'neurotic' behaviour and aggression.

Neurotic behaviours are unconscious behaviours that the individual displays as an attempt to manage its anxiety in the face of an unsolvable problem and uncontrollable situation. Pavlov and subsequent researchers have shown that neurotic behaviour is engendered when an animal cannot differentiate between two stimuli that mean different things – be that using the positive punishment–negative reinforcement axis or the positive reinforcement–negative punishment axis. In Case example 6, positive reinforcement was used, and the animal's neurotic behaviour was based in anxiety and frustration. Where positive punishment is used, neurotic behaviour is based in anxiety and fear. Both routes can result in depression or anxiety.

The importance of cues and clear communication

Pavlov's study (Case example 6) highlights the importance of very clear signals (cues). We need to teach these to the animal and ensure they are used consistently and reliably when we communicate with the animal throughout its life. We should advise owners to have an agreed 'dictionary' of cues and what they mean to the animal and emphasize the need for everyone to use them in the same way. From the author's work [AM] as a Clinical Animal Behaviourist, this lack of consistency in communication is almost always seen as a factor in behaviour problems, from separation issues to aggression. For example, think about the dog who is sometimes allowed on the sofa and sometimes not. Is there any clear signal to tell it when the sofa is 'safe' or when getting on to it may result in punishment? If not, then we may expect the dog to growl or snap at some point when we try to get it off the sofa. Think how you would feel if you had to work or live with someone who was so unpredictable and gave such mixed messages. You too would start to become anxious (sensitized) when that person was around. Being consistent and predictable when communicating is essential if we are to avoid causing anxiety and frustration, or fear and possible aggressive responses. In the dog and sofa example, predictable

Case example 6: Experimental induction of neurosis

Pavlov's 1927 study demonstrates just how easily neurotic behaviours can arise when communication is not clear. First, Pavlov trained a dog to classically associate a projected circle (Figure 3.13a) with food. When this was well established, an ellipse of equal width (Figure 3.13b) began to be presented with the circle and was never accompanied by feeding (Wolpe, 1952). The dog soon learned to discriminate, approaching the circle in expectation of food and moving away from the ellipse. Pavlov then made the ellipse more and more circular until a point was reached when the dog found differentiating extremely difficult (Figure 3.13c).

In Pavlov's own words, "After three weeks of work upon this differentiation not only did the discrimination fail to improve, but it became considerably worse, and finally disappeared altogether. At the same time the whole behaviour

3.13 Pavlov's experimental induction of neurosis. The circle in (a) is classically associated with food, the ellipse in (b) is associated with no food. These are easily discriminated. However, as the ellipse becomes more similar to the circle, as in (c), the dog can no longer discriminate between the two and does not know if food will or will not arrive – this leads to a state of neurotic behaviour.

of the animal underwent an abrupt change. The hitherto quiet dog began to squeal in its stand, kept wriggling about, tore off with its teeth the apparatus… bit through tubes… a behaviour which had never happened before. On being taken to the experimental room the dog now barked violently." (Pavlov, 1927, cited in Wolpe, 1952). This experiment demonstrates how easily anxiety and frustration, and potential for aggression, can be induced. It also shows how increasing sensitization (trigger stacking) results in the considerable worsening of an animal's ability to perform a previously learned response.

communication would mean giving the dog a clear and consistently used signal. A clear signal could be a word cue to invite the dog up or even an object (e.g. if a specific blanket is on the sofa, the dog can get up; if not, it cannot).

It is equally important to always let the animal know when you want to communicate with it and when the interaction is finished. First, say its name. As discussed above, use the dog's name when you are talking to it and want its attention and use a different 'code name' when you are talking about it. At the end of every interaction, the animal should be given a clear release signal, such as the word 'finish'. This goes for all interactions, be they stroking, playing a game, training, or asking for a behaviour, such as sit. When the release signal is given, one should look away from the animal, stop talking to it and stop touching it, so the end of that interaction is clear.

Unintentional punishment

As discussed above, using positive punishment as a training tool is fraught with issues that affect learning, the well-being of the animal and that of those around it. This welfare compromise is not something we would do intentionally, but it is frequently done unintentionally. This is most likely when we do not fully appreciate and account for the animal's ethology and what it is communicating about its emotional state, as observed in the training of horses (Fenner et al., 2019) and interactions with dogs (Shepherd, 2020).

In respect of all sorts of species, too often you will hear the sentence 'he just bit/kicked/butted me, right out of the blue' or similar. However, by not being aware of how our behaviour may be perceived by an animal, not understanding its signals or not listening, we miss these early communications that it is feeling anxious, fearful or frustrated. As a result, we simply teach the animal that this is the way to behave. Regrettably, the animal will be labelled as 'aggressive' and 'unpredictable' and may pay dearly for our unintentional training.

Avoiding the cognitive trap of speciesism

This section has given a minimal introduction to the principles of associative learning and cognition. How associative learning can be applied to captive animals is discussed in Chapter 6. We tend to concentrate on using operant conditioning when we think about training new behaviours, but we have also learned of the power of classical learning and how we can use this to train a desired emotional response (and behaviour). It is important to note that, while classical learning can occur alone, operant learning always involves classical learning. Therefore, we always need to consider other stimuli in the environment when we are teaching animals.

We should not fall into the cognitive trap of categorizing animals by their use, species, breed or how they make us feel (Ostrom, 1969). To do so means we are likely to show perceptual bias. We overestimate the abilities of some animals to understand what we want, even thinking they have some form of telepathic ability, and are shocked when they do not react as we expect. Others, we may consider stupid or more aggressive (Walsh et al., 2007; Gunter et al., 2016). We then do not take the time to communicate but simply handle them in a rougher manner. We may not even consider the emotions they are displaying, or their need for opportunities to feel pleasure, if we have categorized them as having a less rich emotional life (Wilkins et al., 2015).

Whilst you may accept this is not appropriate, the problem with cognitive traps is that we are quite unaware of when we have fallen into them. Just like other animals, we are more likely to fall back on 'tried and trusted' perceptions (prejudices) when we are busy, tired, hungry, anxious or otherwise sensitized. Being aware of this can help you to take a moment to be more attentive to the individual in front of you and the steps to take to have the best interaction possible. Essential steps to help this further and make life easier for all concerned are simple to comprehend but require effort:

Case example 7: The yappy and snappy small dog

Have you ever wondered why small dogs are often yappy and snappy? You may think this is just normal behaviour for them, but actually, it is behaviour they have learned through the inadvertent application of positive punishment by people.

'Oh, he is cute' is often said by strangers, followed by them reaching out to the dog to give it a 'friendly' stroke. This is friendly from a human perspective, but from the dog's it is a threat – a positive punisher. If the dog is on a lead, it may try to move away and this behaviour will be negatively reinforced as the distance from the person increases. However, the owner may not understand the meaning of this move away (Shepherd, 2020), and may drag the small dog forward to interact. A bark ensues, and the stranger backs away. In future, the dog will lunge and bark at people, as that is the behaviour it has now learned is reinforced, and the earlier signals will extinguish. Now we have the yappy dog. But what about the snappy behaviour?

Snapping is just an escalation of the same learning (Figure 3.14). Imagine the dog is picked up in the previous scenario or is already being held by the owner. The stranger approaches and the dog turns its head away. Instead of realizing this is a message of 'leave me alone, you are making me feel uncomfortable', the stranger may interpret it as a request to scratch the dog's neck. The hand just keeps on coming, the bark does not work, but a snap does. Finally, the scary thing, the hand (the positive punisher) goes away. This behaviour works to remove the threat, so it is strengthened through negative reinforcement (i.e. it is rewarded). Next time, the dog will have learned to not bother with turning its head away, but to lunge and snap at the hand. It will also do this earlier in the proceedings, even just as the person starts looking at it. After all, the sooner the punisher is avoided, the quicker the dog can return to a better emotional state. Indeed, the dog will become more confident that this strategy will work, and the original signs of anxiety and fear will be masked to some extent by more confident body language (Figure 3.14). Closer observation will reveal the conflict of emotions, seen for example in repeated barking and retreating, and always keeping an eye on where the scary stimulus is. ▶

Case example 7: The yappy and snappy small dog *continued*

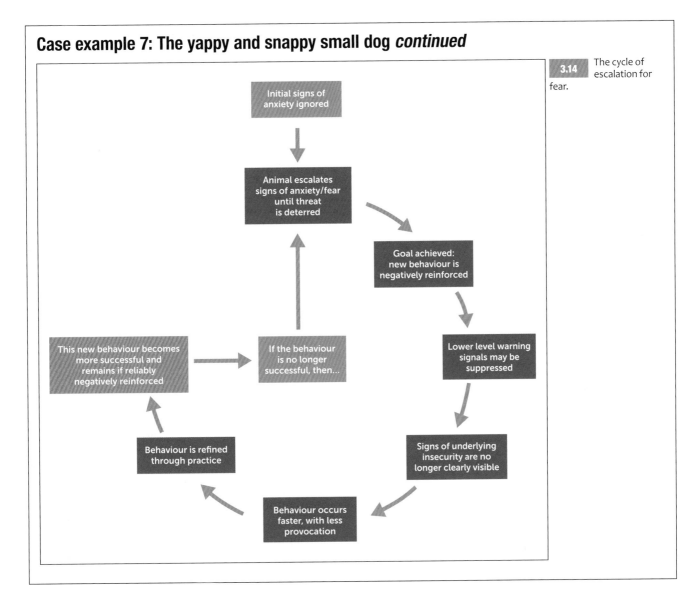

3.14 The cycle of escalation for fear.

Flowchart contents:

- Initial signs of anxiety ignored
- Animal escalates signs of anxiety/fear until threat is deterred
- Goal achieved: new behaviour is negatively reinforced
- Lower level warning signals may be suppressed
- Signs of underlying insecurity are no longer clearly visible
- Behaviour occurs faster, with less provocation
- Behaviour is refined through practice
- This new behaviour becomes more successful and remains if reliably negatively reinforced
- If the behaviour is no longer successful, then...

- Remember each animal is an individual
- Do your 'homework': learn about the species, the breed and the individual's normal environment, behaviour and history
- Apply your knowledge by planning interactions to minimize stress. Ideally, plan as far ahead as possible for eventualities – have a plan A, plan B and plan C
- Advise caretakers on how to prepare the animal for interactions with veterinary and other professionals. Consider useful cues, for example, training all dogs as a matter of course to happily wear a muzzle (just in case they get a grass seed lodged within the ear canal), tigers to lie down and accept an injection, horses to lift each foot on cue to aid the farrier, cats to have their feet held and claws extended, birds to spread each wing or rabbits to feed from a syringe
- Advise owners of the importance of clarity and consistency in their interactions, including having an agreed dictionary of the cues used for different behaviours
- Ensure you can advise caretakers on where to get expert help in training their animal using positive reinforcement
- Ask what cues the animal has been taught and be consistent in using them in your interactions (Figure 3.15). Make a note of these on the animal's record, somewhere prominent, so that everyone is aware.

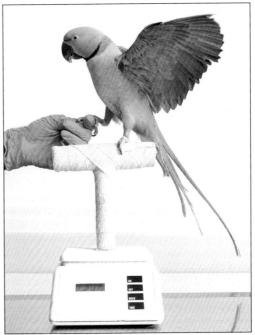

3.15 Parrot whose owner has trained it to perch on a verbal cue, facilitating veterinary examination.
(Shutterstock.com/Susan Schmitz)

Understanding how animals learn and feel, and applying this in their management and training, is a major component to providing good welfare. It helps keep anxiety, fear and frustration to a minimum whilst increasing calmness and encouraging pleasurable anticipation and cooperation even when an animal is unwell or in pain (Vasconsellos *et al.*, 2016; Melfi *et al.*, 2020). We need to be able to 'listen' and interpret what the animal is telling us about how they are feeling and what they intend to do. We need to understand, as best we can, their way of communicating so we can interact appropriately.

Communication

Communication is the transfer of information from a sender to a receiver. This may be intra-specific (between different members of the same species) or inter-specific (between species), and it may be deliberate or unconscious (Knapp *et al.*, 2013). If the receiver receives what the sender intended to send, then communication is successful. If not, then miscommunication has occurred. There is a complex interplay of factors between what is sent and what is received. Humans and animals communicate facts (e.g. I have spotted something that might be dangerous) and social cohesion signals (e.g. you look upset, let me hug/stroke/lick/groom you). We also communicate our emotions and our intentions – i.e. what we will do next, depending on how the receiver responds to our communication. In general, communication is intended to restore homeostasis and feelings of being safe and happy as per Maslow's hierarchy of needs (Maslow, 1987; see above). This is true for humans and non-humans alike.

However, miscommunication (misunderstanding) between humans happens frequently, leading to confusion, upset, mistrust, anger and even aggression between individuals and societies and is all too often the cause of feuds and even wars. It can happen because too little information was provided to facilitate understanding or because mixed messages were sent. When there is inconsistency between verbal and non-verbal communication, humans will pay more attention to the non-verbal signals to try to understand 'what is really being said'. You have likely observed someone say 'it is nice to see you' and thought that is not what they actually feel. An oft-quoted weighting is that 7% of the information comes from words, 38% from how we speak (e.g. tone, pace, pauses, coughs) and 55% from facial expressions and body language (Mehrabian, 1972; Thompson, 2011). Indeed, emojis were invented to try and reduce the potential for misunderstandings in written communication, especially when messages are short and composed quickly with little to no punctuation to add clarity, as in emails and tweets.

Of course, misunderstandings can increase where we have learned different interpretations of words and gestures, as seen with cultural variations. Examples include calling someone 'pet', a friendly term in the Northeast of England, but possibly offensive in the South; or a thumbs up gesture, which means 'OK' in the United Kingdom but is very offensive in some other countries, including parts of the Middle East and Greece. All these communication issues should be remembered when interacting with colleagues and clients, be that face-to-face, on the telephone or in writing (Gray and Moffett, 2013; Simpson *et al.*, 2018).

When it comes to communicating with different species, the possibilities for misunderstanding are greatly increased. We may misinterpret an animal's communication if we have not taken the time to learn how they signal. We may not have been paying full attention and so missed signals. Basically, we miss part of the conversation. Even more often, we will be unaware of the mixed, even unintelligible, messages we are sending to them, such as stroking and saying soothing words whilst our body looms over them and we make eye contact. Then we are surprised by the animal's response.

Communication signals are yet one more part of the jigsaw puzzle of animal behaviour introduced in this chapter. All aspects are interlinked. The ability to communicate clearly requires the physical tools, yet we have compromised this for many by selective breeding for conformation (e.g. brachycephaly, long hair, lop ears, curled tail) or by our choice of grooming styles which some people consider aesthetically pleasing, cute or hilarious (Figure 3.16). Many of these affect the animal's ability to

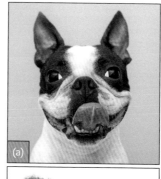
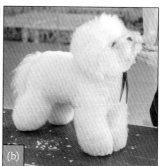
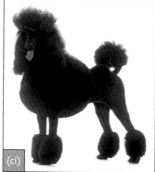
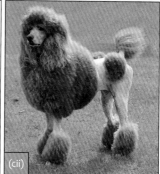
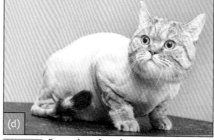

3.16 Examples of conformation and grooming styles that affect communication and thermoregulation. (a) A brachycephalic dog demonstrating staring eyes and a gaping mouth exposing teeth. These are signals of potential threat to another dog, but actually may be the animal trying to breathe or cool down. (b) A grooming style that constricts the dog's visual field and reduces its ability to communicate using subtle body signals, including ear and facial movements. (ci) Common poodle grooming clip that compromises thermoregulation and visual field and, as with (b), impinges on facial and ear communication and enhances the illusion of raised hackles. (cii) This pink version further demonstrates the anthropocentric focus, even though there is a potential welfare cost to the dog. (d) The non-medical grooming cut seen in this cat is a further example of compromised thermoregulation and communication in that it cannot fluff the fur on its body or tail to communicate threat.
(b, Shutterstock.com/Nejron Photo; cii, by Jonner and licensed with CC BY-SA 2.0 (To view a copy of this licence, visit creativecommons.org/licenses/by-sa/2.0); d, Shutterstock.com/lev.studio)

clearly communicate with its own kind and can send mixed messages by, for example, appearing to have raised hackles or a threatening stare. Further, non-medically required grooming cuts can have implications for the individual's ability to maintain thermal homeostasis, with some parts remaining covered in fur and others not, which may affect their mood (see Figure 3.16b–d). In addition, grooming for both medical and non-medical reasons may involve the cutting of whiskers (vibrissae), which are part of both the animal's sensory and communication systems. This should be avoided. Of course, we may ignore all this as we fall into yet another cognitive trap, anthropomorphizing. It looks nice to us and the brachycephalic dog 'looks happy' – its mouth is open, so it must be smiling. If we saw the dog in a different context, we may wonder whether the dog with an open mouth and its tongue out was trying to lose heat or communicate its anxiety.

Being able to communicate clearly also requires socialization and, ideally, experiences that have fostered confidence and calmness. After all, a sensitized individual may not spend time giving signals of its increasing distress but may seemingly jump from 'a bit tense' to 'aggressive'. Of course, this may also happen if they have learned that low-level, early signals are ignored, as seen with the cycle of escalation for fear (see Figure 3.14).

Labels and preconceptions

Our misinterpretation of communication is also affected by our attitudes and the labels we give animals. We may not consider animals able to communicate much if we label them as stupid or as having a limited emotional and cognitive range (Warwick *et al.*, 2013; Wilkins *et al.*, 2015). This is further compounded by myths relating to scientific concepts and data. Regrettably, concepts are sometimes misunderstood and incorrect versions promulgated to the public and to professionals of other disciplines. Important examples include the labelling of animals as 'dangerous', 'dominant', or as having 'bad habits' or 'vices'. All such labels pave the way to assumptions which, unchecked, distort our observations and behaviour, rarely in a manner that enhances welfare (Coleman and Hemsworth, 2014). Such unfortunate attitudes exacerbate poor human–animal interactions when we are sensitized, such as when we are tired, busy, anxious or frustrated (Ceballos *et al.*, 2018).

A quick trawl of the internet shows that the terms 'dangerous', 'dominant' and 'bad habits/vices' are still common currency amongst pet and horse owners and are frequently misused. As discussed above (see 'Nature and nurture'), whilst animals differ, none are inherently evil, bad or dangerous. Certainly, we can make them predisposed to defensive aggression through unfortunate genetics, bad breeding, or inappropriate or inadequate socialization. An individual animal's previous experiences and interactions with people can also predispose them to defensive aggression, as our behaviour will be highly influential in the animal's decision of what to do.

For example, consider the label 'dangerous', as in 'dangerous dogs'. We will react differently if we have decided a dog is of a dangerous 'type' – we will be less relaxed, more tense, and perhaps more aggressive in our movements and tone of voice. What we are communicating is that we are odd, unpredictable and threatening. How do you think this will affect the emotional state of the dog and thus its response? How would you feel (and likely respond) if someone behaved like that toward you? Conversely, when we label something as not dangerous, we may be

Case example 8: Care labels

Care labels are commonly attached to an animal's file and/or kennel in a veterinary setting. Sometimes these may simply say 'aggressive' or 'bites' (Figure 3.17a). The thinking behind these warnings is one of preventative care for humans. Regrettably though, they can also induce unconscious prejudice, heightened fear and/or anxiety and a reluctance to interact with the patient, resulting in increasing miscommunication between human and animal and escalating the risk of physical harm. The importance of being aware of an animal's likely behaviour is not to be underestimated, but it is imperative that the 'why' is understood. Is the animal aggressive, or is it fearful, in pain or scared? Look deeper for the true reasons behind the reactions. Wording labels and notes accordingly will help staff better understand the animal and how best to interact with it, thereby reducing the risk of harm to all parties. A better label may be something such as 'Caution: distressed and defensive', which indicates the animal's emotional state, likely behaviour and appropriate human interaction (Figure 3.17b).

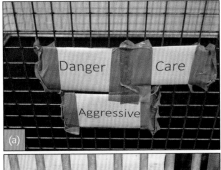

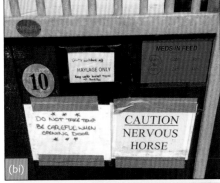

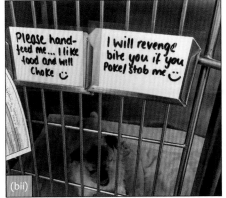

3.17 Examples of care labels. (a) These labels provide a warning but do a poor job of informing the reader. (b) These labels are more informative.

equally blind to the animal's communication and take liberties without thinking. This may lead to learned helplessness, a passive distress response, or a more active response of increasing signalling to the point of a snap, bite or kick (Shepherd, 2020).

Similar issues arise from the label 'dominant'. Whilst dominant–subordinate relationships are part of social living for many species, including humans, they do not rely on aggression. Rather, such a relationship is maintained through appeasement gestures (e.g. exchanging niceties with your boss or teacher). Social hierarchies have evolved to provide stability to groups and thereby reduce aggression. Regrettably, some early work on artificially constructed groups of captive wolves was inappropriately extrapolated to both the wild context and to domestic dogs and other species (Handelman, 2012). This supported perceptions from the 18th and 19th centuries that control of horses, dogs, children and other potentially rebellious 'lesser beings' could only be maintained through forceful, painful positive punishment intended to 'put them in their place' by 'showing them who is boss'. This in turn enhanced perceptions that certain animals were 'mad and bad' or 'dangerous'.

The final example is that of the words 'vices' and 'bad habits'. We have seen that both poor management and poor training techniques that engender anxiety, fear or frustration can lead to repetitive or other unwanted behaviours. Examples include pacing in caged animals, feather plucking in birds (Figure 3.18), persistent barking in dogs, and crib biting, head-throwing and bucking in horses. Regrettably, instead of wondering why the animal needs to behave in this way and listening to what it is communicating, we all too often take the lazy, non-welfare-friendly option and look for the 'quick fix' – the crib collar, the tighter martingale or more severe bit, or the anti-bark collar (Protopopova *et al.*, 2016).

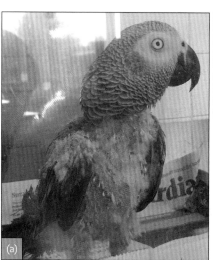
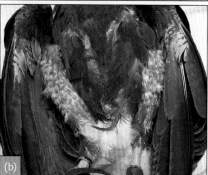

3.18

(a) An African grey parrot and (b) a Harris hawk, showing self-mutilation behaviour (feather plucking).
(© John Chitty)

Observation

On a positive note, research suggests that education about animal communication can significantly improve attitudes, empathy and interactions (Hemsworth and Coleman, 2010; Ceballos *et al.*, 2018). Simply knowing the descriptions of animal behaviour, while important, is not enough to improve welfare and reduce an animal's need to show undesirable behaviour. We also need to know the context in which that behaviour was displayed. The context consists of environmental stimuli, the animal's species, individual history and current arousal level (sensitization).

Importantly, we need to practise our observation skills so we become as fluent as we can in reading and understanding their vocal and physical signals. Take every opportunity you can to watch animals, and people, in as wide a variety of contexts as possible. These may be different locations, times of day, when food is or is not anticipated/present, or when humans are or are not present (webcams and other video recording devices are valuable tools). Readers unable to observe animals live are encouraged to seek out videos; a plethora is available on the internet. Consider the context, watch the individual(s) and predict what they will do next. Then ask yourself why you predicted that, were you right and if not, why not? Finally, practise more and more. You will further hone your observation skills by doing this for a range of individuals and species, not just the ones you are working with. For example, sit in your garden and observe the flying insects, the birds, the ants and the squirrels – practise your observation skills. To help you and clients, information about communication signals in various species is available as downloadable posters and other online resources from reputable sources. See 'References and further reading' for examples.

Some animal communication signals are simply beyond our range of detection, notably ultrasonic and infrasonic sounds (Hillix and Rumbaugh, 2004; Sales, 2012), scent (Nielsen, 2017) and pheromones (Shorey, 2013). Many other signal types are subtle and will only be noticed by humans through practice. We may expect subtlety to be characteristic of prey species or those with more limited musculature inhibiting facial expression (e.g. reptiles, birds and fish), but we may not be aware of some signals used by species we think we know well, including our own (Knapp *et al.*, 2013). The take-home message is that the more you listen, look and wonder why, the greater your understanding will be.

Veterinary professionals should be aware of the pain (grimace) scales that are now available for various species, including rabbits, rats, mice, horses, pigs, sheep, cows, ferrets, cats and dogs (see Chapter 2). Many of the signs involved are very familiar, as we show similar behaviours when in pain (Knapp *et al.*, 2013). However, we find it far more difficult to recognize pain in non-mammalian species. This is true for birds (Gartrell, 2011) and reptiles (Malik, 2018), and even more so for fish, amphibia and invertebrates. While for some the jury is still out as to if and how pain may be felt by these taxa (Rose *et al.*, 2014), this is not the general view amongst scientists. Indeed, the differences that give rise to doubt may simply reflect how we define pain, assess it and thus how we recognize it. Both vertebrates and invertebrates can learn operant responses to events and are known to show behavioural responses to 'painful' events that represent a change in motivational (emotional) state that affects later behaviour (decision making) in similar situations (Sneddon *et al.*, 2014). Behaviour change is an early indicator of an animal not feeling 'well',

Case example 9: Dog barks, tails and eyes

Dogs show a wide range of body signals denoting appetitive (happy, relaxed) and aversive (anxious, frustrated, fearful) emotional states. Shepherd's Ladder of Aggression shows some of the obvious signs of increasing anxiety (Shepherd, 2020; see also Chapter 7), but canine communication is much more complex. Let us consider barks, tails and eyes.

A bark is not just a bark. We may recognize differences in play, threat and fear barks, and the quiet warning woof that tells you 'something is there'. But dogs use barks far more creatively. The author's [AM] dog uses different barks to convey 'let me out', 'let me in', 'get up, it is morning' and 'let's play', and to specify if a cat, squirrel or fox has been in the garden. He also has a double repeated bark, known as the 'hurry up, help me' bark, used when he cannot reach something – often a squirrel up a tree or a rat under a pile of wood. It is likely that he is trying to convey even more meaning through pitches inaudible to human ears.

Dogs also convey nuanced messages with their tails. Commonly recognized signals include: the 'friendly' sweeping wag, the 'excited' windmill wag, the tucked-under 'anxious' wag and the stiff 'beware' wag where the tip of the upright tail vibrates. Studies show that asymmetrical wagging provides another depth to this communication: a left- and right-biased wag do not mean the same thing (Quaranta *et al.*, 2007). Right bias communicates a pleasant emotion; left bias, that the dog is less happy (Figure 3.19). Seeing the asymmetrical wags from another dog also produces a different emotion and behaviour in the observer dog (Leaver and Reimchen, 2008; Artelle *et al.*, 2011; Siniscalchi *et al.*, 2013).

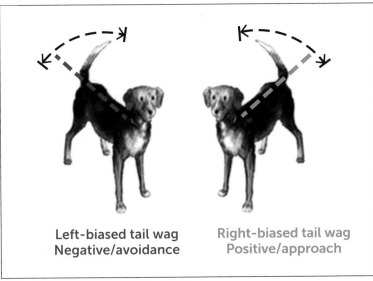

3.19 The asymmetrical wag of the dog: right bias indicates a pleasant emotion and left bias a degree of anxiety.

Left-biased tail wag
Negative/avoidance

Right-biased tail wag
Positive/approach

Recent work suggests that how dogs use their inner eyebrow may have been influenced by human selection pressures during domestication (Kaminski *et al.*, 2019). Dogs can follow our gaze messages, though this can vary between breeds and is based on what the individual dog has learned (Jakovcevic, 2010). This ability is reduced if the dog is trained to focus too much on human faces (Wallis *et al.*, 2015). Perhaps not surprisingly, dogs also use gaze messages with each other and with us. They indicate the location of something they want or that is interesting by looking between the receiver and the object or location of interest. This is known as gaze alternation and constitutes a visual conversation (Marshall-Pescini *et al.*, 2013). We can unwittingly teach dogs that gaze alternation with us is a waste of their time. Much is missed when we walk or spend time 'with' our dogs, yet focus on our phones, television or conversation with another person. The dog will soon learn there is no outcome to communicating with its owner, so the behaviour becomes extinguished. Basically, they learn their human is boring and rude as they do not take part in the dog's conversations or engage in the adventure of a walk. This weakens the human–animal bond. Then owners wonder why their dog shows so little interest in them and tends not to come back when called. The eventual outcome may be that the dog will be permanently constrained on a lead when on a walk. This highlights the importance of observing, listening and engaging when interacting with or spending time around animals.

that is to say being in an aversive emotional state and not in homeostasis. All this may be considered as evidence of pain, especially if changes are seen when analgesia is provided (Brown *et al.*, 2019; Elwood, 2019; Hedley *et al.*, 2019; Sneddon and Wolfenden, 2019; Winlow and Di Cosmo, 2019). It is the authors' contention that we should err on the side of good ethics, regardless of species, and presume all animals can feel pain.

Whilst recognizing pain is important, equally important to the provision of good welfare is the recognition of signals of distress (anxiety, fear, frustration), eustress (anticipation, pleasure) and relaxation. It is not possible to describe all the behavioural indicators for all species in a chapter and, if it were, it would soon be out of date. We are continually learning, for example, the ultrasonic sounds of pleasure (laughter) emitted by rats (Panksepp, 2007) went undiscovered for some time, and work is ongoing to assess how different species understand and respond to the emotions expressed by others (empathy) (Špinka, 2012; Briefer, 2018). What this chapter provides is some examples across taxa and consideration of some general principles (see 'Behaviour commonalities', below).

Animals that are anxious show inhibited variation in behaviour. They will reduce exploration, movement, self-care (grooming) and social interaction. If very anxious, especially in the presence of a perceived immediate threat, they may try to hide or become small, as in the case of the hedgehog, pill beetle and ball python curling up, or the dog or person cowering in the corner. Behavioural inhibition, including not playing, is a sign of both depression and fear of threat (anxiety).

Alert/alarm calls and body movements signal an acute threat and often have similarities across species and taxa. Think of the 'chink chink' of the blackbird who has spotted an owl in the tree, the staccato chatter (and flicking tail) of the squirrel at the sight of the prowling cat, or the dog's rapidly repeated bark at the night-time passer-by. Animals respond to the alarm calls of their own species but also those of others, and this is true across taxa including between reptiles and birds (Vitousek *et al.*, 2007; Suzuki, 2018; Russell and Bauer, 2021).

Signals of pleasurable relaxation tend to be 'long' – relaxed muscles, long sighs, stretched limbs and relaxed sleep. Animals are also curious when relaxed, they will explore their environment, venture further and investigate more intensively.

Alternatively, signals of pleasure may be more active, as in play – be it solitary object play or social play (Burghardt, 2005). Play, of course, has both immediate and long-term benefits for the development and maintenance of good physical and mental health. However, play further reminds us that behaviour must be interpreted holistically, considering all the display signals and the context. To quote Held and Špinka (2011):

"As a welfare indicator, play may signal both the absence of bad welfare and the presence of good welfare, thus covering a wide range of the welfare spectrum. However, play can also increase in stressful situations, in response to reduced parental care, or as a rebound after a period of deprivation and therefore does not consistently reflect favourable environmental conditions. A better fundamental understanding is needed of the varied ultimate functions and proximate mechanisms of play, and the species-specific play patterns of captive animals, in order to be able to explain exactly what an animal's play behaviour tells us about its welfare state, and whether and how play might be applied as a tool to improve welfare."

Animals sometimes display apparently contradictory signals simultaneously. These are often of approach-and-avoidance or approach-threat-withdraw. These animals are experiencing conflicting emotions, for example, wanting to approach whilst experiencing anxiety or physical discomfort. Conflict can occur in social and non-social situations and in wild, captive and domesticated species, as illustrated in work on dogs and horses (Győri *et al.*, 2010; Kienapfel *et al.*, 2014; Kuhne, 2016). We need to be aware of the complex message the animal is imparting when we see such signals and respond gently.

Clearly, we still have much to learn about how animals communicate and how they interpret our communication. Happily, there is an ongoing surge of research interest in animal communication and cognition. Therefore, it is important that we frequently reflect on our knowledge and how we are applying it. Further, evidence serves to undermine any defence for using the uncivilized methods of persuading animals through pain and fear. After all, 'Jaw, Jaw' (communication) is far better than 'War, War'.

The Three Rules of Life

All the behaviours and learning mechanisms covered in this chapter are core to an individual animal's survival and its chances of passing its genes on to the next generation. Different species have evolved to survive in different environments where they need to overcome the challenges of getting enough to eat, avoiding being killed and reproducing successfully – the 'Three Rules of Life'. Human and non-human behaviour and communication continues to evolve in response to the best (most successful) ways to meet the demands associated with acquiring food, constructing safe homes, being alert to threats, defending oneself and one's resources, and the courtship, mating and parenting requirements for successful reproduction. All three rules are intertwined, as outlined below.

Getting enough to eat

Getting enough to eat and knowing what to eat is not simple. Food in nature is a variable resource whose quality, abundance and accessibility alters with the seasons. This explains both behaviour around food and the tendency to obesity in captivity. Animals are attracted to highly calorific foods (sugars and fats) as these are naturally seasonal and essential to survival during the energy-intense times of reproduction and maintaining physiological homeostasis in harsh weather (McBride, 2014a–d). Humans and captive animals, be they wild or domesticated species, are still attracted to these foods even though food is easily available all year round and shelter, rugs and central heating reduce the need to burn calories to keep warm.

Apart from a few hunter-gatherer and subsistence living groups, the relationship most of us have with food is one we share with our pets, intensively kept livestock, laboratory animals and zoo animals. We do not have to work for food, it simply arrives – in the bowl, the hay rack, the shop or the restaurant. Indeed, many people have little or no idea (or interest in) how these foods are grown or processed. All is well until there is unreliability in the system: the classically learned pleasant association between shops and food begins to extinguish. We feel anxiety and may become confrontational in order to get what we want be it food or other resources. This is synony-mous with the behaviour of the dog who is anxious that someone will take away its food, toy or other resource. This increase in anxiety also happens when food is limited in the wild, and those best able to attain and maintain resources are more likely to survive.

Species that fight over food in the wild tend to be hunters – carnivorous predators and carnivorous scavengers. Making a kill takes effort and energy expenditure and most hunting attempts fail. When hunting is difficult or the numbers of prey animals has decreased, as seen in a drought or flood, then an animal will risk injury and fight over food rather than expose itself to the greater certainty of starvation.

Omnivores, particularly rodents, and some herbivores and seed eaters, including birds, will hoard food in preparation for winter. This may be as simple as an underground store of seeds (e.g. for mice, rats and hamsters) or an underwater collection of leafy branches in the case of beavers. Some species, such as the rabbit's relative the Pika, cut and dry grasses in the sun (i.e. make their own hay) to store in rock crevices and burrows (Dearing, 1997). It would be reasonable to hypothesize that having such a store engenders pleasant emotions and that its removal would result in anxiety. Unfortunately, owners often remove the hoard when they clean the cage, for reasons of hygiene. Perhaps a more natural and less stressful feeding strategy would be to feed sufficient food to let the animal build up a small hoard, then feed less so they use up some/most of their hoard and repeat the cycle. This advice follows the same principle as advice to leave some used bedding in the cage so that it still smells familiar and represents safety (McBride, 2017).

Regardless of the diet, acquiring food takes time as well as physical and mental energy. This is most obvious in respect of carnivores or the busy behaviour of omnivores, such as pigs and rodents, as they climb and dig and search for insects, eggs, meat, seeds and fruits (Berdoy, 2002). Yet it is equally true for herbivores (e.g. deer, horses, sheep, cows, guinea pigs, chinchillas and rabbits) who spend many hours a day foraging, covering significant distances as they wander from one patch of vegetation to another. The herbivore diet is not boring. Grasslands are not comprised of a single species but are a mixed salad that changes in composition as the year progresses and different grasses, herbs, leaves and flowers become available. Herbivores are selective feeders, not simply indiscriminate mowing machines.

We may wish to consider how these factors, particularly variety and the use of time in acquiring food, apply to other taxa we keep, not least birds, fish, reptiles and cephalopods. For all, we can make food more interesting in terms of variety and in acquisition. To put it simply, puzzle feeding, scatter feeding and hiding foods are not just for dogs and cats. They are ways of providing natural occupation and pleasure to all animals (see Chapter 4).

Avoiding being killed

Avoiding being killed also relates to food and knowing what to eat. Animals belonging to many species across taxa learn this from their parents and/or others in the group. For insects and reptiles, this may be through items left for them to feed on when they hatch, or emerge as larvae/caterpillars, such as leaves, dead insects or other meat. Young birds and mammals spend time with adults learning what to eat and how to acquire it, and what to avoid. When exposed to human activity, the natural evolved systems to ensure survival can be tricked, as seen in birds eating plastics and herbivores eating plants that they would never come across in their native wild habitats. This can spell a slow or a rapid death.

Where death is slow and insidious, even the more adaptable omnivores may be deceived, as seen in dogs eating chocolate and rats eating poisoned bait. As omnivores are opportunistic feeders, they will try anything and that puts them at greater risk of eating something potentially deadly. As mentioned earlier, taste aversion is the exception to the 'close in time' rule of classical conditioning (see 'Classical and operant conditioning', above). It is specific to omnivores (including humans) and means that if an individual feels ill after trying a new food, they will avoid it in future and can inform others of the danger. We may tell others to avoid a food or restaurant using words, rats do this through scent. Smelling the breath of an unwell rat informs others to avoid the food it ate (Berdoy, 2002).

For predators, especially of larger prey, learning how to hunt safely is important as fatal injuries can occur. Apart from a few 'top' predators, most predator species also have potential predators of their own that they need to avoid, and thus require means by which they can escape attack.

For these and prey species, strategies to avoid being caught and eaten are essential. This requires being alert and social species have an additional advantage as more eyes, ears and noses mean less chance of being surprised by a predator, and less chance of being the target of the predator's hunt. For those that depend on speed to outrun predators, open space is necessary, with long views so predators can be detected and no dead ends in which one can be trapped. Hence why horses, deer, ostriches and sheep, for example, do not like confined spaces such as trailers and stalls. The opposite is true for small species whose first response is to stay still, rely on camouflage and hope to avoid notice. If the danger comes too close, their good spatial abilities enable them to swiftly return to the safety of a dark burrow, rock crevice or deep thicket (McBride and Magnus, 2022).

All species have various strategies for evading capture if chased. One is to bedazzle the predator with changes of direction – leaping and twisting. Practising such techniques in play is important in keeping fit. Examples include stotting in gazelle, 'binking' in rabbits and 'popcorning' in guinea pigs.

If caught, evasion of death means fighting or, *in extremis*, playing dead. Known as tonic immobility, this behaviour is seen across taxa and is a final attempt to avoid being killed (McBride, 2015). When the prey is dead, predators relax their grip and back away for a moment or two to clean themselves and recover from the exertions of the hunt. This gives an opportunity to the animal in tonic immobility to try and escape. This is what happens when cats 'play with' their prey. The prey is not playing, it is trying to live. The prey is alternately going into tonic immobility and taking an opportunity to escape when the cat seems to have lost interest, only to be caught again and the cycle repeated until it succeeds in escaping or the cat finally delivers a kill bite. Animals can be put into tonic immobility quite easily – often by simply placing them on their back and applying gentle pressure, as used by alligator wranglers and uninformed rabbit owners or handlers. These animals are not in a relaxed trance but are fully conscious and very stressed.

It is not sufficient to keep an animal safe, they need to feel safe too (Magnus and McBride, 2022). To help animals feel safe, we need to provide them with suitable accommodation. This entails provision of lookout places for all, truly dark places with tunnel entrances for burrowers and wide vistas for runners. For the latter, especially if stalled or stabled, the judicial use of mirrors may be helpful to extend their view.

Successful reproduction

Finally, consider the ultimate life goal in the wild – successful reproduction. This means successfully raising enough young to adulthood so that one's genes continue to pass down the generations.

The initial part of this process is courtship and mating. Interest in the opposite sex starts in adolescence, which, as discussed earlier, is a time of substantial physical and psychological change. For males, this is the onset of adult behaviours such as scent marking, territoriality and roaming, especially if there is a likelihood of meeting a receptive female. Female behaviour around times of receptivity (heat) may also be perceived as problematic. Neutering has long been established as a routine means of controlling sexual behaviour in male livestock. More recently it has become routine for dogs and cats of both sexes. There are good reasons to neuter, predominately negating unwanted litters as in outdoor cats, male–female pairs of rabbits or households with multiple dogs of different sexes. There are also adverse physical and psychological consequences to neutering which may be related to the individual's age, breed and personality, as research is evidencing for the dog (Fattah and Abdel-Hamid, 2020; Hart and Hart, 2021). Neutering during psychologically sensitive growth periods, including adolescence, may have unintended repercussions for anxiety levels and later resilience to stress, due to both changes in hormonal status and the stress of the hospitalization experience. Some countries have incorporated these welfare concerns into legislation regarding dogs. In Norway, dogs can be neutered for health reasons or if required by their role (e.g. assistance dog) or if it helps give the dog a justifiable quality of life, including social contact with other dogs. Thus, the authors encourage veterinary professionals to advise dog owners on a case-by-case basis, and ideally delay the decision until maturity as it may not be needed. The adolescent period regardless requires owners to keep up training, be consistent with cues and rules and at times restrict freedom (e.g. by walking on the leash more during those 'difficult weeks'). This advice is similar to that given to parents of adolescent humans.

Courtship rituals enable a pair to form a relationship and to ensure the female is primed for the best chance of a successful mating. Depending on species, courtship may involve displays or building attractive structures such as piles of stones, mutual grooming, offering of food and play. This does not happen where the female is fertilized through artificial insemination (AI) or by forced mating. Forced mating is used in dog and horse breeding and, as with AI, the female is restrained and is not a relaxed and willing partner. The process is therefore likely to be both painful and fear provoking, especially as the male is frequently highly sexually aroused by the time he reaches the female, as he will have made classical associations with aspects of the environment. Indeed, it is classical learning that enables males to be trained to mate with 'dummies' for semen collection for AI. Many breeding males, such as stud stallions and bulls, may be further aroused as this is a 'highlight' in their day since many are kept alone even though they are social species, with little other cognitive stimulation.

Across both vertebrates and invertebrates, there is a wide range of different strategies employed in providing for young animals, starting with who is involved. In some species, single parenthood is the norm and is not always left to the female, in others, the work is shared between the parents, who may pair for life or just for a season, while for some species rearing the young is a more communal affair involving members of different generations (Royle et al., 2012). Pair bonding can also lead to problematic animal–human interactions, especially with birds. Many, such as some parrot species, pair for life and this can have repercussions for owners of single birds. Owners may unwittingly stroke the bird in ways that mimic courtship preening or reinforce the bird's 'romantic' overtures. The bird can become quite possessive and aggressive towards other people, including other human members of the family (Luescher, 2006).

How much time is spent directly with the offspring varies between species, as does the state of development at birth/hatch. Animals may be precocial or altricial. This will affect both how they are cared for and their early life chances. A nest of altricial blackbird chicks raided by a rat, magpie or cat will likely have no survivors, whereas some precocial ducklings will be more likely to escape such an attack.

We are obliged to understand as much as we can about the parenting strategies of animals we breed and to provide suitable resources (Dalmau et al., 2020). We need to also understand that for most animals, parenting does not end with weaning. Like us, birds, mammals and species of other taxa continue to learn lessons of survival from their elders at least until they reach social maturity. In captivity they often are denied this extended time with adults. We perhaps need to reflect on this because early life experiences, including parenting, provide a foundation for the development of confident, well-balanced individuals (see 'Developmental stages', above).

Behaviour commonalities

Figures 3.20–3.23 show some common behaviours that can be observed in a range of species. These figures are intended as quick reference guides and are not a replacement for in-depth learning about individual species. However, the figures do illustrate that some considered generalizations can be made about species you have not seen before. For example, if the animal has ears with external pinnae and is holding them flat against their head, then it is highly likely that they are experiencing fear or pain. On comparing the figures you will notice that many species display the same behaviours for a variety of reasons – for example, rabbits will circle each other when happy and excited but also as part of a mating ritual. It is vital that the observed behaviours are analysed in conjunction with physiological, physical and social environmental parameters to ensure a holistic view is achieved and, thus, a more accurate interpretation of what the animal is communicating.

Pain

Human pain scales tend to focus heavily on the face, particularly on the eyes; it is well documented that humans have a recognizable 'pain face' and this has been extrapolated to animal studies. Of the 11 animal scoring systems that the authors have reviewed, all but one (dogs) include eye changes and, generally, these are seen as some of the most obvious and easy to read indications of pain. In the authors' opinion, dogs also show orbital tightening when they are experiencing pain. Though not included as part of the species coverage in this manual, there are behavioural studies on farm animals such as pigs and sheep, which may be of interest, especially as these species are sometimes kept as pets.

There are a wide range of grimace scales, pain questionnaires and other behavioural tools available to help assess the animal in front of you (see Chapter 2). However, interpreting the findings is never simple! For example, as well as orbital tightening, animals can also exhibit a wide-eyed stare when in pain or distress, as seen in dogs and horses, or show more 'whites of their eyes', as seen in cows and rabbits (Sandem et al., 2002). Cats are known to squint (ocular tightening) and slow blink at their caregivers as a sign of affection, so a lack of slow blinking may be a cue that pain is being experienced in this species. This example highlights the need to know species-specific signals. Another example is that rabbits may grind their teeth when in pain or when happy (similar to how cats use purring).

Of course, when assessing pain or other emotions we need to remember that some breeds have physical restrictions that limit their expressions. Notable are brachycephalic animals whose head shape means they are unable to alter their eye positions fully and/or have seemingly abnormal eye positions (e.g. Pugs with bulging eyes or wall-eyed Chihuahuas).

Further, different species have different abilities to show facial expressions. When a bird is in pain, there is normally a change or absence of one or more normal behaviours (Paul-Murphy and Hawkins, 2015). Reptiles can be tricky to assess for many reasons, including a lack of external pinnae and the fact that they tend to have very rigid facial skin if they have scales. Snakes do not have eyelids nor much soft tissue over their nares and their lips tend to be rigid. Temperature plays a huge part in assessing cold-blooded species such as amphibians, fish and reptiles. These species will act differently if they are comfortably warm or too cold. All of this increases the difficulty in identifying and assessing the levels of pain felt by them (Reid, 2018). Some studies have investigated pain assessment methods in reptiles (Ayers, 2016) and this field will continue to grow.

The Animal Facial Action Coding System (FACS) website provides guides for chimpanzees, gibbons, macaques, orangutans, dogs, cats and horses (Parr *et al.*, 2010; see 'Useful websites', below). These guides highlight the importance of species-specific knowledge and multiparameter monitoring in accurately assessing animals to the best of our ability.

We need to consider our handling methods too as capture and restraint can result in the animal displaying pain-like behaviours. This may be why the dog scale includes parameters such as demeanour and reaction to wounds, humans and palpation, as dogs are generally very comfortable with human interactions. Other species should be considered to be uncomfortable with human interactions. Rabbits, for example, are a prey species and, as such, will mask their discomfort and distress to the best of their ability. This results in very subtle changes to their appearance and behaviour that can be hard for an inexperienced person to identify. The sheer act of handling a fit and healthy rabbit can cause it to display behaviour and

facial changes that correlate strongly with an acute pain response – even when the rabbit is not experiencing any physical pain. This clearly illustrates why we need to bear in mind the capture and restraint methods used when conducting behavioural assessments, as these will vary for each species and each individual animal. It is also important to remember that if the animal is displaying signs of ocular, aural or oral pain these can be mistaken by the assessor as fear/anxiety behaviour markers. Therefore, the authors recommend using a more holistic approach that includes pain scoring but also takes into account the animal's behaviour and current environment (see Chapter 2 for more information).

Conclusion

We have an ethical and moral duty to provide for the welfare of all animals we keep. It is not quantity of life that is important, but its quality. Regardless of an animal's taxon, why it is kept or its expected lifespan, we should aim to give it a life worth living. Fundamental to that is understanding its behaviour and providing for its cognitive and emotional needs. Animal behaviour is a complex and fascinating subject and research continues to extend our knowledge base apace. Consequently, as professionals, we should aim to increase our own knowledge and reflect on, and alter, our management and interaction practices accordingly, and likewise educate owners and those who care for animals. We should try to make that education relevant to them, so they do not just know but understand. This can be achieved by using analogy to human experiences, as in this chapter, or animal-related examples. As professionals, we must remember that what we do is as much a teaching tool as what we say, if not more so. Thus, we need to ensure we practise what we preach by planning and reviewing handling of animals during clinical procedures and sharing best practise (see Chapter 7). This is important not only for the welfare of animals but also for the safety of the handlers and others who may interact with the animals later.

Behaviour	Dog	Cat	Rabbit	Rat	Mouse	Ferret	Reptile	Chelonian	Bird	Horse	Seal
Orbital tightening[a]		✓	✓	✓	✓	✓	✓	✓	✓	✓	✓
Ear flattening[a]		✓	✓	✓	✓	✓				✓	
Open mouth[a]		✓					✓	✓	✓	✓	✓
Lip tightening/curling[a]							Not included			✓	Not included
Cheek flattening/bulging			✓	✓	✓		Not included	Not included	Not included	✓	Not included
Nares flattening/bulging			✓				Not included			✓	✓
Nose bulging				✓	✓	✓	Not included				
Whiskers forward[a]		✓	✓	✓	✓	✓					Not included
Head down[b]	✓	✓							✓		
Vocalization[b]	✓						✓	✓	✓		✓
Altered body position[b]	✓								✓		✓
Altered demeanour[b]	✓						✓	Not included	✓		✓
Negative (defensive) reaction to human[b]	✓						✓	Not included	✓		Not included
Wound interference[b]	✓						Not included	Not included	Not included		Not included
Negative (defensive) reaction to palpation[b]	✓						Not included	Not included	Not included		✓

3.20 Common pain responses and the species that can exhibit them, based on a selection of current published scoring guides. [a] = applicable to dogs in authors' opinion; [b] = potentially applicable to all species in authors' opinion.

Behaviour	Dog	Cat	Rabbit	Rat	Mouse	Ferret	Reptile[a]	Chelonian[a]	Bird[a]	Horse	Seal[a]
Mild anxiety/fear											
Tail – tucked under body	✓	✓									
Tail – low/slow wagging	✓	✓									
Low head position	✓	✓	✓							✓	
Eyes – avoiding eye contact	✓									✓	
Eyes – slow blinking	✓	✓								✓	
Mouth – yawning/lip licking	✓							n/a		✓	
Ears – held sideways/back	✓	✓	✓	✓	✓		n/a	n/a		✓	
Lifting limb/foot	✓	✓	✓				✓		✓	✓	✓
Pacing	✓									✓	
Cowering/crouched	✓	✓	✓	✓	✓		✓				
Vocalization – whimpering	✓										
Eyes – dilated pupils	✓		✓								
Eyes – 'whale eye' (sclera visible)	✓	✓	✓							✓	
Hiding	✓	✓	✓	✓	✓		✓				
Erratic grooming/plucking/barbering/scratching	✓	✓	✓				✓		✓	✓	
Quivering/shaking	✓	✓	✓						✓		
Puffing up to look bigger	✓	✓			✓	✓			✓		
Urinating/defecating	✓	✓	✓								
Escalated anxiety/fear											
Strike pose/S shape (snakes)	n/a	n/a	n/a	n/a	n/a	n/a	✓	n/a	n/a	n/a	n/a
Stiffened body posture/freezing	✓	✓	✓	✓	✓				✓	✓	
Flattening body/feathers		✓	✓						✓		
Sitting on hind legs			✓								n/a
Pawing the ground		n/a	✓							✓	
Pushing/nudging threat away			✓	✓	✓			✓			
Ears – held forward/flat	✓	✓	✓				n/a	n/a			
Erect fur/feathers/scales	✓	✓		✓	✓	✓			✓		
Eyes – staring at perceived threat	✓		✓	✓	✓					✓	✓
Tail – held up/stiff/extended	✓	✓	✓			✓		✓			
Tail – flicking side to side		✓	✓								
Wrinkled nose	✓							n/a	n/a		
Mouth – open (may be for thermoregulation)		✓	✓			✓	✓		✓		✓
Vocalization – growling/snarling/snorting/squeaking	✓		✓	✓	✓	✓				✓	
Tense facial muscles	✓	✓	✓	✓	✓					✓	
Eyes – narrowed				✓	✓		✓			✓	
Severe anxiety/fear											
Mouth – lips drawn back	✓							n/a	n/a		
Mouth – baring teeth	✓	✓	✓			✓		n/a	n/a		✓
Mouth – biting/pecking	✓	✓	✓	✓	✓	✓	✓	✓	✓	✓	✓
Mouth – teeth chattering	n/a	n/a	✓	✓				n/a	n/a		
Head held upwards	✓		✓						✓		✓
Neck extended								✓			
Eyes – wide open	✓	✓	✓	✓	✓						
Eyes – flashing/pinning/pinpointing	n/a	n/a	n/a						✓		

3.21 Common signs that animals use to express fear and anxiety and the species that can exhibit them. A single behaviour (as listed in the table) should be considered in conjunction with other physiological, physical and social parameters, as well as the other behaviours being expressed by the animal. The behaviours are grouped to show how they may be assessed in an unfamiliar species. [a] = different species may react differently.
☐ = very low-level anxiety/fear; ☐ = mild anxiety/fear; ▨ = moderate anxiety/fear; ▨ = escalated anxiety/fear; ■ = severe anxiety/fear; ■ = extreme anxiety/fear. (continues)

▶

Behaviour	Dog	Cat	Rabbit	Rat	Mouse	Ferret	Reptile[a]	Chelonian[a]	Bird[a]	Horse	Seal[a]
Severe anxiety/fear continued											
Vocalization – barking/hissing/screaming/wailing	✓	✓	✓	✓		✓	✓	✓			✓
Position – standing with bodyweight back	✓		✓								
Position – standing with arched back		✓		✓				✓			
Position – standing side-on to threat		✓								✓	
Running/backing away			✓	✓		✓				✓	
Charging/kicking/boxing/headbutting/lunging towards the threat		✓	✓	✓			✓	✓		✓	✓
Thumping back feet	n/a	n/a	✓	n/a	n/a	n/a	n/a	n/a	n/a	n/a	n/a
Head tossing/twirling/prancing	n/a	n/a							✓	✓	
Spreading out wings/feathers	n/a	n/a	n/a	n/a	n/a	n/a	n/a	n/a	✓	n/a	n/a
Tail – slapping	n/a			✓							
Foot tapping	n/a	n/a	n/a						✓		n/a

3.21 (continued) Common signs that animals use to express fear and anxiety and the species that can exhibit them. A single behaviour (as listed in the table) should be considered in conjunction with other physiological, physical and social parameters, as well as the other behaviours being expressed by the animal. The behaviours are grouped to show how they may be assessed in an unfamiliar species. [a] = different species may react differently. ☐ = very low-level anxiety/fear; ☐ = mild anxiety/fear; ☐ = moderate anxiety/fear; ☐ = escalated anxiety/fear; ■ = severe anxiety/fear; ■ = extreme anxiety/fear.

Behaviour	Dog	Cat	Rabbit	Rat	Mouse	Ferret	Reptile[a]	Chelonian[a]	Bird[a]	Horse	Seal[a]
Relaxed posture	✓	✓	✓	✓	✓	✓	✓	✓	✓	✓	✓
Position – play bow	✓										
Position – exposed abdomen	✓	✓	✓								✓
Position – prone with legs extended			✓						n/a		
Position – circling		✓	✓								
Relaxed muscles	✓	✓	✓	✓	✓	✓	✓	✓	✓	✓	✓
Smooth fur/feathers/scales	✓	✓	✓	✓	✓	✓	✓	✓	✓	✓	✓
Ears – normal position	✓	✓	✓	✓	✓	✓	✓	✓	✓	✓	✓
Eyes – normal shape	✓	✓	✓	✓	✓	✓	✓	✓	✓	✓	✓
Eyes – slow blink	✓	✓									
Eyes – small pupils	✓	✓									
Eyes – bulging/boggling				✓							
Whiskers – relaxed	✓	✓	✓	✓	✓	✓	n/a	n/a	n/a		
Tail – high/quick wagging	✓			✓							
Tail – held upright with curved tip		✓									
Tail – held upright and quivering		✓									
Vocalization – friendly barking	✓										
Vocalization – chirp/trill/purr		✓		✓							
Tooth/beak grinding	n/a	n/a	✓	✓					✓		
Mouth – relaxed open	✓										
Mouth – relaxed closed	✓	✓	✓	✓	✓	✓	✓	✓	✓	✓	✓
Head rubbing/chinning		✓	✓	✓							
Kneading	n/a	✓	n/a	n/a	n/a	n/a	n/a	n/a	n/a	n/a	n/a
Binkying/popcorning/jumping and twisting	n/a	n/a	✓	✓	n/a	n/a	n/a	n/a	n/a	n/a	n/a
Bottom twitching	n/a	n/a	✓	n/a	n/a	n/a	n/a	n/a	n/a	n/a	n/a
Relaxed grooming	✓	✓	✓	✓	✓	✓	✓	✓	✓	✓	✓

3.22 Common signs that an animal is happy or relaxed and the species that can exhibit them. Note that context is important – animals may use 'happy behaviours' to reduce perceived threats (appeasement). [a] = different species may react differently.

Behaviour	Dog	Cat	Rabbit	Rat	Mouse	Ferret	Reptile	Chelonian	Bird	Horse	Seal
Mounting	✓	✓	✓	✓	✓	✓	✓	✓	✓	✓	✓
Circling/dancing			✓	✓		✓ a	✓ a	✓ a	✓	✓	
Ears – quick waggling			✓	✓			n/a	n/a			n/a
Ears – pinking/flushing with colour				✓	✓		n/a	n/a			n/a
Eyes – flashing/pinning/pinpointing	n/a	n/a	n/a	n/a	n/a	n/a	n/a	n/a	✓	n/a	n/a
Position – mating posture	✓	✓	✓	✓	✓	✓	✓	✓	✓	✓	✓
Nesting			✓	✓			✓ a	n/a	✓		
Whisker barbering				✓	✓		n/a	n/a	n/a		
Scent marking	✓	✓	✓	✓	✓	✓	✓ a	✓ a	✓ a	✓ a	
Thumping	n/a	n/a	✓	n/a	n/a	n/a	n/a	n/a	n/a	n/a	n/a
Vocalization – barking/honking/yowling/screeching	✓	✓	✓					✓ a	✓ a		
Feathers – tail fanning/wing lifting	n/a	n/a	n/a	n/a	n/a	n/a	n/a	n/a	✓	n/a	n/a
Allogrooming	✓	✓	✓	✓	✓	✓			✓	✓	
Regurgitation	n/a	n/a	n/a	n/a	n/a	n/a	n/a	n/a	✓	n/a	n/a
Masturbation		n/a	n/a	n/a	n/a	n/a	n/a	n/a	✓	n/a	n/a
Head bobbing/butting							✓ a	✓	✓ a		

3.23 Common sexual and territorial behaviours and the species that can exhibit them. a = authors' opinion.

References and further reading

Ahola MK, Vapalahti K and Lohi H (2017) Early weaning increases aggression and stereotypic behaviour in cats. *Scientific Reports* **7**, 1–9

Alcock J (2013) *Animal behavior: An evolutionary approach, 10th edn.* Sinauer Associates, Sunderland

Amat M, Manteca X, Mariotti VM, de la Torre JLR and Fatjó J (2009) Aggressive behavior in the English cocker spaniel. *Journal of Veterinary Behavior* **4**, 111–117

Ambrose SH (2001) Paleolithic technology and human evolution. *Science* **291**, 1748–1753

Artelle KA, Dumoulin LK and Reimchen TE (2011) Behavioural responses of dogs to asymmetrical tail wagging of a robotic dog replica. *Laterality* **16**, 129–135

Asher L, England GCW, Sommerville R and Harvey ND (2020) Teenage dogs? Evidence for adolescent-phase conflict behaviour and an association between attachment to humans and pubertal timing in the domestic dog. *Biology Letters* **16**, 20200097

Atkinson T (2018) *Practical feline behaviour: Understanding cat behaviour and improving welfare.* CABI, Wallingford

Ayers H (2016) Pain recognition in reptiles and investigation of associated behavioural signs. *The Veterinary Nurse* **7**, 292–300

Azrin NH and Holz WC (1966) Punishment. In: *Operant behavior: Areas of Research and Application*, ed. WK Honig, pp. 380–447. Appleton-Century-Crofts, New York

Bailey G (2008) *The Perfect Puppy, revised edn.* Hamlyn, London

Berdoy M (2002) *The Laboratory Rat: a natural history.* Available from: norecopa.no

Blakemore SJ (2008) The social brain in adolescence. *Nature Reviews Neuroscience* **9**, 267–277

Bradshaw J and Ellis S (2017) *The Trainable Cat.* Penguin, London

Braun K and Champagne FA (2014) Paternal influences on offspring development: behavioural and epigenetic pathways. *Journal of Neuroendocrinology* **26**, 697–706

Briefer EF (2018) Vocal contagion of emotions in non-human animals. *Proceedings of the Royal Society B: Biological Sciences* **285**, 20172783

Broom DM and Fraser AF (2015) *Domestic Animal Behaviour and Welfare, 5th edn.* CABI, Wallingford

Brown C, Wolfenden D and Sneddon L (2019) Goldfish (*Carassius auratus*). In: *Companion Animal Care and Welfare: The UFAW Companion Animal Handbook*, ed. J Yeates, pp. 467–478. John Wiley and Sons, Chichester

Brunton PJ and Russell JA (2010) Prenatal social stress in the rat programmes neuroendocrine and behavioural responses to stress in the adult offspring: Sex-specific effects. *Journal of Neuroendocrinology* **22**, 258–271

Burch MR and Bailey JS (1999) *How dogs learn.* Howell Book House, Turner Publishing, Nashville

Burghardt GM (2005) *The genesis of animal play: Testing the limits.* MIT Press, Cambridge

Ceballos MC, Sant'Anna AC, Boivin X *et al.* (2018) Impact of good practices of handling training on beef cattle welfare and stockpeople attitudes and behaviors. *Livestock Science* **216**, 24–31

China L, Mills DS and Cooper JJ (2020) Efficacy of dog training with and without remote electronic collars *versus* a focus on positive reinforcement. *Frontiers in Veterinary Science* **7**, 508

Coleman GJ and Hemsworth PH (2014) Training to improve stockperson beliefs and behaviour towards livestock enhances welfare and productivity. *Revue Scientifique et Technique* **33**, 131–137

Cooper J, Mills D and China L (2021) Response: Commentary: Remote Electronic Training Aids; Efficacy at Deterring Predatory Behavior in Dogs and Implications for Training and Policy. *Frontiers in Veterinary Science* **8**, 675005

Costa ED, Minero M, Lebelt D *et al.* (2014) Development of the Horse Grimace Scale (HGS) as a Pain Assessment Tool in Horses Undergoing Routine Castration. *PLoS One* **9**, e92281

Czerwinski VH, Smith BP, Hynd PI and Hazel SJ (2016) The influence of maternal care on stress-related behaviors in domestic dogs: What can we learn from the rodent literature? *Journal of Veterinary Behavior* **14**, 52–59

Daleswartzentruber (2007a) *Habituation of a startle response.* Available from: www.youtube.com

Daleswartzentruber (2007b) *Dishabituation of a rat's startle response.* Available from: www.youtube.com

Daleswartzentruber (2007c) *Spontaneous recovery.* Available from: www.youtube.com

Dalmau A, Moles X and Pallisera J (2020) Animal welfare assessment protocol for does, bucks, and kit rabbits reared for production. *Frontiers in veterinary science* **7**, 445

Dearing M (1997) The Function of Haypiles of Pikas (*Ochotona princeps*). *Journal of Mammalogy* **78**, 1156–1163

Doherty O, Casey V, McGreevy P and Arkins S (2017) Noseband Use in Equestrian Sports – An International Study. *PLoS One* **12**, e0169060

Domjan M (2015) *Principles of Learning and Behavior, 7th edn.* Cengage Learning, Boston

Domjan M (2017) *The Essentials of Conditioning and Learning, 4th edn.* APA Books, Washington

Dybkjaer L (1992) The identification of behavioural indicators of 'stress' in early weaned piglets. *Applied Animal Behaviour Science* **35**, 135–147

Ebbesen CL and Froemke RC (2021) Body language signals for rodent social communication. *Current Opinion in Neurobiology* **68**, 91–106

Elwood RW (2019) Assessing the Potential for Pain in Crustaceans and Other Invertebrates. In: *The Welfare of Invertebrate Animals*, ed. C Carere and J Mather, pp. 147–177. Springer Nature Switzerland AG, Cham

Evangelista MC, Watanabe R, Leung VSY *et al.* (2019) Facial expressions of pain in cats: the development and validation of a Feline Grimace Scale. *Scientific Reports* **9**, 19128

Fagen A, Acharya N and Kaufman GE (2014) Positive reinforcement training for a trunk wash in Nepal's working elephants: demonstrating alternatives to traditional elephant training techniques. *Journal of Applied Animal Welfare Science* **17**, 83–97

Fattah AFA and Abdel-Hamid SE (2020) Influence of gender, neuter status, and training method on police dog narcotics olfaction performance, behavior and welfare. *Journal of Advanced Veterinary and Animal Research* **7**, 655

Fenner K, Mclean AN and McGreevy PD (2019) Cutting to the chase: How round-pen, lunging, and high-speed liberty work may compromise horse welfare. *Journal of Veterinary Behavior* **29**, 88–94

Fraser D (1978) Observations on the behavioural development of suckling and early-weaned piglets during the first six weeks after birth. *Animal Behaviour* **26**, 22–30

Gartrell BD (2011) *Science with feeling: animals and people – The recognition and relief of pain in birds.* Proceedings of the ANZCCART Conference 26–28 June 2011, 21–23

Gibsone SH, McBride EA, Redhead ES, Cameron KE and Bizo LA (2021) The Effectiveness of Visual and Auditory Elements of a Compound Stimulus in Controlling Behavior in the Domestic Dog (*Canis familiaris*). *Journal of Veterinary Behavior* **46**, 87–96

Gray C and Moffett J (2013) Handbook of Veterinary Communication Skills. John Wiley and Sons, Chichester

Groves PM and Thompson RF (1970) Habituation: a dual-process theory. *Psychological Review* **77**, 419–450

Grundwald NJ and Brunton PJ (2015) Prenatal stress programs neuroendocrine stress responses and affective behaviors in second generation rats in a sex-dependent manner. *Psychoneuroendocrinology* **62**, 204–216

Gubernick DJ and Klopfer PH (1981) *Parental Care in Mammals.* Plenum Press, New York

Gunter LM, Barber RT and Wynne CD (2016) What's in a name? Effect of breed perceptions and labeling on attractiveness, adoptions and length of stay for pit-bull-type dogs. *PloS One* **11**, e0146857

Győri B, Gácsi M and Miklósi Á (2010) Friend or foe: Context dependent sensitivity to human behaviour in dogs. *Applied Animal Behaviour Science* **128**, 69–77

Handelman B (2012) *Canine Behavior: A Photo Illustrated Handbook.* Dogwise Publishing, Wenatchee

Hart LA and Hart BL (2021) An Ancient Practice but a New Paradigm: Personal Choice for the Age to Spay or Neuter a Dog. *Frontiers in Veterinary Science* **8**, 244

Haselgrove M (2019) Learning. In: *Psychology*, ed. G Davey, pp. 382–428. John Wiley and Sons, Chichester

Hayward T (2015) *A Deaf Dog Joins the Family: Training, Education, and Communication for A Smooth Transition.* CreateSpace, Scotts Valley

Hazel SJ, Jenvey CJ and Tuke J (2018) Online relinquishments of dogs and cats in Australia. *Animals* **8**, 25

Hedley J, Johnson R and Yeates J (2019) Reptiles (Reptilia). In: *Companion Animal Care and Welfare: The UFAW Companion Animal Handbook*, ed. J Yeates, pp. 371–394. John Wiley and Sons, Chichester

Held SD and Špinka M (2011) Animal play and animal welfare. *Animal Behaviour* **81**, 891–899

Hemsworth PH and Coleman GJ (2010) *Human-livestock interactions: The stockperson and the productivity of intensively farmed animals.* CABI, Wallingford

Herzog H (2010) *Some we love, some we hate, some we eat: Why it's so hard to think straight about animals.* Harper, New York

Heyes C (2012) Simple minds: a qualified defence of associative learning. *Philosophical Transactions of the Royal Society B: Biological Sciences* **367**, 2695–2703

Hillix WA and Rumbaugh D (2004) *Animal Bodies, Human Minds: Ape, Dolphin, and Parrot Language Skills.* Springer, New York

Hradecká L, Bartoš L, Svobodová I and Sales J (2015) Heritability of behavioural traits in domestic dogs: A meta-analysis. *Applied Animal Behaviour Science* **170**, 1–13

Ijichi C, Tunstall S, Putt E and Squibb K (2018) Dually Noted: The effects of a pressure headcollar on compliance, discomfort and stress in horses during handling. *Applied Animal Behaviour Science* **205**, 68–73

Jakovcevic A, Elgier AM, Mustaca AE and Bentosela M (2010) Breed differences in dogs' (*Canis familiaris*) gaze to the human face. *Behavioural Processes* **84**, 602–607

Jones AC and Gosling SD (2005) Temperament and personality in dogs (*Canis familiaris*): A review and evaluation of past research. *Applied Animal Behaviour Science* **95**, 1–53

Kaminski J, Waller BM, Diogo R, Hartstone-Rose A and Burrows AM (2019) Evolution of facial muscle anatomy in dogs. *Proceedings of the National Academy of Sciences* **116**, 14677–14681

Kienapfel K, Link Y and Borstel UKV (2014) Prevalence of different head-neck positions in horses shown at dressage competitions and their relation to conflict behaviour and performance marks. *PLoS One* **9**, e103140

Knapp ML, Hall HJA and Horgan TG (2013) *Nonverbal communication in Human Interaction, 8th edn.* Cengage Learning, Boston

Kuhne F (2016) Behavioural responses of dogs to dog-human social conflict situations. *Applied Animal Behaviour Science* **182**, 38–43

Kukekova AV, Oskina IN, Kharlamova AV et al. (2008) Fox farm experiment: hunting for behavioral genes. *Вестник ВОГиС* **12**, 50–62

Leaver SDA and Reimchen TE (2008) Behavioural responses of *Canis familiaris* to different tail lengths of a remotely-controlled life-size dog replica. *Behaviour* **145**, 377–390

Levitis DA, Lidicker WZ Jr and Freund G (2009) Behavioural biologists do not agree on what constitutes behaviour. *Animal Behaviour* **78**, 103–110

Lezama-García K, Mariti C, Mota-Rojas D et al. (2019) Maternal behaviour in domestic dogs. *International Journal of Veterinary Science and Medicine* **7**, 20–30

Locke P (2006) *History, practice, identity: An institutional ethnography of elephant handlers in Chitwan, Nepal.* Doctoral dissertation, University of Kent, Canterbury

Løtvedt P and Jensen P (2014) Effects of Hatching Time on Behavior and Weight Development of Chickens. *PLoS One* **9**, e103040

Luescher AU (2006) *Manual of Parrot Behavior.* Blackwell, Oxford

MacRae AM, Makowska IJ and Fraser D (2018) Initial evaluation of facial expressions and behaviours of harbour seal pups (*Phoca vitulina*) in response to tagging and microchipping. *Applied Animal Behaviour Science* **205**, 167–174

Magnus E and McBride A (2022) What every rabbit and rodent owner should know. In: *Companion Animal Behaviour Problems: prevention and management of behaviour problems in veterinary practice*, ed. H Zulch, R Casey and S Heath. CABI, Wallingford

Mahoney A, Lalonde K, Edwards T et al. (2014) Landmine-detection rats: An evaluation of reinforcement procedures under simulated operational conditions. *Journal of the Experimental Analysis of Behavior* **101**, 450–456

Malik A (2018) Pain in reptiles: a review for veterinary nurses. *Veterinary Nursing Journal* **33**, 201–211

Malik A and Valentine A (2018) Pain in birds: a review for veterinary nurses. *Veterinary Nursing Journal* **33**, 11–25

Marshall-Pescini S, Colombo E, Passalacqua C, Merola I and Prato-Previde E (2013) Gaze alternation in dogs and toddlers in an unsolvable task: evidence of an audience effect. *Animal Cognition* **16**, 933–943

Maslow AH (1987) *Motivation and personality, 3rd edn.* Pearson Education, Delhi

McBride A (2014a) The Year of the Rabbit: Autumn. *Rabbiting On* **Autumn 2014**, 25–25

McBride A (2014b) The Year of the Rabbit: Spring. *Rabbiting On* **Spring 2014**, 10–11

McBride A (2014c) The Year of the Rabbit: Summer. *Rabbiting On* **Summer 2014**, 11–12

McBride A (2014d) The Year of the Rabbit: Winter. *Rabbiting On* **Winter 2014**, 10–11

McBride A (2015) Animals in trances: peace of mind or panic? *Rabbiting On* **Winter 2015**, 10–12

McBride A (2017) Small prey species' behaviour and welfare: implications for veterinary professionals. *Journal of Small Animal Practice* **58**, 423–436

McBride A (2019) Lifelong Welfare – teaching older animals new tricks. *BVNA Congress Times* **2019**, 6–8

McBride A and Baugh S (2022) Animal Welfare in context: historical, scientific, ethical, moral and One Welfare perspectives. In: *Human/Animal Relationships in Transformation – Scientific, Moral and Legal Perspectives*, ed. A Vitale and S Pollo, pp. 119–147. Palgrave Macmillan, London

McBride A and Magnus E (2022) Rabbit and rodent behaviour. In: *Companion Animal Behaviour Problems: prevention and management of behaviour problems in veterinary practice*, ed. H Zulch, R Casey and S Heath. CABI, Wallingford

McBride A and Montgomery DJ (2018) Animal Welfare: A Contemporary Understanding Demands a Contemporary Approach to Behavior and Training. *People and Animals: The International Journal of Research and Practice* **1**, Article 4

McCune S (1995) The impact of paternity and early socialisation on the development of cats' behaviour to people and novel objects. *Applied Animal Behaviour Science* **45**, 109–124

McCune S, McPherson JA and Bradshaw JW (1995) Avoiding problems: the importance of socialisation. In: *The Waltham Book of Human–Animal Interaction*, ed. I Robinson, pp. 71—86. Pergamon Press, Oxford

McGreevy P and Boakes R (2011) *Carrots and sticks: principles of animal training.* Darlington, Prestatyn

McGreevy P, Grassi TD and Harman AM (2004) A strong correlation exists between the distribution of retinal ganglion cells and nose length in the dog. *Brain, Behavior and Evolution* **63**, 13–22

McLean AN and McGreevy PD (2010) Horse-training techniques that may defy the principles of learning theory and compromise welfare. *Journal of Veterinary Behavior* **5**, 187–195

McMillan FD (2017) Behavioral and psychological outcomes for dogs sold as puppies through pet stores and/or born in commercial breeding establishments: Current knowledge and putative causes. *Journal of Veterinary Behavior* **19**, 14–26

Mehrabian A (1972) *Nonverbal Communication.* Aldine Transaction, New Brunswick

Mejdell CM, Jørgensen GH, Buvik T, Torp T and Bøe KE (2019) The effect of weather conditions on the preference in horses for wearing blankets. *Applied Animal Behaviour Science* **212**, 52–57

Melfi VA, Dorey NR and Ward SJ (2020) *Zoo Animal Learning and Training.* Wiley-Blackwell, Chichester

Mellersh CS (2014) The genetics of eye disorders in the dog. *Canine Genetics and Epidemiology* **1**, 3

Mellor DJ (2016) Updating animal welfare thinking: Moving beyond the 'Five Freedoms' towards "a Life Worth Living". *Animals* **6**, 21

Mikulincer M and Shaver PR (2012) An attachment perspective on psychopathology. *World Psychiatry* **11**, 11–15

Miller RM (1991) *Imprint Training of the Newborn Foal*. Western Horseman Inc., Colorado Springs

Nicol CJ and Badnell-Waters AJ (2005) Suckling behaviour in domestic foals and the development of abnormal oral behaviour. *Animal Behaviour* **70**, 21–29

Nielsen BL (2017) *Olfaction in Animal Behaviour and Welfare*. CABI, Wallingford

O'Donnell K, O'Connor TG and Glover V (2009) Prenatal stress and neurodevelopment of the child: focus on the HPA axis and role of the placenta. *Developmental Neuroscience* **31**, 285–292

Olsson IAS, Nevison CM, Patterson-Kane EG *et al.* (2003) Understanding behaviour: the relevance of ethological approaches in laboratory animal science. *Applied Animal Behaviour Science* **81**, 245–264

Oltenacu PA and Broom DM (2010) The impact of genetic selection for increased milk yield on the welfare of dairy cows. *Animal Welfare* **19**, 39–49

O'Neill DG, Church DB, McGreevy PD, Thomson PC and Brodbelt DC (2013) Longevity and mortality of owned dogs in England. *The Veterinary Journal* **198**, 638–643

Ostrom TM (1969) The relationship between the affective, behavioral, and cognitive components of attitude. *Journal of Experimental Social Psychology* **5**, 12–30

Panksepp J (2007) Neuroevolutionary sources of laughter and social joy: Modeling primal human laughter in laboratory rats. *Behavioural Brain Research* **182**, 231–244

Parr LA, Waller BM, Burrows AM, Gothard KM and Vick SJ (2010) MaqFACS: A muscle-based facial movement coding system for the rhesus macaque. *American Journal of Physical Anthropology* **143**, 625–630

Paul-Murphy JR and Hawkins MG (2015) Bird specific considerations: Recognizing pain behaviour in pet birds. In: *Handbook of veterinary pain management, 3rd edn*, ed. JS Gaynor and WW Muir, pp. 536–554. Elsevier, St. Louis

Pollock C (2019) *Reading Bird Body Language*. Available from: lafeber.com/vet

Powell SB, Mitchell LJ, Phelan AM *et al.* (2021) A five-channel LED display to investigate UV perception. *Methods in Ecology and Evolution* **4**, 602–607

Protopopova A, Kisten D and Wynne C (2016) Evaluating a humane alternative to the bark collar: Automated differential reinforcement of not barking in a home-alone setting. *Journal of Applied Behavior Analysis* **49**, 735–744

Quaranta A, Siniscalchi M and Vallortigara G (2007) Asymmetric tail-wagging responses by dogs to different emotive stimuli. *Current Biology* **17**, R199–R201

Rahim MA (2010) *Managing conflict in organizations*. Transaction Publishers, New Jersey

Rankin CH, Abrams T, Barry RJ *et al.* (2009) Habituation revisited: an updated and revised description of the behavioral characteristics of habituation. *Neurobiology of Learning and Memory* **92**, 135–138

Reader SM, Morand-Ferron J and Flynn E (2016) Animal and human innovation: novel problems and novel solutions. *Philosophical Transactions of the Royal Society B: Biological Sciences* **371**, 20150182

Reid J, Nolan AM, Hughes JML *et al.* (2007) Development of the short-form Glasgow Composite Measure Pain Scale (CMPS-SF) and derivation of an analgesic intervention score. *Animal Welfare* **16**, 97–104

Reid SA (2018) Identifying pain in reptiles. *Veterinary Practice Today* **6**, 58–62

Reijgwart ML, Schoemaker NJ, Pascuzzo R *et al.* (2017) The composition and initial evaluation of a grimace scale in ferrets after surgical implantation of a telemetry probe. *PLoS One* **12**, e0187986

Reither K, Jugheli L, Glass TR *et al.* (2015) Evaluation of giant African pouched rats for detection of pulmonary tuberculosis in patients from a high-endemic setting. *PLoS One* **10**, e0135877

Ristau CR (1991) *Cognitive ethology: The minds of other animals: Essays in honor of Donald R. Griffin*. Taylor and Francis, London

Roberts M (1997) *The Man Who Listens to Horses*. Arrow Books, London

Rogers S (2018) *Equine behaviour in mind: applying behavioural science to the way we keep, work and care for horses*. 5M Publishing, Sheffield

Rose JD, Arlinghaus R, Cooke SJ *et al.* (2014) Can fish really feel pain? *Fish and Fisheries* **15**, 97–133

Rose MP and Williams DL (2014) Neurological dysfunction in a ball python (*Python regius*) colour morph and implications for welfare. *Journal of Exotic Pet Medicine* **23**, 234–239

Royle NJ, Smiseth PT and Kölliker M (2012) *The evolution of parental care*. Oxford University Press, Oxford

Russell AP and Bauer AM (2021) Vocalization by extant nonavian reptiles: A synthetic overview of phonation and the vocal apparatus. *The Anatomical Record* **304**, 1478–1528

Rutherford KM, Piastowska-Ciesielska A, Donald RD *et al.* (2014) Prenatal stress produces anxiety prone female offspring and impaired maternal behaviour in the domestic pig. *Physiology and Behavior* **129**, 255–264

Sales G (2012) *Ultrasonic communication by animals*. Springer, Berlin

Samhita L and Gross HJ (2013) The 'Clever Hans Phenomenon' revisited. *Communicative and Integrative Biology* **6**, e27122

Sandem AI, Braastad BO and Boe KE (2002) Eye white may indicate emotional state on a frustration–contentedness axis in dairy cows. *Applied Animal Behaviour Science* **79**, 1–10

Sargisson RJ and Mclean IG (2021) Commentary: Efficacy of Dog Training With and Without Remote Electronic Collars vs. a Focus on Positive Reinforcement. *Frontiers in Veterinary Science* **8**, 184

Schalke E, Stichnoth J, Ott S and Jones-Baade R (2007) Clinical signs caused by the use of electric training collars on dogs in everyday life situations. *Applied Animal Behaviour Science* **105**, 369–380

Schilder MB and van der Borg JA (2004) Training dogs with help of the shock collar: short and long term behavioural effects. *Applied Animal Behaviour Science* **85**, 319–334

Scott JP and Fuller JL (1974) *Genetics and the Social Behaviour of the Dog*. University of Chicago Press, Chicago

Seligman ME and Maier SF (1967) Failure to escape traumatic shock. *Journal of Experimental Psychology* **74**, 1–9

Shepherd K (2020) *Demystifying dog behaviour for the veterinarian*. CRC Press, London

Shorey HH (2013) *Animal communication by pheromones*. Academic Press, Cambridge MA

Simpson BS (2002) Neonatal foal handling. *Applied Animal Behaviour Science* **78**, 303–317

Simpson L, Robinson P, Fletcher M and Wilson R (2018) *E-Communication Skills – a guide for primary care*. CRC Press, London

Siniscalchi M, Lusito R, Vallortigara G and Quaranta A (2013) Seeing Left- or Right-Asymmetric Tail Wagging Produces Different Emotional Responses in Dogs. *Current Biology* **23**, 2279–2282

Sneddon L and Wolfenden D (2019) Ornamental Fish (Actinopterygii). In: *Companion Animal Care and Welfare: The UFAW Companion Animal Handbook*, ed. J Yeates, pp. 440–466. John Wiley and Sons, Chichester

Sneddon LU, Elwood RW, Adamo SA and Leach MC (2014) Defining and assessing animal pain. *Animal Behaviour* **97**, 201–212

Somppi S, Törnqvist H, Hänninen L, Krause C and Vainio O (2012) Dogs do look at images: eye tracking in canine cognition research. *Animal Cognition* **15**, 163–174

Špinka M (2012) Social dimension of emotions and its implication for animal welfare. *Applied Animal Behaviour Science* **138**, 170–181

Squibb K, Griffin K, Favier R and Ijichi C (2018) Poker Face: Discrepancies in behaviour and affective states in horses during stressful handling procedures. *Applied Animal Behaviour Science* **202**, 34–38

Stapleton N (2021) Guide to behavioural issues in rabbits. *In Practice* **43**, 18–25

Strain GM (2011) *Deafness in dogs and cats*. CABI, Wallingford

Sturman DA and Moghaddam B (2011) The neurobiology of adolescence: changes in brain architecture, functional dynamics, and behavioral tendencies. *Neuroscience and Biobehavioral Reviews* **35**, 1704–1712

Summers JF, Diesel G, Asher L, McGreevy PD and Collins LM (2010) Inherited defects in pedigree dogs. Part 2: Disorders that are not related to breed standards. *The Veterinary Journal* **183**, 39–45

Suzuki TN (2018) Alarm calls evoke a visual search image of a predator in birds. *Proceedings of the National Academy of Sciences of The United States of America* **115**, 1541–1545

Thompson J (2011) *Is Nonverbal Communication a Numbers Game?* Available from: www.psychologytoday.com

Timberlake W and Silva FJ (1994) Observation of behavior, inference of function, and the study of learning. *Psychonomic Bulletin and Review* **1**, 73–88

Toda K and Watanabe S (2008) Discrimination of moving video images of self by pigeons (*Columba livia*). *Animal Cognition* **11**, 699–705

Troscianko J and Rutz C (2015) Activity profiles and hook-tool use of New Caledonian crows recorded by bird-borne video cameras. *Biology Letters* **11**, 20150777

Universities Federation for Animal Welfare (2018) *Genetic Welfare Problems of Companion Animals: An information resource for prospective pet owners*. Available from: www.ufaw.org.uk

University of Glasgow and University of Edinburgh Napier (2015) *Glasgow Feline Composite Measure Pain Scale: CMPS – Feline*. Available from: www.newmetrica.com

Vasconcellos ADS, Virányi Z, Range F *et al.* (2016) Training reduces stress in human-socialised wolves to the same degree as in dogs. *PLoS One* **11**, e0162389

Vitousek MN, Adelman JS, Gregory NC and St Clair JJH (2007) Heterospecific alarm call recognition in a non-vocal reptile. *Biology Letters* **3**, 632–634

Wallace D, Greenberg DS, Sawinski J *et al.* (2013) Rats maintain an overhead binocular field at the expense of constant fusion. *Nature* **498**, 65–69

Wallis LJ, Range F, Müller CA *et al.* (2015) Training for eye contact modulates gaze following in dogs. *Animal Behaviour* **106**, 27–35

Walsh EA, McBride A, Bishop F and Muser Leyvraz A (2007) Influence of breed, handler appearance and people's experience of dogs on their perception of the temperament of a breed of dog in Ireland. *Proceedings of the 16th Annual Meeting of the International Society for Anthrozoology*, 32

Warwick C, Arena P, Lindley S, Jessop M and Steedman C (2013) Assessing reptile welfare using behavioural criteria. *In Practice* **35**, 123–131

Waters AJ, Nicol CJ and French NP (2002) Factors influencing the development of stereotypic and redirected behaviours in young horses: findings of a four year prospective epidemiological study. *Equine Veterinary Journal* **34**, 572–579

Weinstock M (2008) The long-term behavioural consequences of prenatal stress. *Neuroscience and Biobehavioral Reviews* **32**, 1073–1086

Wilkins AM, McCrae LS and McBride EA (2015) Factors affecting the human attribution of emotions toward animals. *Anthrozoös* **28**, 357–369

Winlow W and Di Cosmo A (2019) Sentience, Pain and Anesthesia in Advanced Invertebrates. *Frontiers in Physiology* **10**, 1141

Wolpe J (1952) Experimental neuroses as learned behaviour. *British Journal of Psychology* **43**, 243–268

Wynne CD and Udell MA (2013) *Animal cognition: evolution, behavior and cognition*. Macmillan International Higher Education, London

Yang Z, Bertolucci F, Wolf R and Heisenberg M (2013) Flies cope with uncontrollable stress by learned helplessness. *Current Biology* **23**, 799–803

Yeates J (2019) *Companion Animal Care and Welfare: The UFAW Companion Animal Handbook*. John Wiley and Sons, Chichester

Yerkes R and Dodson JD (1908) The relation of strength of stimulus to rapidity of habit-formation. *Journal of Comparative Neurology and Psychology* **18**, 459–482

Young RW (2003) Evolution of the human hand: the role of throwing and clubbing. *Journal of Anatomy* **202**, 165–174

Ziv G (2017) The effects of using aversive training methods in dogs – A review. *Journal of Veterinary Behavior* **19**, 50–60

Useful websites

Animal Facial Action Coding System
www.animalfacs.com

Cats Protection
www.cats.org.uk/help-and-advice/cat-behaviour/cat-body-language

Lafeber Company – Pet Bird and Parrot Behaviour
lafeber.com/pet-birds/bird-behavior

National Centre for the Replacement, Refinement and Reduction of Animals in Research (NC3Rs)
www.nc3rs.org.uk

Rabbit Welfare Association and Fund
rabbitwelfare.co.uk/behaviour

Rat Behaviour
lafeber.com/mammals/category/rat/rat-behavior

Royal Society for the Prevention of Cruelty to Animals
www.rspca.org.uk/adviceandwelfare

Studying seals
sealbehaviour.wordpress.com

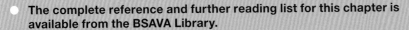

Further reading

● The complete reference and further reading list for this chapter is available from the BSAVA Library.

Access via QR code or: bsavalibrary.com/pvw_3

Chapter 4

Animal enrichment

Molly Varga Smith and Craig Tessyman

Introduction

Most people working directly with animals understand that enrichment (e.g. making an *ad hoc* toy for a stray kitten or using a Kong® toy to occupy an anxious dog in a hospital ward) makes a difference to the lives of the individuals under their care. The provision of environmental enrichment is also directly associated with attempts to improve animal welfare.

It should be remembered that a captive animal's experience of life is not the same as that of its wild counterparts. Captivity is inevitably accompanied by compromises in terms of nutrition, environmental conditions, social interaction and the ability to display normal behaviours. There are positive and negative aspects to both captive and wild states that impact welfare, manifesting as changes in behaviour, alterations in reproductive success and the viability of an individual to succeed when released into or living in the wild. Understanding what is available to animals in the wild is key to enriching a captive environment.

In some instances, domestication has sufficiently altered a species such that its behaviour is very different from that of its wild counterparts. In these cases, captivity has a different impact on individual animals of that species than it does for newly captured wild animals. This is not to suggest that life as a domesticated animal cannot be negatively impacted by poor welfare. Enrichment may mean different provisions when applied to domesticated species, such as dogs, cats and rabbits, compared with captive wild animals (e.g. injured animals undergoing rehabilitation) or those in zoological collections, but the principles remain the same.

The 'Five Freedoms' (the aspects of captive animal welfare that are under human control) should inform the way that all animals are kept in captivity (see also Chapter 1):

- Freedom from hunger and thirst
- Freedom from discomfort
- Freedom from pain, injury and disease
- Freedom to express normal behaviour
- Freedom from fear and distress.

It should be borne in mind that enrichment is not a replacement for basic care but is provided in addition to these fundamental requirements. Thus, in order for an animal's environment to be truly enriched, the animal should be able to easily access food and water in a manner that is behaviourally appropriate, the environment should not cause damage to the animal when it is exhibiting normal behaviours, and it should allow the animal to protect itself from fear and distress, whilst allowing the owner or keeper sufficient access to be able to notice if the animal becomes unwell.

The relative importance of each Freedom may change, depending upon the situation. This means that the way in which environmental enrichment is approached will alter. For example, in a clinical situation, observation of the patient may take precedence and for a 'shy' species this means a reduced ability to be removed from fear and distress (i.e. a prey species in a hospital ward may not have as much ability to remove itself from perceived threats as would be ideal for the animal in the home environment). Similarly, performing normal exercise activities may be discouraged to reduce pain in postoperative patients or trauma cases, even though it reduces an animal's ability to display normal behaviour.

The way that welfare is measured also needs to be evaluated (see Chapter 2). The exhibition of stereotypical behaviours (i.e. the persistent repetition of an act by an animal for no obvious purpose) has traditionally been associated with animals kept in conditions that do not adequately meet their welfare needs. However, these behaviours need to be accurately characterized. For example, in one group of kennelled working dogs, repetitive behaviour was noted and assumed to be stereotypical; however, on closer observation the behaviour was associated with the presence of kennel staff who inadvertently reinforced the behaviour and thereby caused it to become a learned response (Denham *et al.*, 2014). It is beyond the scope of this chapter to provide a list of behaviours that are always associated with a poor environment, due to the variety of animals that are kept, but a suggested reading list is provided at the end of the chapter (see 'References and further reading').

Enrichment types

Definitions of enrichment are as varied as the species to which they refer. In general terms, enrichment is a combination of environmental factors (with or without the presence of humans) that tend to increase the amount of time a captive animal spends exploring, foraging in and/or manipulating its environment. Enrichment encourages mental engagement and physical mobility, as well as normal behaviour patterns (see Chapter 3). The presence or absence of humans can also produce interesting effects; pet animals often benefit from the presence of humans, whilst wild animals may become stressed by human contact. Habituation of both wild and zoological species in order to reduce this stress is well reported. Training of both domestic and zoological animals can serve enrichment goals by promoting desired behaviours and reducing stress in adverse situations (see Chapter 6).

Definitions of enrichment

National Animal Welfare Trust

The National Animal Welfare Trust (NAWT) defines (canine) enrichment "enrichment improves and enhances your dog's mental state using a range of activities designed to challenge and exercise their brains. These activities encourage your dog to problem solve, learn new skills and become more confident" (NAWT, 2022). Puzzle feeders are an example of simple enrichment tools that follow the principles of the NAWT definition (see 'Feeding enrichment', below).

International Cat Care

International Cat Care (ICC) has a slightly different take on enrichment, defining it as "making provisions within a cat's confined environment that stimulate and challenge and enable it to perform natural behaviour" (ICC, 2018). Many forms of play, such as encouraging cats to engage in natural predation behaviours to attain rewards, meet the ICC definition of enrichment (see 'Play', below).

Association of Zoos and Aquariums

The Association of Zoos and Aquariums (AZA) defines environmental enrichment as a "process for improving or enhancing animal environments and care within the context of their inhabitants' behavioural biology and natural history. It is a dynamic process in which changes to structures and husbandry practices are made with the goal of increasing behavioural choices available to animals and drawing out their species-appropriate behaviours and abilities, thus enhancing welfare" (Behavior and Husbandry Advisory Group, 1999). See 'Zoological collections', below, for examples that reflect the AZA definition of enrichment.

Summary

Other species-specific organizations provide definitions, but they are all variations on a theme and are dependent on the species being considered and the complexities of its natural behaviour. Despite the variation between definitions, the ultimate message is that enrichment tends to bring about a positive change to the welfare of captive animals. The important point is to address enrichment within the constraints of the situation and to recognize that not enriching an environment because there is conflicting information is worse than at least trying.

It is important to consider how enrichment can be provided. Changes to the animal's environment, provision of conspecific company, alterations to how food is presented (in particular the use of foraging toys/puzzle feeders), provision of human company, use of training to achieve certain ends and play (whether autonomous or with human/conspecific interaction) can all be part of an enrichment programme. Enrichment programmes are informed by the species involved; they should be dynamic and ever-evolving and may take countless forms.

Social enrichment

Social enrichment relates to the provision of companionship for captive animals. An example of this is keeping social animals together in groups (such as bonded pairs of rabbits, meerkats in zoological collections and friendly horses when turned out to the field). Animals that are not social in nature (e.g. Syrian hamsters, pandas and many reptile species) should not be housed together as they may become stressed or even fight when kept in groups.

Environmental enrichment

Different species have different basic requirements in terms of the environment/enclosure that should be provided. Providing an interesting, appropriate and varied environment is one of the most common forms of enrichment that augments these fundamental requirements. Examples include the provision of hide boxes and toys for small rodent species and the use of puzzle feeders for a variety of species, from pet parrots to large felids in zoological collections. Interaction with the environment (e.g. cat trees for domestic homes or platforms in large cat enclosures within a zoo) can provide the animal with an opportunity to display an increased range of normal behaviours.

Feeding enrichment

Food-related toys (e.g. puzzle feeders) are commonly used to provide feeding enrichment for pet animals such as dogs, cats, rabbits and small rodents. These toys are one method of providing positive reinforcement of a behaviour, providing occupation and increasing the amount of time spent engaged in the activity of feeding. In larger captive species, the method of food provision itself can become the enrichment; for example, the use of whole carcasses and placing these in elevated or hidden positions within an enclosure is a common strategy to provide enrichment for carnivores in zoological collections.

Exercise

Most animals benefit from moving and exercising their bodies in the normal course of their lives. Captivity can negatively impact the amount of exercise an animal undertakes, leading to problems such as obesity (see Chapter 5). Encouraging exercise, often in combination with social and environmental enrichment, can be very helpful. For example, two dogs will often play together, horses will often gallop around a field with a friendly conspecific, and hamsters and other small rodents may choose to run in activity wheels if they are provided.

Training

Many species that are kept in captivity are trained for both work and safety reasons. Positive reinforcement training should be encouraged and can be applied to many species in a variety of different situations; for example, guinea pigs can be 'clicker' trained to come when called, parrots can be trained to present a foot or wing for clinical examination, and elephants can be trained to present their feet for clinical care and their ears for blood sampling. When implemented correctly, training utilizes the natural behaviours of an animal to achieve the desired outcome. See Chapter 6 for further information on welfare-focused animal training.

Training can also be beneficial in a clinical setting. For example, training a dog to tolerate a clinical examination (including checking of the eyes, ears and feet) from an early age can help when that animal is presented to the veterinary clinic with a clinical problem or painful condition. The Fear Free® initiative, which is increasingly gaining acceptance within the veterinary profession, advocates positive reinforcement training and the use of minimal restraint for most animals within a clinical setting. The initiative aims to reduce the stress and anxiety an animal feels during a visit to the veterinary practice. The veterinary team should work with owners to implement training plans that will minimize patient stress (see Chapters 6 and 7).

Play

Play is an important part of the development of young animals. It can define and inform hierarchy within a group (as seen with boxing in hares), it can test and develop strength and coordination, and it can teach animals how to behave, survive and thrive within their environment. Adult animals often play less autonomously (unless interacting with their young), although dogs are an exception to this rule. However, play can be used as a form of enrichment in captive adult animals; for example, cats playing with laser pointers, elephants playing with tractor tyres and adult langurs swinging on vines. Essentially, animals interacting with their environment where there is not an outcome of positive reinforcement are playing.

Enrichment in clinical settings

In a clinical setting, even simple attempts at enrichment can be helpful and reduce stress in patients (see Chapter 7). Clinical enrichment can encompass several of the types described above, including play, training, social and environmental. For example, providing hide boxes for timid cats or prey animals such as rabbits, allowing a bonded companion to attend veterinary appointments with the patient (rabbits and guinea pigs) and training zoological species to present themselves for clinical examination or blood sampling can all be useful in a clinical setting.

Domestic species

For the purposes of this chapter, 'domestic species' refers to dogs, cats and rabbits.

Dogs

Those who keep or work with dogs will recognize behaviours that are reminiscent of wild dogs or wolves and these traits can vary depending on the breed. Retrievers will naturally retrieve, whilst herding dogs will naturally herd. Domestic dogs, however, are not animals that are a single degree away from their wild counterparts; several thousand years of domestication have inevitably altered the species in terms of behaviour.

In recent years, there has been a lot of controversy around how dogs are kept and how humans interact with them. Dogs can display a variety of behaviours when their physical or psychological wellbeing is suboptimal. It can be difficult to determine whether expression of a particular behaviour is indicative of poor welfare and, therefore, it is hard to know whether enrichment efforts have been successful or not.

Enrichment for pet dogs should include human interaction and training. Owning a dog (or any pet) should be enriching for both the animal and human, and spending time bonding with the pet benefits both parties. The amount of time that dogs can be left alone depends on the individual; physical needs such as toileting and the provision of food and water need to be taken into account. To an extent, this will also depend on the age of the dog; younger and geriatric individuals often require more attention than healthy adults to address their physical needs. Some individuals may have psychological needs (such as separation anxiety) that require more attention. The Royal Society for the Prevention of Cruelty to Animals (RSPCA) recommends that dogs should be left for no longer than 4 hours without being attended (RSPCA, 2015). The use of dog walkers and 'doggy day care' allows busy and working owners to meet the needs of their pets in ways that suit the modern lifestyle.

Social enrichment

Dogs are pack animals, meaning that in the wild they live socially and benefit from interaction with conspecifics. Living as a pack brings advantages in terms of food acquisition, avoidance of threats and rearing of young. In a domestic situation, there may be advantages and disadvantages of having more than one dog in a home. Many dogs will benefit from positive interactions with other dogs (Figure 4.1), although most dogs will form strong bonds with their owners that fulfil the need for social interaction. In households with multiple dogs, competition for resources can cause conflict. Whilst this can be managed, even 'stable' packs can fight, which is detrimental and can potentially cause physical trauma.

Feeding enrichment

In the wild, dogs are opportunistic feeders, which is hard to replicate in captivity. Providing a bowl of dog food once or twice daily removes the need for locating, stalking and killing prey. Filling this time with alternative activities such as walks and play provides enrichment, as does the use of puzzle feeders (Figure 4.2), foraging bowls and toys that can be filled with various types of foods that take longer to access than in a bowl (e.g. Kong® toys).

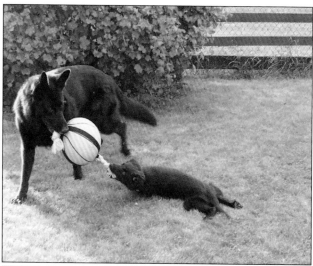

4.1 Puppies benefit from engaging in play with well socialized adult dogs.
(Reproduced from the *BSAVA Manual of Canine and Feline Behavioural Medicine*)

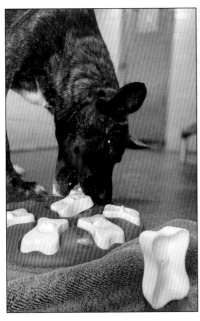

4.2 This puzzle feeder provides physical and mental stimulation to the dog using it.
(Shutterstock.com/Ryan Brix)

Exercise

Exercise is crucial for the physical and mental wellbeing of dogs. The breed (especially if bred for a specific purpose), demeanour of the individual dog and the size of its home environment should all be taken into account when determining how much exercise is required. An assessment regarding the appropriate type and amount of exercise should be made on an individual basis and should also take into account any underlying medical conditions. Most dogs display high levels of exploratory behaviour (Siwak *et al.*, 2001), and it is important that this be factored in to both the home environment and exercise routine.

Over the past few years, there have been concerns raised about how dogs are exercised, in particular the use of repetitive movements (e.g. retrieving a ball) or participation in agility training/events. In a natural setting, dogs will instinctively chase after prey in order to eat. This instinct has not been lost and both retrieving and agility in some ways capitalize on this instinct. It is clearly unacceptable to put an animal in a position where it could potentially damage itself; however, the judicious use of some of these exercise techniques positively benefits many individuals, providing they are fit, the equipment and obstacles are appropriate and the dogs participating have been properly trained.

Training

Training is also important for pet dogs and can take many different forms. At a minimum, it allows owners to have a degree of confidence when dealing with their dogs both inside and outside the home. Training should be reward based (positive reinforcement should be paired with negative punishment; see Chapter 3). Aversive training methods, such as the use of shock collars, are not recommended. The reader is referred to Chapter 6 and the 'References and further reading' at the end of this chapter for examples of positive reinforcement training.

Play

Time for play is as important as training and should be viewed positively as a form of enrichment. Many dogs enjoy playing with toys, either autonomously or with their owners. Chew toys are especially popular as most dogs are highly motivated to chew. Many dogs also enjoy retrieving balls or bumpers (often playing on their natural instincts), although in some circles this is now viewed as potentially damaging as it can predispose dogs to abnormal joint loading and either acute or chronic injury if the same action is repeated for too long and/or too often.

Enrichment in clinical settings

Providing enrichment for canine patients in a clinical setting is vitally important, because there will be compromises in what can be provided in the veterinary practice compared with what may be provided in the animal's normal home environment. Human interaction (outside of physical examination and the administration of medication) is positive for most canine patients and can take the form of grooming, encouragement to eat and short walks to allow toileting, if the animal is well enough. These interactions allow better evaluation of an individual's condition, particularly with regard to general mentation and pain scoring (see Chapter 2), and can be helpful in determining an accurate clinical assessment.

However, not all animals are confident and friendly, and recognizing the different needs of individual patients is also important. Some dogs will benefit from being able to hide away from practice staff, either behind a barrier or in a hide box. Whilst this helps the animal, it may compromise the ability of the staff to visually monitor the patient and to access it within or remove it from the kennel; this may lead to an increased prominence of behaviours such as cage guarding. Those canine patients whose behaviour presents a physical risk to staff may benefit from muzzle training. Muzzle training should be a positive experience for the dog (associated with positive reinforcement) and, ultimately, allows staff to be safe whilst handling the animal (see Chapter 6).

A muzzled dog should be handled with the same respect for its psychological welfare as any other animal, ideally with positive reinforcement as appropriate, and it must be remembered that an aversive event will still be aversive, regardless of whether or not a muzzle is fitted. Basket muzzles are preferred because they allow dogs to eat, drink, pant and display some social signals (such as a curled lip as a warning sign). Open-ended fabric muzzles may be appropriate for short-term use, but they still compromise panting and the ability to display social cues, and do not always prevent dogs from biting. In an emergency, a tape muzzle can be useful, but these muzzles should not be left *in situ* for extended periods of time. Figure 4.3 provides examples of the different types of muzzles available.

The provision of toys can also provide enrichment in a clinical setting; for example, the use of size-appropriate Kong® toys provides safe entertainment and engagement for many dogs during stressful situations. The advantage of using a Kong® toy is that it can be adequately disinfected and reused with subsequent patients.

Working dogs

The considerations for working dogs are slightly different to those for pet dogs. Human interaction and training are still both vitally important, but the animal is required to perform a set job. Working dogs and their handlers are often intensely bonded and, as is the case with military working dogs, lives may depend on the understanding between dog and handler. ▶

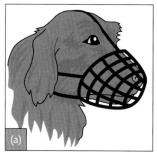 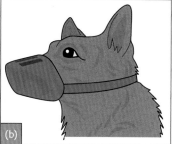 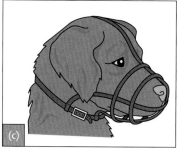 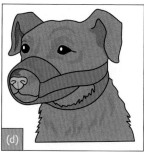

4.3 Examples of muzzles. (a) Closed basket type. (b) Closed plastic type. (c) Semi-closed leather type. (d) Open-ended fabric type.
(Reproduced from the BSAVA Textbook of Veterinary Nursing)

Working dogs *continued*

Working dogs are often kept in outdoor kennels (rather than in a home environment) and may be housed in the same facility with many other animals. Working dogs also benefit from enrichment strategies, such as being housed with another animal and the use of puzzle feeders, in addition to human contact and training. Working dogs that are not stressed have been shown to work more effectively.

Cats

It is believed that feline domestication occurred in a process not directly instigated by humans. When farming became more popular, 8000 years ago, mice moved into the fields to eat the grains being cultivated and cats moved closer to human dwellings in order to eat the mice. Cats and humans developed a mutually beneficial relationship, as the cats reduced the mouse population and humans provided the cats with warmth and security. When the Egyptians started to migrate across into the Mediterranean and Old World, 3500 years ago, they brought cats with them. It is believed that they were attracted to traits such as sociability and tameness in these cats.

There are many different ideas on how domestic cats should be kept, each with potential advantages and disadvantages. The main points for consideration include:

- Should cats be kept indoors all the time or have access to the outside?
- Should cats be kept in single-animal households or can multiple cats be housed together?

Social enrichment

Single cats will have a larger territory and potentially be less stressed than cats in multi-cat households. However, in multi-cat households, if the animals get along well then they will have companionship during the hours that the owners are not at home and can engage in play together. This may have the added advantage of preventing the cats from becoming overweight due to sleeping during the hours they are alone.

Environmental enrichment

Cats with access to the outside have a larger territory in which to roam and engage in natural behaviours, but this can be detrimental to the local wildlife, especially if the cat has free access to the outdoors. There is also the potential for cats to stray, fight with other cats that encroach on their territory and become involved in road traffic accidents. Indoor cats have protection from many potentially harmful situations and the environment in which they live is their own. However, if there is little enrichment provided in the home, indoor cats are more likely to lead a sedentary lifestyle and may become obese.

Owners of both indoor and outdoor cats need to focus on creating an environment that exceeds the needs of the inhabitants. This involves looking at both the horizontal and vertical spaces available in the home; making use of vertical space is advantageous especially in multi-cat households and smaller homes, as the more vertical space that is available, the more territory the cats have to share. Vertical space can be created using cat trees (Figure 4.4), shelves or wall-mounted beds; these come in a variety of shapes and sizes, with some extending to the ceiling, and there are different options depending on budget.

There should be more beds and resting places than there are cats in the environment. This is because cats will change the location that they wish to sleep in a number of times a day, as it is unsafe in the wild to be in the same place all the time and all together in a group.

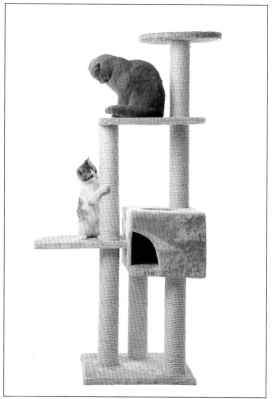

4.4 Cat trees are an efficient way to provide meaningful enrichment with a small area of floor space.
(Shutterstock.com/Africa Studio)

Feeding enrichment

As with dogs, feeding enrichment can be provided for cats. The use of puzzle feeders (e.g. Kong® toys), food cubes or even hiding food in paper bags will provide enrichment via play and hunting (Figure 4.5).

Play

Small cat toys such as fabric mice and balls can be used as hunting items, but oversized toys may be needed to help express natural behaviours such as 'bunny' kicking and killing. The use of flying and stick toys encourages cats to leap and pounce as they would in the wild. These are particularly effective for energetic breeds or for tiring cats out before bedtime. The use of laser pointers has advantages and disadvantages. Cats will hunt on average 5–8 times a day and use of a laser pointer can provide some of the mental and physical stimulation that they need to replicate this activity. Unfortunately, the use of a laser pointer does not provide the same satisfaction as hunting, as the laser can never be caught, and this may lead to frustration, which the cat may take out on their owner or another cat in the household. To prevent this frustration, an item that can be physically caught, such as a toy or treats, should be used at the end of the play session.

Enrichment in clinical settings

In the veterinary practice, the use of multi level cages with shelves will give the cat control over where it chooses to sleep. A box half covered with a towel can be used to provide a place to hide. It is advisable to ask the owner whether the cat uses a litter tray, whether it is open or closed and what substrate is used, in order to replicate these provisions within the hospital. If the cat is willing to engage in play, suitably sized balls of dressing material can be used as a play item or tied to a length of bandage and suspended from the top of the enclosure or the kennel door.

Rabbits

Of the three 'domesticated' species discussed in this chapter, rabbits have retained behaviours that are most closely aligned with those of their wild counterparts. This is because rabbits have been bred for traits other than

specific behaviours. In contrast to dogs and cats, rabbits are a prey species and this informs the ways in which enrichment should be provided.

Social enrichment

Rabbits are an intensely social species (McBride, 1988) and it is recommended that they should not be kept singly if this can be avoided. The presence of a *compatible* conspecific is a very beneficial type of enrichment, allowing normal social behaviours such as mutual grooming to occur (Varga, 2013; see also 'Useful websites'). The authors do not advocate keeping rabbits with guinea pigs as companions; guinea pigs are often bullied due to their smaller size, their food requirements are different, and rabbits may carry *Bordetella bronchiseptica* asymptomatically, which can cause pneumonia in guinea pigs. However, where there is an established bond between a guinea pig and a rabbit, it is not suggested that this be disrupted. In some cases, where bonding with other rabbits has repeatedly failed and where owners are dedicated enough to become part of the rabbit's social structure, a rabbit can be kept as a singleton.

Environmental enrichment

Rabbits can be kept either as house rabbits (Figure 4.6) or outside (Figure 4.7). In either case, the enclosure provided should be of sufficient size to allow normal behaviours to be performed. In the wild, rabbits are territorial and may range over an area the size of several football pitches in order to obtain food and defend territory. In recent years, research has been performed to evaluate space usage in pet rabbits and a minimum space requirement has been suggested (Rooney *et al.*, 2014). In addition, the Rabbit Welfare Association and Fund (RWAF) 'A hutch is not enough' campaign publicized the need for rabbits to have adequately sized indoor and outdoor environments. The current RWAF recommendation for a pair of average sized rabbits is an enclosure with a minimum footprint of 3 m by 2 m, which should include a sheltered area of 1.8 m by 0.6 m (see 'Useful websites').

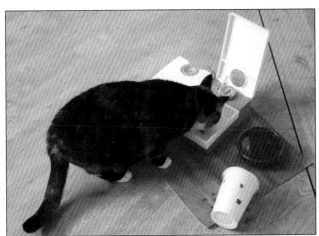

4.5 An automated feeder can be used to offer a cat small meals during the day when the owner is absent. When rolled, the white plastic container delivers the daily dry food ration through cut-out holes – this is a form of feeding enrichment and requires the cat to spend more time eating.

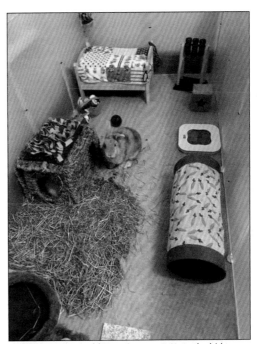

4.6 Indoor rabbit environment. Note the hide areas and tunnels, puzzle feeders and toys with food rewards.

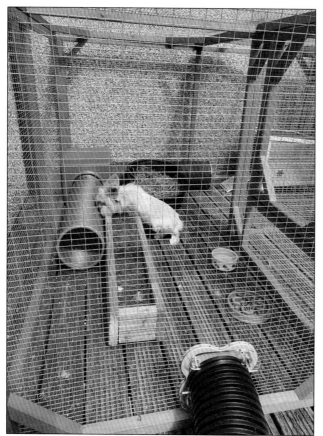

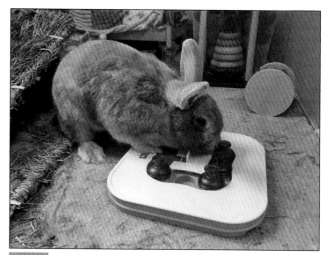

4.8 Rabbit playing with a puzzle feeder.

4.7 Outdoor rabbit environment that has been enclosed to prevent predation. Note the provision of both tunnels and hides, enough space to allow normal mobility and growing weeds to encourage foraging behaviour.

As rabbits are prey animals, they will benefit from having refuge areas within their enclosure. These may take the form of hide boxes or tunnels. In most situations, the authors recommend that the enclosure housing a pair or group of rabbits has one more hide box than there are inhabitants, so that each animal can hide in a separate box and also be able to run from one hide box to an empty one should they wish to do so. Each hide box should only be large enough to contain a single animal, so if there is conflict they can escape. Additional larger hide boxes and tunnels can also be provided. It should be noted that a tunnel is not equivalent to a hide box as there is no protection from predators at either end; however, they are useful for allowing a rabbit to move safely from one place to another within the enclosure. A wide range of proprietary rabbit hide boxes and tunnels is commercially available; however, a cardboard hide box can be replaced easily and rabbits often appear to enjoy both hiding in and demolishing these types of hide.

Feeding enrichment

Wild rabbits spend several hours each day foraging and eating. For pet rabbits that are provided with a bowl of concentrated feed, this requirement is removed, meaning that a lot of the time that would ordinarily be occupied by foraging and eating is left free. Rabbits should primarily be fed on hay, with concentrated food comprising only a small portion of the ration. This in itself increases the amount of time the rabbit spends feeding. Rabbits also benefit from being able to forage and eat growing plants and grass. The use of puzzle feeders (Figure 4.8), strategies such as scatter feeding, and the use of food-based toys (such as hay or sisal

mats that can be destroyed and then eaten) can increase the amount of time the rabbit spends expressing foraging and eating behaviours. In addition, presenting hay or herbs in an elevated position encourages rabbits to periscope (stand on their hind legs); this is an effective way of making use of vertical space within the enclosure.

Training and play

Many pet rabbits enjoy human interaction and play time; the use of toys and even some training can be viewed as positive enrichment. However, it should be remembered that rabbits are inherently fearful of being lifted off the ground, so play that involves direct handling should take place on the floor. Toys for rabbits should encourage natural behaviours, such as running, jumping and digging. Digging trays are a good source of enrichment and access to outdoor areas where digging is permitted can be valuable. Balls and other objects that can be thrown are also popular as toys for rabbits; willow balls, in particular, are useful because they can be chewed as well as thrown. Often rabbits will interact with balls and throw them around of their own accord. Cardboard play structures are also available and allow expression of several behaviours, including hiding, jumping and chewing. In addition, rabbits can be trained to accept certain health procedures, such as nail trimming or checking teeth, using positive reinforcement (see Chapters 3 and 6). This is beneficial as it allows owners to check the health of their rabbits on a regular basis without causing undue stress.

Enrichment in clinical settings

In the veterinary practice, it is very important that rabbits are recognized as prey animals and that the practice team understands the potentially significant adverse effects associated with stress due to hospitalization. Ideally, rabbits (and other prey species) should not be housed in the same ward as predators (e.g. dogs and cats) and, if possible, they should be located outwith the sight, smell and sounds of predatory species. All prey animals should be provided with some form of hide box within their enclosure; this may compromise direct observation of the rabbit by the team, but the benefits to the patient's wellbeing outweigh this concern.

Rabbits are a social species, and therefore the authors always advocate keeping bonded pairs together within the veterinary practice in order to reduce the stress on both individuals. Whilst having two animals within an enclosure can make observation of parameters such as food intake, volume of urine output and faecal production more challenging, this is not an insurmountable problem (time spent encouraging and allowing observation is valuable in these circumstances) and companionship will be positive in terms of welfare. It should be borne in mind that the patient's welfare is likely to be compromised by its clinical condition, so admittance to the veterinary practice should have a positive impact. Whereas, for the companion animal that is brought into the practice healthy, the hospitalization experience must not compromise its welfare.

Enrichment for non-domesticated species

The basic principles and different types of enrichment are constant and can be applied equally to domesticated and non-domesticated species. The level of detail provided above for dogs, cats and rabbits is made possible by a longer history of recognition of their needs and cognitive abilities, but the methods described can be modified to provide a better captive environment for any animal.

The following sections take into account the natural history and unique needs of various groups of non-domesticated animals. Species-specific guidance is also given for some key species that are commonly kept. The reader is encouraged to adapt this information for use with the animals in their care.

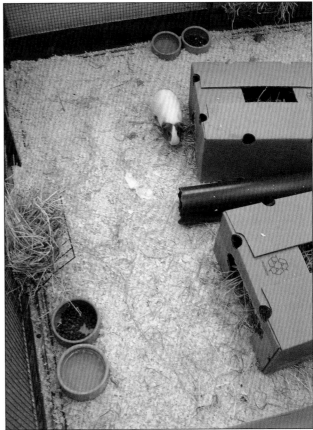

4.9 Typical guinea pig housing. Cardboard boxes facilitate gnawing and multiple sources of food and water are available.

Exotic pets

Small mammals

The trend of increasing interest in exotic pets shows no sign of slowing and the number of small mammals kept as pets continues to grow. Although many small mammals have very specific requirements, their needs can be met with the correct husbandry. In terms of the environment provided, this should take into consideration the design of the enclosure, building materials, size, substrates, temperature, humidity, light, ventilation, furniture, water, ease of cleaning and social structure of the species being kept. For detailed information on the basic requirements for the captive maintenance of small mammals, the reader is referred to the *BSAVA Manual of Exotic Pets* and the *BSAVA Manual of Rodents and Ferrets*.

Guinea pigs

Guinea pigs are increasingly commonly kept as pets and are much less likely to be viewed as a child's pet than previously. Guinea pigs are a social species and, as such, keeping two or more animals together is positive in terms of enrichment, as long as they are compatible. The authors do not advocate keeping guinea pigs with rabbits as companions (see 'Rabbits', above).

Guinea pigs are typically housed in pens, cages, aquaria or hutches made of wood, plastic, concrete, stainless steel or wire (Figure 4.9). The flooring should be smooth and covered with hardwood shavings, shredded or pelleted recycled paper, or hay. Guinea pigs are sensitive to heat and humidity, so their environment must be well insulated and ventilated. The space required will depend on the number of guinea pigs to be housed together. Guinea pigs do not tend to burrow themselves but will seek refuge in the burrows of other animals. Guinea pigs are prey animals and benefit from hide boxes; the rule of one hide box per animal, plus one applies. Guinea pigs also enjoy tunnels, but these are not equivalent to hide boxes as they can allow individuals to be chased.

In the wild, a large amount of a guinea pig's time is spent foraging for food and eating. Strategies such as scatter feeding and the use of puzzle feeders can increase the amount of time they spend interacting with food and thereby reduce boredom. As a rodent species, guinea pigs are adapted to gnaw and provision of suitable toys in the environment can help promote this activity.

Guinea pigs also enjoy interaction with their owners and toys, suitable treats and even training can reinforce this. It must be remembered that some individuals may be shy or find human interaction aversive and their desire to be left alone should be respected.

In a hospital environment, the authors advocate keeping bonded companions together where possible. If an owner has a group of several guinea pigs, then bringing two together is a practical compromise that will benefit the patient and be minimally disruptive to the group. Provision of hide boxes in a clinical situation is beneficial even though it can compromise observation. Provision of suitable food and things to gnaw on can also reduce stress. As with other prey species, guinea pigs should be kept separately from predators and clinical staff should remember that they themselves may be perceived as predators in this situation. Guinea pigs can become stressed very easily in a hospital situation and in particular appear to find injections aversive.

Hamsters

There are 12 species of hamster and their social enrichment needs vary. Some should be kept alone (e.g. Syrian hamsters), some may be kept with or without conspecifics (e.g. Chinese hamsters) and others are highly sociable and should not be without company (e.g. Campbell's dwarf hamsters).

Hamsters are naturally inquisitive and typically kept in small wire or plastic cages, or aquarium-style tanks, which should be a minimum size of 75 cm × 30 cm × 30 cm. The addition of levels and tube networks reduces stress levels and keeps hamsters from getting bored (Figure 4.10). In the wild, hamsters dig and make tunnels, so an area to allow them to perform this natural behaviour is encouraged (Figure 4.11). If this is not possible, then the inclusion of tunnels and pipes will keep them entertained. Wheels are a great addition to keep a hamster entertained and also to exercise; hamsters will travel up to 9 kilometres (5.6 miles) in a 24-hour period in the wild. Wheels should have a solid back and sides to prevent injuries and must be of sufficient diameter (the hamster's back should be straight during use); saucer style wheels are one design that removes the risk of back arching (see Figures 4.10 and 4.12). Taking care to keep the wheel clean will prevent damage to the feet of the hamster that could lead to infections of the skin and feet.

There are different opinions about the use of hamster balls. As hamsters are unable to remove themselves from the ball, hide or stop when they are tired, it is the authors' opinion, and that of the RSPCA, that they should be avoided where possible due to the added stress and potential chance of injury if left unsupervised.

Scatter feeding will encourage foraging; providing food in a bowl can lead to a lazy, bored hamster.

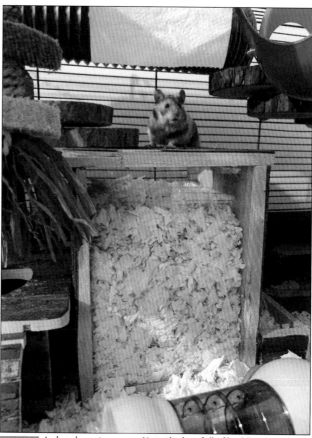

4.11 Indoor hamster space. Note the box full of bedding to encourage burrowing.

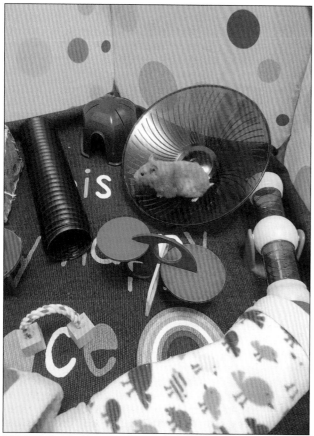

4.10 Enriched hamster play area including toys, hides and tunnels, along with areas of different textures to add interest. The saucer style wheel allows the hamster to run without arching its back.

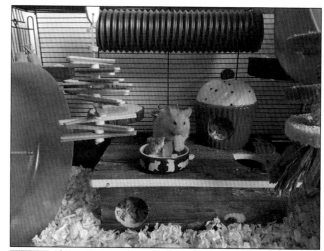

4.12 This environment includes lots of different levels, textures and cage furniture to encourage mobility and interaction with the environment. The wheel provided is large enough for the hamster to run comfortably and has a solid back and sides.

Rats

Laboratory rats are kept singly in small cages with no furniture and are handled two or three times a week; this is a boring life, and they have been shown to be less engaged and perform worse on memory tests than rats that have enrichment (Hullinger *et al.*, 2015).

In the wild, rats live in large groups and seek out companionship. It is advised that rats are housed in single-sex groups to stop unwanted breeding. Rats should be provided with large cages made of metal (they will gnaw through wood or plastic). Wood chips, shavings and sawdust are appropriate bedding materials. Rats make good use of vertical space; areas to climb, different levels and multiple sleeping areas are advised so the rats can choose to spend time together or alone (Figures 4.13 and 4.14). Providing boxes, balls and tubes that are rotated every few days encourages play and prevents boredom. A wheel is beneficial but not necessary and should always be made of a solid material that is easy to clean. Wire wheels are not recommended as feet and tails can get caught in rungs.

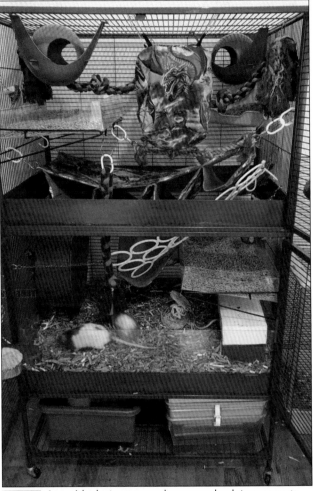

4.13 An enriched rat cage spread over many levels to encourage climbing and exploration. A variety of textures and substrates are available as well as hide areas.

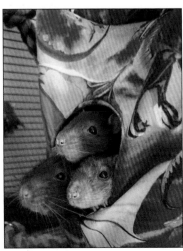

4.14 Rats huddled together in a hammock. Rats prefer to sleep in suspended hammocks and the presence of conspecifics can contribute to social enrichment.

A minimum play space of 1.5 m x 1.5 m where the rats can have supervised time with the owner is advised; this area should have capacity for climbing and playing to encourage exercise and should be regularly moved around to prevent boredom. Rats should have access to their play area daily for a minimum of 45 minutes a day and should handled during this time. Food-oriented play can also feature with items that the rats only get during this play time (e.g. bowls of water with floating 'islands' of food or frozen peas).

Rats can be clicker trained and should be rewarded with healthy treats, such as corn and peas.

Mice

Laboratory mice have poorer memories and interest levels than mice that have enrichment. Single-sex groups are advisable, and littermates are preferred over different age pairings as the latter may fight over territory. The housing requirements of mice are similar to those of rats (see above). Scatter feeding, rather than feeding in a bowl, is more interesting to mice. Mice can be clicker trained and should be rewarded with healthy treats that they do not get in their daily feed (see Chapter 5).

Daily handling and giving the mice places to interact with owners during supervised times is advised, but care should be taken as mice are incontinent and leave a trail of urine wherever they go.

Gerbils

Wild gerbils live in colonies and, as such, it is not advised to house gerbils on their own; single-sex groups should be housed together and ideally be littermates. Gerbils should be housed in a gerbilarium so they can exhibit natural behaviours such as digging and making a burrow. Burrowing material such as wood shavings or aspen should be compacted down so that tunnels and burrows retain their shape.

It is important to provide items to gnaw on. Fruit tree branches can be exercised on as well as gnawed. Used cereal boxes and toilet roll tubes are cheap additions to the enclosure; these provide a plaything and gerbils will also gnaw them and use them as a burrowing material. Too many items at the same time can overexcite gerbils – two or three items at a time is ideal, and these can be changed every few days.

Chinchillas

Chinchillas are a social species and should be kept in compatible pairs where possible. Chinchillas may be housed in a room in the house or in a cage. If housed in a cage, this should be large (at least 2 m x 2 m x 1 m) and ideally made of wire since they will chew wooden furniture. Chinchillas are more agile and climb more readily than many rodent species, so providing them with vertical as well as horizontal space is important. In the wild, chinchillas (and many other rodent species) use dust baths to aid in grooming – these should be readily available within the captive environment.

Chinchillas are a prey species and, as such, should be provided with refuges so that they can hide from perceived predators as well as from companions during times of conflict. Cardboard boxes can be useful and allow a range of behaviours as they can be manipulated and shredded. Chinchillas often chew on wood within their enclosures, so wooden hide boxes can serve a dual purpose.

Changing how food is presented can provide interest and challenge within a chinchilla's environment. Scatter feeding, food-oriented toys and some puzzle feeders can be useful.

In a clinical situation, chinchillas should be treated in much the same way as other social prey animals – i.e. kept separate from predatory species and with a bonded companion. Often, the companion is the most important form of enrichment in the hospital environment, followed by a place to hide. In appropriate cases, the ability to dust bathe should also be allowed.

African pygmy hedgehogs

African pygmy hedgehogs are generally best housed individually. They are very prone to obesity and inactivity, thus enrichment and the opportunity to exercise and engage in play are vital. Large cages with multiple levels that are accessible via ramps and with different interesting items on each level are important to encourage movement. Large solid-walled wheels are frequently used by African pygmy hedgehogs but they will toilet on them, so care should be taken to keep the wheels clean. A box to dig in with substrate (e.g. shredded newspaper, aspen shavings) can also be provided.

A large play area is advised and daily interaction with the owner will keep hedgehogs entertained. Food hidden around the play area and toys (such as balls or Kong® toys) that can be rolled and played with will keep hedgehogs entertained. Before returning the hedgehog to its cage, items can be moved around and food/treats hidden so that the enrichment continues after 'play time'. Puzzle boxes with pulleys and levers designed for parrots can also be used, and hidden treats can be hung in the enclosure.

Ferrets

Ferrets have been domesticated for around 2500 years, historically as working animals in the UK; however, they are now more commonly kept as pets. In the wild, polecats (the wild ancestors of ferrets) are solitary animals that spend 14–18 hours sleeping every day. While modern ferrets still sleep for a large portion of the day, they can happily be kept in small compatible groups. Ferrets are naturally territorial, like to burrow and prefer to sleep in enclosed spaces. Ferrets may be kept outdoors in purpose-built wooden units (Figure 4.15) or housed indoors in tall wire cages similar to those used for chinchillas, as they appreciate vertical space.

Until recently, very little research had been undertaken on the impact of enrichment on ferret welfare. Sleeping enrichment items, for example ferret hammocks, are a key form of enrichment. Hammocks seem to be preferred to sleeping at ground level and can be positive in terms of social interaction as ferrets like to sleep together. However, ferrets are also territorial and intraspecific conflict can occur even in stable pairs/groups, particularly at times of stress (Rejigwart *et al.*, 2018).

Ferrets naturally like to burrow and in the wild have to hunt for food; therefore, foraging toys are popular. Ferrets will interact with foraging toys even when they are not hungry. Foraging toys made for cats are generally suitable.

Ferrets also seem to enjoy interacting with tunnels, particularly flexible systems; those made specifically for rabbits can be very useful to provide opportunities for exercise. As they are not prey animals, ferrets, while liking enclosed spaces for sleeping, have less need for hide boxes to avoid predation.

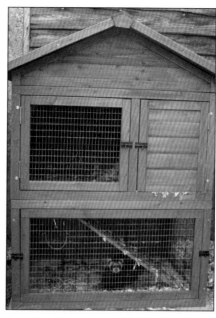

4.15 Basic ferret unit with sleeping quarters (upstairs) and a play area.

In clinical situations, where stress is a common factor, ferrets are less likely to benefit from having a companion than other small mammal species. In fact, the presence of a conspecific may cause conflict. Ferrets may be kept in a quiet cat ward if necessary but should be kept away from prey animals. In hospital, providing a ferret with suitable sleeping accommodation is an important enrichment factor: allowing them to have a hammock, particularly a familiar one, will encourage sleeping. Giving the ferret the opportunity to burrow, perhaps in soft bedding, is also helpful. Feeding enrichment can be provided for ferrets in hospital using toys that can be disinfected.

Reptiles

The number and type of reptiles being kept has exponentially increased over the past 10 years and, although there have been many positive improvements to reptile keeping over this time, a number of clinical conditions seen are still directly related to deficiencies in basic husbandry. It is perfectly possible to provide a good captive environment for many species of reptiles, allowing freedom from disease and encouraging normal behaviour. In terms of the environment provided, this should take into consideration the design of the enclosure, building materials, size, substrates, temperature, humidity, light, ventilation, furniture, water, ease of cleaning and social structure of the species being kept. Particular attention must be paid to the provision of ultraviolet (UV) light and a temperature gradient that allows animals to remain within their preferred optimal temperature zone (POTZ). For detailed information on the basic requirements for the captive maintenance of reptiles, the reader is referred to the *BSAVA Manual of Reptiles*.

Lizards

Lizards can be found on every continent except Antarctica, with different species adapted to living in all types of environment with the exception of areas of extreme cold and the oceans. Providing the correct environment for these animals is easily achieved in both home and zoological collections, but care should be taken to research the correct ambient temperatures, humidity, lighting and substrates required for each individual species. The size of the enclosure provided is important, and it should be noted that bigger is not necessarily better; large enclosures for small lizards such as leopard geckos may induce stress as the animals find it more difficult to catch their prey, whereas a small enclosure for a green iguana is not suitable as they grow rapidly and a large amount of space is required to be able to provide the necessary temperature and humidity gradients. The height of the enclosure is another important consideration; terrestrial species will not benefit from a tall vivarium and this will be wasted space, whereas arboreal species, such as green anoles and crested geckos, will benefit from a tall enclosure as they can utilize the vertical space (Figure 4.16). Vertical space can also be furnished to provide larger surface areas for these animals to explore and can be used for protection and hunting.

Bearded dragons: Bearded dragons are a commonly kept lizard species (Figure 4.17). They are naturally found in arid to semi-arid areas of Australia, where the vegetation ranges from woodland areas to rocky outcrops. Bearded dragons should be provided with an enclosure that contains a variety of basking areas (e.g. rocks, branches and hammocks), as well as areas to hide. This allows them to replicate the behaviour of their wild counterparts (basking during the morning and evening hours and hiding during the hottest part of the day). Tunnels that are designed for small cats and kittens can be provided when the bearded dragon is exercising outside of its enclosure and act as hides to escape if the animal becomes fearful or overexcited. Bearded dragons have been known to play

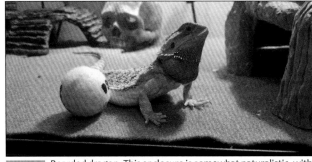

4.17 Bearded dragon. This enclosure is somewhat naturalistic, with the use of sand and hides, but also contains ornamentation for the owner's enjoyment and a tennis ball as a play item.
(Shutterstock.com/Brett Upshaw)

with small cat toys, such as lightweight balls and crinkle toys, or pieces of rolled up paper. Engagement begins by rolling the item towards the bearded dragon in order to get their attention; they learn that the item is a plaything and will run, jump and push the ball around. Bearded dragons are also known to sit in front of windows when out of their enclosure and the provision of a television or laptop may provide additional enrichment. It is important to remember not to have the volume too loud if the animal is unable to escape and hide.

Leopard geckos: Another commonly kept lizard is the leopard gecko (Figure 4.18). They are naturally found in the highlands of Asia and throughout Afghanistan to parts

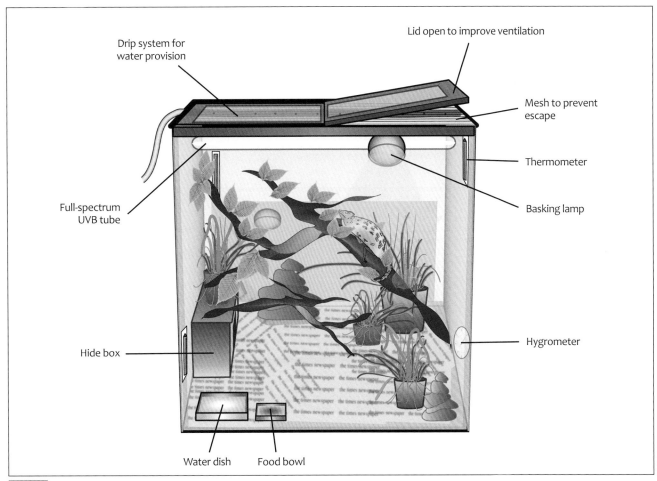

4.16 Arboreal environment for a lizard.

- Drip system for water provision
- Lid open to improve ventilation
- Mesh to prevent escape
- Thermometer
- Basking lamp
- Full-spectrum UVB tube
- Hide box
- Hygrometer
- Water dish
- Food bowl

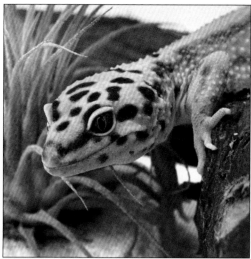

4.18 A leopard gecko. This species will make good use of logs as climbing frames.
(Shutterstock.com/Nyvlt-art)

of northern India. They are crepuscular and active mostly at twilight. Leopard geckos should be provided with an enclosure that contains shelves or elevated areas to allow them to move between areas containing different substrates and to select the environmental temperature they prefer. Both dry and moist hides should be provided; this allows the leopard gecko to choose an area with their preferred humidity when shedding their skin. As geckos are live feeders, they get some of their exercise and enrichment from hunting prey, but this activity will only constitute a small amount of the time they are awake. Placing live food into a cat Kong® toy or small puzzle box feeder will keep them interested in feeding for longer. Balls can be used to provide enrichment and leopard geckos will move these around their enclosure.

Snakes

Snakes can be found almost anywhere in the world, with the exception of Antarctica, Iceland, Ireland, Greenland and New Zealand. Commonly kept species include those belonging to the families Boidae (boa constrictor, royal python, Burmese python) and Colubridae (corn snake, kingsnake, garter snake). Snakes can be kept in either a plain clinical environment (i.e. a single substrate, a hide box and a water area) (Figure 4.19) or a well planted enriched environment.

With an enriched environment, the enclosure often features real or artificial planting, multiple hides, leaf litter coverage and different substrates. Providing more than one type of substrate (e.g. dry leaves, wood chips and soil) provides stimulation for the snake and allows the animal to choose where it wants to rest or sleep. The enclosure may also have variations in both terrestrial and arboreal levels. Adding levels to the enclosure interconnected with cork bark, branches or jungle vines provides the snake with more variation in terms of location and can help with thermoregulation. The provision of large water bowls, situated away from heat sources, gives the snake the opportunity to submerge itself in water and exercise by swimming.

In some instances, snake drawers are used. These are stacked small drawers that each house a single snake. The benefit to this type of set-up is that it allows owners to keep multiple snakes in a confined space. However, regardless of the type of enclosure selected, it should be of sufficient size so that the snake can fully extend its body. In addition, although snakes do not appear to prefer a clinical or enriched environment, this does not mean that they should not be provided with both physical and mental stimulation. Regular handling and interacting with snakes provides enrichment and exercise.

In clinical practice, it is important that the enclosure provided mimics the environment that the owners keep the snake in. This will provide the animal with familiarity and help to reduce stress levels.

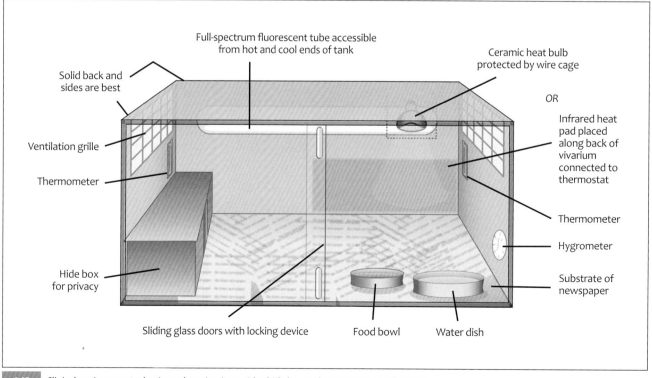

Full-spectrum fluorescent tube accessible from hot and cool ends of tank

Ceramic heat bulb protected by wire cage

Solid back and sides are best

OR

Ventilation grille

Infrared heat pad placed along back of vivarium connected to thermostat

Thermometer

Thermometer

Hygrometer

Hide box for privacy

Substrate of newspaper

Sliding glass doors with locking device

Food bowl

Water dish

4.19 Clinical environment: plastic or glass vivarium with a hide box and newspaper as substrate.

Chelonians

The order Testudines represents all modern chelonians and there are two types that are commonly kept:

* Tortoises
* Terrapins.

Tortoises are routinely kept in vivaria, specially designed tortoise tables or (for larger species) in large tortoise rooms. Provisions within the enclosure should be varied regularly to prevent boredom; it is a good idea to have more cage furniture than can fit into the enclosure, so that it can be rotated to keep tortoises stimulated. It is advisable to provide an area of substrate that tortoises can dig in as they would in the wild to make nests and lay eggs. The substrate provided should be digestible as it may be eaten (hay, peat and bark mulch are all suitable). Tortoises also engage with their environment and will look out of windows/doors at birds, cats and humans walking past. Ramps and tunnels that are available for cats can provide an opportunity for tortoises to play and hide, but these should only be used under supervision as they can tip a tortoise.

The diet of tortoises varies significantly depending upon the species and its natural environment, but it is important to vary the type and size of food given (e.g. sometimes whole food should be provided so that they have to break it apart, and other times the food should be cut into more manageable pieces). Foraging should be encouraged by hiding food under the substrate and planting food within the enclosure. Kong® or boomer balls (for larger tortoises) and other food-based puzzle toys commonly marketed for dogs can be used to hide food and make eating more of a challenge; this will keep the tortoise occupied for a longer time than if food is simply placed into a bowl, but time with these toys must be supervised.

Terrapins are all at least semiaquatic, so an appropriate environment should be provided (Figure 4.20). As with tortoises, terrapins also benefit from regular changes to their environment and in the method of feeding. For feeding enrichment, floating food items or floating islands with food items placed on them can be used. Kong® toys float in water and can be used to hide food and provide enrichment.

Amphibians

Amphibians are a class of ectothermic vertebrates that comprises frogs, toads, salamanders, axolotls and caecilians. They inhabit a wide variety of environments in the wild, with most species living within terrestrial, fossorial, arboreal or freshwater ecosystems. Thus, in terms of captive environment, the type of species to be housed should be taken into consideration, as well as the design of the enclosure, building materials, substrates, temperature, humidity, light, ventilation, furniture, water and ease of cleaning. As with reptiles, amphibians generally need to be kept within their POTZ. Animals kept at temperatures above their POTZ may show inappetence, weight loss, immunosuppression, agitation and changes to skin colour. Those kept below their POTZ may demonstrate lethargy and inappetence, become immunocompromised and develop bloating due to bacterial overgrowth from poorly digested food within the gastrointestinal tract. They will also have poor growth rates. For detailed information on the basic requirements for the captive maintenance of amphibians, the reader is referred to the *BSAVA Manual of Exotic Pets*.

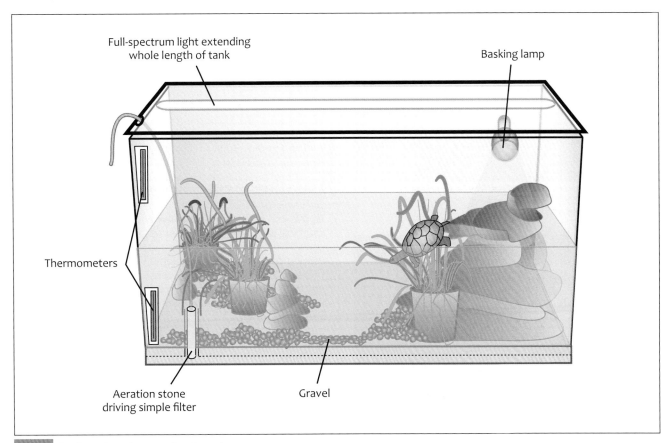

4.20 Semiaquatic environment for a terrapin.

Frogs and toads

Frogs and toads constitute the order Anura, which contains over 4000 species. Anurans are distinguished from other amphibians by the absence of a tail and the presence of long back legs designed for jumping. Frogs and toads are often kept individually; however, if a number of animals are to be housed together it should be remembered that males are territorial and will plague other males if the vivarium does not provide enough space for them to escape, causing stress to both parties. Females are not as territorial but will eat eggs laid by other individuals within the enclosure. Different species should not be housed together.

Terrestrial frogs and toads require an enclosure with a deep substrate into which they can burrow; it should be compact and able to hold the structure of a burrow. Coconut fibre is a suitable substrate for many species and bark can be added to improve drainage. Arboreal species (e.g. red-eyed tree frogs; Figure 4.21) require a larger enclosure with branches and leaves that can support their weight; driftwood, small stones and pebbles can also be provided for additional enrichment. All frogs and toads require lots of areas to hide; providing more hides than the number of inhabitants in the vivarium is ideal. Areas for egg laying should also be provided (e.g. half a coconut with a hole cut in it placed on a dish can be useful for smaller species such as poison dart frogs). The ground level should have areas of higher humidity containing moss and also places to climb and hide (e.g. driftwood, small stones and pebbles) (Figure 4.22).

Care should be taken that any non-food items that are used for enrichment are larger than the animal's head, as they will try to eat anything smaller.

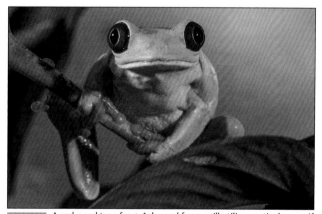

4.21 A red-eyed tree frog. Arboreal frogs will utilize vertical space if it is populated with branches for them to climb.
(Shutterstock.com/Rosa Jay)

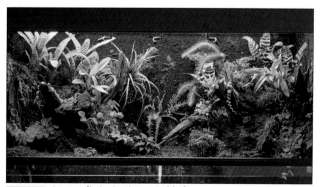

4.22 A naturalistic vivarium suitable for anurans. The moss and other plants maintain a good moisture level throughout and provide opportunities for hiding and climbing.
(Shutterstock.com/Dirk Ercken)

Axolotls

Axolotls are aquatic amphibians with a very limited natural habitat. A lack of knowledge of their ecology presents a challenge in terms of creating a naturalistic enclosure, but their basic requirements are well understood from extensive use in laboratories. Axolotls require a cold environment of 14–18°C (60–64°F). They are nocturnal and will shy away from harsh lighting. Housing at a ratio of 20 gallons to a single axolotl helps prevent fighting over territory and is necessary to maintain good water quality due to the amount of waste that they can produce. The substrate provided should be easy to clean but have a texture so that the axolotl can grip when on the bottom of the aquarium. The substrate should also be bigger than the axolotl's head as they will try and eat anything that will fit into their mouths – large slates can be appropriate.

Enclosure furniture can consist of live or artificial plants; live plants should be hardy as axolotls can be quite clumsy and will knock anything over that is not securely fixed. Bogwood, slate and large pebbles can be used to add texture and hiding places, and to make the environment more aesthetically pleasing to the owner. Changing the environment during the weekly clean will encourage the axolotls to explore and will help prevent boredom. Axolotls should not be handled unless absolutely necessary, so tactile play is not appropriate, but hand feeding lessens the risk of the axolotl accidentally ingesting non-food items.

Fish

Fish naturally inhabit an incredibly wide range of environments, and the basic needs and enrichment of different species vary accordingly. Water quality is a vitally important aspect of fish husbandry. Fish tend to thrive in stable environments and any change in parameters such as temperature, salinity or light can cause stress and illness, which must be borne in mind when designing and implementing enrichment. Tanks come in a range of sizes and care must be taken to avoid overstocking; a ~40 litre tank (30 cm × 30 cm × 45 cm) should be regarded as the bare minimum in which to keep even a small number of fish. Bowls are not acceptable as they do not provide enough space, are hard to filter and provide a poor surface for gas exchange. For detailed information on the basic requirements for the captive maintenance of fish, the reader is referred to the *BSAVA Manual of Ornamental Fish*.

There are multiple ways in which a fish tank or pond can be enriched. Varying the substrate and aquarium furniture will provide fish with a variety of places to hide. Bogwood can provide shelter and retreats; gluing large pebbles and stones together with aquarium sealant can provide more variety and dimensions for the fish to swim around and through. Live plants can be included, adding more hiding places and also shade and protection from any aquarium lighting; live plants that grow above the water level provide additional protection from light. Artificial plants are a good substitute for real plants and are easy to maintain. Feeding enrichment should be species appropriate (e.g. tailored to bottom or surface feeders) and may include an appropriate variety of fresh fruit and vegetables that are suspended in the aquarium.

Aquatic invertebrates

The environment that has been described for an aquarium for most fish species will be adequate for aquatic invertebrates. Lobsters will solve basic puzzle toys for food and

Kong® toys can be used as a feeding aid. Octopuses will solve puzzle toys as well as open jars and squeeze into small spaces, so tubes and small hides should be added to their enclosures. Octopuses fair better in enclosures with clear walls as they will watch what is going on outside their enclosure.

Birds

As with all groups, it is key for keepers and carers of birds to understand how each species has adapted to, and interacts with, its natural environment. For a discussion of the ethology of a range of avian species and detailed information on the basic requirements for the captive maintenance of birds, the reader is referred to the *BSAVA Manual of Avian Practice*.

Parrots

Parrots are incredibly intelligent and can become bored easily. Keeping them entertained in their caged and play areas can take time and patience, as wild parrots will spend over half of their waking hours eating and foraging (Koutsos *et al.*, 2001). Cockatiels are one of the smallest parrot species and are the second most popular bird kept in captivity, after the budgerigar (see below). Cockatiels originated in Australia, where they are found in arid or semi-arid areas in pairs or small flocks. Many parrots are flock animals and, as such, are highly sociable and can benefit from being kept in opposite-sex pairs (Figure 4.23). Solo parrots will often form very strong bonds with their human caregivers, sometimes to the detriment of their relationship with other humans.

If caged, a parrot requires a minimum space of 1.5 times the bird's adult wingspan in all directions. The cage should be constructed of a chew-resistant metal and should be kept at human eye level or higher to make the bird feel more secure. In addition to this space, the parrot should have access to play areas that are interesting not only to the owner but more importantly to the parrot. A boring play area can make the parrot more destructive, thus leading the owner to keep the parrot in the cage for longer periods of time, leading to a cycle of boredom and destructive behaviour. If the play area is not interesting enough to the parrot but the cage is, then the parrot may choose to return to the cage as they have more to entertain themselves.

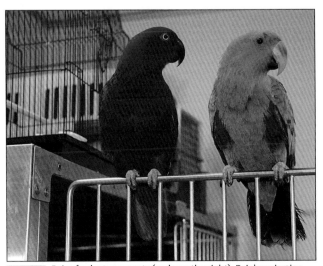

4.23 Pair of eclectus parrots (male on the right). Pair housing is a practical way to provide social enrichment in this species.

Introducing chew toys does not need to be expensive; these can be made out of paper towel rolls, cereal boxes, old phone books or newspaper with treats (such as good quality nuts) hidden inside. These toys are meant to be destroyed, so should be cheap and quick to make out of items that would normally be thrown away. It is a good idea to hang these chew toys from the cage and not place them on the base of the cage or play areas, otherwise they will become soiled with faeces if below feeding stations and could also be seen as nesting materials to sexually mature parrots. Care should be taken to avoid overcrowding the cage, as this could inhibit the bird's movement.

Parrots can be taught to do tricks and will also quickly learn to solve puzzle feeders; these can be simply paper inside a box with a treat or more complex with pulleys, levers and removable (parrot safe) nuts and bolts that take more dexterity but will keep the parrot entertained for longer as they work out how to use the item. See the *BSAVA Manual of Avian Practice* for more information about parrot behaviour and teaching tricks.

Toys, puzzle feeders and play areas should be moved around frequently to keep the parrot entertained and some items should be removed for a period of time and then reintroduced.

In clinical practice, using newspaper and paper rolls is an inexpensive and quick way to create foraging toys. Placing the patient's normal feedstuff inside these items will keep them entertained and distracted when in an unfamiliar environment. It is advised to bring small parrots in their own cage for hospitalization, if possible. Cage mates should also be hospitalized together where possible and if it will not be detrimental to the treatment being provided to the patient. (Chapter 6 provides a scale training plan that could act as enrichment and facilitate the weighing of parrots in a clinical setting.)

Budgerigars

Budgerigars (budgies) originated in Australia and can live in a range of habitats from rainforest to desert, although they primarily live in grassland areas. Budgies will travel hundreds of kilometres a day in search of food. Wild budgies live in flocks, with numbers varying from two to thousands, with higher numbers seen after rainfall.

Budgies are relatively easy to tame but a companion or two is advisable, especially if they are to spend a large proportion of their time in a cage. This will keep budgies entertained when their owners are away and help prevent boredom.

Budgies have lots of energy and require both physical and mental stimulation – this can be achieved by encouraging foraging or through play. The caged area should be as large as possible but minimum size requirements should allow the occupants to spread their wings in all directions. The cage should be decorated with perches, toys, and food and water bowls. The same techniques used for encouraging foraging in parrots can be modified and used with smaller birds.

Their natural diet consists of seeds, shoots and other plant materials and this should be replicated in the home with commercially available budgie food and access to fresh greens, shoots and seeds. Water should be available at all times and should be monitored for quality as budgies will bathe and defecate in water bowls.

In clinical practice, if possible, a budgie should be hospitalized in its own cage to keep some normality in its environment. It is also advisable to hospitalize budgies with cage companions for familiarity and to reduce stress levels.

The patient should have an area and/or time to exercise and display normal play behaviour. Just as a dog should be walked in a clinical setting, a bird should be allowed to spread its wings and fly if it is able to do so. Feeding the same diet that is fed in the home environment will provide the patient with some normality and routine.

Birds of prey

Many species of birds of prey are kept for various purposes. Most falcons and hawks are kept as hunting birds, whereas owls are more likely to be kept as pets. Working hawks and falcons will generally be tethered to a block or perch during the flying season and moved to a free-flying aviary outside of this time. For these birds, training and flying regularly is vital enrichment. In the UK, it is a requirement that tethered birds are flown at least five out of seven days, and training is needed in order to fly a bird (and to get it back).

Raptors are intelligent animals and training does not need to be limited to hunting. Raptors can be trained to perform basic behaviours (in a similar way to parrots), as well as also 'tricks'. Depending on the species, aviaries should provide both access to and shelter from wind, rain and sun, thus providing enrichment by increasing the bird's ability to choose its environment (Figure 4.24). Some species, such as kestrels, are fairly shy and benefit from a lot of cover (e.g. live planting or sheets within the aviary, or around some of the sides, to reduce observation), while more confident species, such as Harris hawks, are comfortable with less cover.

Enrichment can also take the form of toys or foraging strategies to provide occupation and entertainment. Birds will benefit from puzzle feeders (these could be as simple as a pine cone with mealworms hidden inside for a young owl, or a puzzle feeding toy suitable for a small dog containing chick pieces for a buzzard). Other popular enrichment toys include things that a bird can shred or destroy; for example, a phone directory that has pieces of food between some of the pages. Alternatively, many birds enjoy a 'foraging box' – a cardboard box containing a variety of natural/non-harmful materials with some food treats hidden inside.

Poultry

Poultry are prone to a range of behavioural disorders, most of which result from being unable to appropriately express normal behaviours. Simple measures such as scatter feeding, giving birds access to a dust bath and providing the opportunity to choose to go out in the rain can enhance welfare and prevent several problem behaviours.

For information on the husbandry needs of poultry, and a detailed consideration of behavioural disorders, see the *BSAVA Manual of Backyard Poultry Medicine and Surgery.*

Wildlife

There are legal and ethical aspects to be considered when caring for and releasing wildlife. The reader is encouraged to review appropriate legislation when dealing with these animals (see Chapter 1). In all instances, wildlife should be moved to a rehabilitation centre as soon as possible as they will have more equipment and experience in dealing with different species. See the *BSAVA Manual of Wildlife Casualties* for further information on housing hospitalized British wildlife.

Small mammals

Small British wildlife should be housed in a quiet, dimly lit area of the hospital. Animals such as field mice, rabbits and hedgehogs are crepuscular and will spend large parts

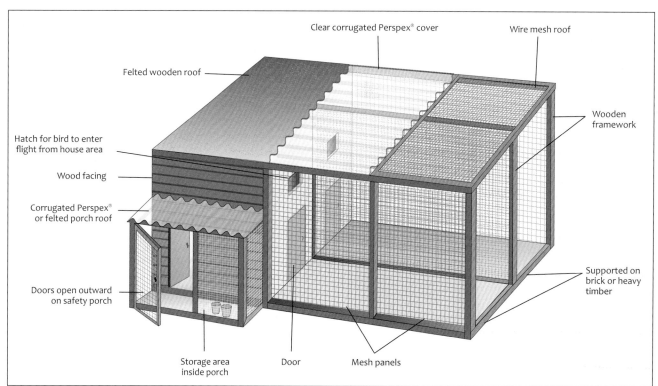

4.24 A 'three-thirds' aviary set-up provides birds with the security of an indoor area and the option to spend time in an outside flight. While in the outside flight, occupants can shelter under the roofed area from hot sun or heavy rain or snow, but may choose to stay in the open area in fine weather or light showers.

of the day sleeping. This needs to be taken into consideration when monitoring and administering medication to avoid disturbing their normal pattern.

Animals such as otters, badgers and foxes can give a nasty bite and will defend themselves if they feel threatened, so care should be taken with unfamiliar species.

In practice, enclosures should be easy to clean or disposable; more than one hide with different bedding material should be provided. A designated ward away from predators should be used to reduce stress levels from sight, sound and smell.

As these patients are not familiar with human contact, offering puzzles, balls and other forms of entertainment that may be used by cats and dogs will only cause more stress and discomfort to the animal; trying to keep the area traffic-free and minimizing human contact are key in treating most of these patients.

Bats should be housed individually to monitor behaviour. A box with a snap-top lid and lots of ventilation is a good enclosure for a short-term stay; a towel should be placed into the box down one wall and held in place with the lid. This will provide an area for a bat to climb and hide within the folds of the towel, giving warmth and protection. Once the bat is able to or trying to fly, a larger enclosure should be used, such as a pop-up butterfly enclosure (pop-up laundry baskets can also be used). Pop-up enclosures are only suitable for short-term use, as bats need to have access to a flighted area to build up muscle strength prior to release.

Large mammals

Large wild mammals likely to be in a captive situation in the UK are limited to deer species. Deer are generally found in woodland habitats near arable land, but they are adaptable and are increasingly found in urban environments. Despite this adaptability, deer remain very shy and flighty animals and close proximity to humans causes stress. Stress often manifests as self-trauma in deer, which can delay release. Wild deer should be housed away from dogs and cats, in a quiet area with minimal human traffic. Padding the interior of the holding pen and providing deep bedding makes this safer for the animal. Deer benefit from being able to hide from perceived predation, so full walls and doors are useful, as are areas of plant or tree cover in larger enclosures. Shelters made of straw bales or small sheds can provide even more cover.

As deer are so shy, and wild deer should be destined for release, enrichment strategies should not involve human interaction. Deer are often group housed towards the end of the rehabilitation period, so social enrichment is addressed. Feeding enrichment can take the form of making browse feeding more challenging by hanging bunches of branches in a tree or making bundles of browse that the deer must interact with in order to eat. Those deer that have been in a captive environment for any length of time may have learned to eat ruminant pellets. These pellets can be used to provide enrichment, for example, by scatter feeding or encouraging the deer to find pellets in man-made foraging areas (areas with lots of natural objects in which the pellets can be hidden). Most wild deer are relatively neophobic and 'toys' are less accepted.

Wild birds

Enrichment for wild birds is very species dependent. General guidelines for other avian species should be followed in terms of providing hides and cover, as well as nesting opportunities (see 'Birds', above). Enrichment strategies should guard against too much human contact and should emphasize behaviours that will serve the particular species in the wild. For example, birds of prey can be rehabilitated using falconry techniques, including training them to fly well using a creance and lure. Similar techniques have been employed with other bird species, particularly corvids. However, these techniques are controversial because they require fairly intense human involvement.

Feeding enrichment can be useful for many wild bird species to encourage foraging and food acquisition behaviours. For example, the use of forage boxes (boxes containing a range of natural/non-toxic commonly encountered objects in which are hidden some high value food items) will encourage investigation and foraging behaviours.

Marine species

Marine species likely to be seen in a rehabilitation setting in the UK are primarily pinnipeds (grey and harbour/common seals). There are no dedicated facilities available to rehabilitate cetaceans (whales, porpoises and dolphins) in the UK. Most pinnipeds should be sent to a specialist rehabilitation facility prior to release. Any enrichment strategies should focus on retaining normal behaviours and emphasizing abilities that are required in the wild, such as diving and catching food. British Divers Marine Life Rescue and the Cetacean Research & Rescue Unit offer advice and training on rescuing marine animals (see 'Useful websites').

Zoological collections

Felids

In the wild, big cats and wildcats are predominantly solitary, with the exception of lions; family groups will stay together for the early stages of life but will separate into smaller groups or solitary individuals.

In captivity, boredom is a problem as the large areas of territory these animals occupy in the wild are impossible to replicate. Changing the feed station or area that food is offered in will encourage exploration and sometimes play. Placing food in different areas of the enclosure, on different levels or even on pulley systems will make the cats have to work for their prey.

Using boxes and large hessian sacks with perfumes, essential oils or smells from prey animals will also promote play and exploration. Movement of soiled bedding from prey species into the cats' enclosure will spark interest and can keep cats entertained for long periods of time.

Target training and keeper training can be used as enrichment and entertainment, which could help develop a human–animal bond that is essential when needing to treat or medicate these animals (see Chapter 6).

Canids

Wild canids can be either solitary or pack animals and are kept as such in the zoological setting. There are 35 canine species, and they display a wide variety of natural behaviours. Canids also inhabit most of the globe, so environmental requirements of different species can vary significantly. It is nearly impossible to standardize housing requirements for all species. The presence of conspecifics is the primary form of enrichment. Often these animals are relatively shy, so exposure to human contact needs to be minimized; refuges/hides and viewing windows, rather than open enclosures, can all contribute to making these animals more comfortable in their environment. Having extensive space allows these animals to behave in a way that is closer to how they would in the wild, and particularly it allows them to move out of their flight zone if humans are in the area.

Feeding whole prey items or partial carcasses as part of a balanced diet can help to stimulate pack behaviours and combines social and feeding enrichment.

Primates

With species as evolved and complex as primates, enrichment becomes of paramount importance. There are many examples of good enrichment visible in zoological collections all over the world. Enclosure size gives enrichment opportunities in terms of groups of animals being able to be active within their environment. Adding vertical space with platforms, branches and ropes effectively increases the enclosure size. Use of different substrates can provide different foraging and manipulation opportunities.

Hamadryas baboons in the National Zoo of South Africa

The National Zoo of South Africa instigated an enrichment plan for its hamadryas baboons and measured activity levels before and after the introduction of enrichment (Cloete et al., 2008). Enrichment accessories added to the enclosure included hammocks, feeding tables, areas of woodchip substrate and tree stumps with hiding places. Feeding enrichment included changing the way food was presented (whole instead of chopped), wrapping food in newspaper, putting food in pine cones and hiding food, sometimes in woodchip substrate. Following these changes, the baboons demonstrated an increase in activity levels, particularly foraging activity, and a reduction in stereotypical behaviour and aggression.

A very different method of enrichment is the use of television, video and computer games. Chimpanzees that were shown videotapes of chimpanzees and other animals watched the monitors for a third of the time available, and chimps housed singly watched the monitors for longer than those that were group housed. While behaviour was not significantly changed, time budgets were, suggesting that the use of video images could be a good form of enrichment.

Ungulates

Ungulates are large mammals with hooves. The group can be divided into odd-toed ungulates, such as horses, rhinoceros and tapirs, and even-toed ungulates, such as cattle, pigs, giraffes, camels, sheep, deer and hippopotamuses.

Providing a paddock large enough to foster normal behaviour can be difficult for some species; for example, hippopotamuses require a large pool to express normal behaviour within the water, as well as a large land area that is heavily planted to provide cover and protection. Many ungulates are prey species; a stable or some form of shelter should be provided for protection from environmental elements and as a hide from the public for animals on display. Some zoological collection enclosures use walls to restrict public viewing to small windows for shy animals such as okapi, which spend their time in the wild hidden in forests away from predators and humans.

A variety of food should be offered in different ways, such as in ground nets and on pulley systems to emulate both shrubs and trees that food would be sourced from in the wild; scatter feeding of non-leafy food will also encourage exploration and interest in food. Large, durable balls that require the animal to move around to release the food can also be used to provide feeding enrichment and exercise.

Movement of bedding from other enclosures can be useful if there are no known parasites within the collection.

It is difficult to house or treat large ungulates within the practice and this will primarily be done on site with the owner or keeper.

Birds

The principles that apply to domestically kept birds also apply to those kept in zoological collections (see 'Exotic pets', above). Provision of enrichment in the zoological setting can be complicated by the tendency to keep more than one species in an enclosure. What can be viewed as positive enrichment for one species may not work for another. However, these enclosure types tend to provide a naturalistic and very heterogeneous environment, perhaps negating the requirement for additional enrichment (e.g. toys).

Reptiles

The principles that apply to domestically kept reptiles also largely apply to those kept in zoological collections (see 'Exotic pets', above); for example, puzzle style feeders and hiding food in the enclosure provide enrichment for reptiles and visitors alike. Training also provides excellent enrichment in a zoological setting and most zoological collections now clicker train their larger reptiles.

Where there is known parasitic testing and all animals have passed quarantine, then bedding from other enclosures can be moved between different animals to allow for scent marking and exploration of new smells. This can also be used to lay a trail in the enclosure for the inhabitants to find and follow to a reward.

The stimulation that visitors in a zoological setting bring should not be discounted as most reptiles will people-watch; they often spend a lot of their time at the front of their enclosures watching humans pass by.

Invertebrates

The key to terrestrial invertebrate enrichment is the enclosure: this should be large enough to accommodate the animal, but not so large as to create a void of space that will not be utilized and thus cause stress to the animal that is enclosed. A place to burrow or create a scrape should be included, as well as areas to hide with the use of cork hides, leaves, rocks or stones, depending on the environmental needs of the animal that is being kept in the enclosure. Shade from light should be provided with the use of live or artificial plants and leaves. An arboreal set-up with the use of textured walls and large pieces of cork or tree branches can provide not only height but places to hide and burrow. Changing the location of food and water stations will encourage exploration and exercise.

Fish

Zoological collections are better placed than domestic owners in terms of space and facilities to provide a naturalistic environment for fish to live in. Multi-species enclosures with varying depth and size create a more natural ecosystem and provide a more enriching setting. Variety, including different substrates and moving aquarium furniture periodically, will prevent boredom and encourage exploration.

A range of feeding methods will also help prevent boredom and encourage exploration of the enclosure. Food can be suspended from the top of the water or allowed to drop to the substrate layer. Target training can be used for feeding and also for health checks; a reward-based system can increase the enrichment that the animal will experience.

Rescue animals

Rescue animals of any species can present challenges in terms of providing enrichment, because their previous history and experiences are very often unknown. Things that are positive for other individuals may be negative if they are associated with aversive events; for example, a rescue dog that has had a negative experience whilst on a lead may not view an on-lead walk as a positive experience. In particular, human interaction can initially be very aversive for some rescue animals. Recognizing signs of physical and psychological distress and acting upon these on an individual case basis is key to providing positive enrichment for any rescue animal.

Many animals in a rescue situation are kennel housed rather than fostered in a home. This environment can be intensely stressful, so enrichment is very important. Introducing animals to a kennelling environment gradually has been shown to reduce behavioural signs of stress in dogs, as has providing adequate contact time with carers. Reducing the length of time animals are left alone can also be a positive enrichment factor.

In some rescue centres, particularly for dogs, the pair housing of compatible animals and group exercise has been shown to improve measures of good welfare and reduce behaviours associated with poor welfare. This is more problematic when considering rabbits and rodents, because the bonding process can be long and time intensive.

Psittacines, especially large parrots, benefit from training enrichment in a rescue situation.

References and further reading

Behavior and Husbandry Advisory Group (1999) *A scientific advisory group of the American Zoo and Aquarium Association Workshop at Disney's Animal Kingdom*, Orlando

Brouwer K, Jones ML, King CE and Schifter H (2000) Longevity records for Psittaciformes in captivity. *International Zoo Yearbook* **37**, 299–316

Chitty J and Monks D (2018) *BSAVA Manual of Avian Practice: A Foundation Manual*. BSAVA Publications, Gloucester

Cloete C, Mogogane O and Sebati M (2008) A change in perspective: providing enrichment for hamadryas baboons. *The Shape of Enrichment* **17**, 1–3

Cooper B, Mullineaux E and Turner L (2020) *BSAVA Textbook of Veterinary Nursing, 6th edn*. BSAVA Publications, Gloucester

Denham HDC, Bradshaw JWS and Rooney NJ (2014) Repetitive behaviour in kennelled domestic dog: stereotypical or not? *Physiology and Behaviour* **128**, 288–294

Gaines SA, Rooney NJ and Bradshaw JWS (2008) The effect of feeding enrichment upon reported working ability and behaviour of kenneled working dogs. *Journal of Forensic Sciences* **53**, 1400–1404

Girling S and Raiti P (2019) *BSAVA Manual of Reptiles, 3rd edn*. BSAVA Publications, Gloucester

Hearne T (2017) *The Official RSPCA Pet Guide: Care for Your Gerbil*. Harper Collins, London

Hediger H (1965) *Wild Animals in Captivity – An Outline of the Biology of Zoological Gardens*. Dover Publications, New York

Horwitz DF and Mills DS (2009) *BSAVA Manual of Canine and Feline Behavioural Medicine, 2nd edn*. BSAVA Publications, Gloucester

Hosey G (2013) Hediger revisited: How do zoo animals see us? *Journal of Applied Animal Welfare Science* **16**, 338–359

Hullinger R, O'Riordan K and Burger C (2015) Environmental enrichment improves learning and memory and long-term potentiation in young adult rats through a mechanism requiring mGluR5 signaling and sustained activation of p70s6k. *Neurobiology of Learning and Memory* **125**, 126–134

ICC (2018) *Making your Home Cat Friendly*. Available from: icatcare.org/advice

Johnson-Bennett P (2018) *What is Environmental Enrichment and Why Does Your Cat Need it?* Available from: www.catbehaviorassociates.com

Keeble E and Meredith A (2009) *BSAVA Manual of Rodents and Ferrets*. BSAVA Publications, Gloucester

Koutsos EA, Matson KD and Klasing KC (2001) Nutrition of birds in the order Psittaciformes: A review. *Journal of Avian Medicine and Surgery* **15**, 257–275

McBride A (1988) *Rabbits and Hares*. Whittet Books Ltd, London

Meredith A and Johnson-Delaney C (2010) *BSAVA Manual of Exotic Pets, 5th edn*. BSAVA Publications, Gloucester

Mullineaux E and Keeble E (2016) *BSAVA Manual of Wildlife Casualties, 2nd edn*. BSAVA Publications, Gloucester

NAWT (2022) *7 DIY canine enrichment ideas with NAWT*. Available from: www.nawt.org.uk/blog

Poland G and Raftery A (2019) *BSAVA Manual of Backyard Poultry Medicine and Surgery*. BSAVA Publications, Gloucester

Raftery A (2002) *Pet Owner's Guide to the Bearded Dragon*. Ringpress Books Ltd, Lydney

Rees PA (2011) *An Introduction to Zoo Biology and Management*. Wiley-Blackwell, Chichester

Rejigwart M, Vinke CM, Hendriksen C *et al*. (2018) An explorative study on the effect of provision of preferred and non-preferred enrichment on behavioural and physiological parameters in laboratory ferrets (*Mustela putorius furo*). *Applied Animal Behaviour Science* **203**, 64–72

Rooney NJ, Blackwell EJ, Mullan SM *et al*. (2014) The current state of welfare, housing and husbandry of the English pet rabbit population. *BMC Research Notes* **7**, 942

Rooney N, Gaines S and Hiby E (2009) A practitioner's guide to working dog welfare. *Journal of Veterinary Behaviour* **4**, 127–134

RSPCA (2015) *Learning to be left alone*. Available from: www.rspca.org.uk

Sherwin CM (1998) Voluntary wheel running: A review and novel interpretation. *Animal Behaviour* **56**, 11–27

Siwak *et al*. (2001) Effect of age and level of cognitive function on spontaneous and exploratory behaviours in the beagle dog. *Learning and memory* **8**, 317–325

Trocino A, Majolini D, Tazzoli M and Fillou E (2012) Housing of growing rabbits in individual, bicellular and collective cages: Fear level and behavioural patterns. *Animal* **7**, 1–7

Varga MJ (2013) *Textbook of Rabbit Medicine, 2nd edn*. Elsevier, Oxford

Wildgoose WH (2001) *BSAVA Manual of Ornamental Fish, 2nd edn*. BSAVA Publications, Gloucester

Useful websites

Animal Training – Disney's training and enrichment programmes
www.animaltraining.org

British Divers Marine Life Rescue
bdmlr.org.uk

Cetacean Research & Rescue Unit
www.crru.org.uk/rescue.asp

Fear Free® Initiative – resources on emotional wellbeing, enrichment and the reduction of fear, stress and anxiety in pets
www.fearfreepets.com

Problem Parrots – parrot training and enrichment resources
www.problemparrots.co.uk

Rabbit Welfare Association & Fund
www.rabbitwelfare.co.uk

UC Davis Koret Shelter Medicine Program – canine and feline enrichment in a shelter situation
www.sheltermedicine.com

Chapter 5

Nutritional welfare

Rachel Lumbis and Chloe White

Introduction

Nutrition is fundamental to the health and wellbeing of animals and is an aspect of husbandry in which the owner or caregiver, along with the veterinary healthcare team, plays a critical role. However, according to the People's Dispensary for Sick Animals (PDSA) Animal Wellbeing (PAW) Report published in 2019, 9% of owners surveyed did not feel wholly confident that they were fulfilling their pets' nutritional needs. In addition, a Dutch Zoo Federation survey found that nutritional education and understanding amongst captive animals' primary keepers was lacking and many were acting on out-of-date information (Nijboer et al., 2011). It is the responsibility of the veterinary team to equip owners with the knowledge to enable them to make informed decisions about what and how to feed the animals in their care.

Nutritional assessment

A nutritional assessment should be considered as part of the minimum standard of care and conducted at every patient examination. The World Small Animal Veterinary Association (WSAVA) recognizes nutrition as the fifth vital assessment following temperature, pulse, respiration and pain (Freeman et al., 2011). Following on from the publication of the WSAVA Global Nutrition Guidelines in 2011, the WSAVA Global Nutrition Committee has developed a suite of support materials and practical aids as part of a 'Global Nutrition Toolkit' (WSAVA, 2022). A basic nutritional assessment comprises:

- Weighing the animal
- Body condition scoring
- Muscle condition scoring
- Obtaining a dietary history
- Calculating caloric requirements.

A full nutritional assessment should also cover (Bissell et al., 2019):

- Holistic evaluation to ensure that the diet is meeting the animal's needs
- Analysis of how food is presented and how that influences the animal's behaviour
- Determining whether the diet is fulfilling the needs of the animal with consideration given to its environment.

> ### Body and muscle condition scoring
> The veterinary team should undertake body condition scoring for every patient. The WSAVA nutritional assessment guidelines are the accepted standard in small animals (Freeman et al., 2011; WSAVA, 2022). Similar guidance is available for captive animals (AZA Nutrition Advisory Group, 2017). Muscle condition scoring is also becoming a more accepted protocol in small animal practice and should be encouraged in all captive animals as it can identify sarcopenia and cachexia in animals who may have a normal or obese bodyweight. See Chapter 2 for more information on body and muscle condition scoring.

Once a nutritional assessment has been completed, an appropriate feeding plan and exercise regime should be created, and specific nutritional recommendations provided. This plan needs to take into consideration the life stage of the animal and any concurrent clinical conditions (Debraekeleer et al., 2010). Each life stage of an animal (growing, adult, senior) has very different nutritional requirements and these need to be taken into account when discussing nutrition with clients and formulating a plan. Pregnant and lactating animals require a significantly higher energy and nutrient intake and should be closely monitored. Animals with concurrent diseases are likely to be more vulnerable to nutrient excesses and deficiencies, so it is vital that owners of animals with chronic conditions are advised on the correct nutrition to mitigate this risk. It should be borne in mind that malnutrition (see below) can worsen the impact of some clinical conditions (e.g. obesity has a negative impact on osteoarthritis). For more information on calculating nutritional requirements for different life stages and clinical conditions, see the BSAVA Textbook of Veterinary Nursing.

The National Research Council (NRC) has set minimum nutrient requirements for domestic animals and exotic pets, and those species that have close relatives in captivity, such as ungulates, mustelids, canids, felids, primates, rodents, lagomorphs, birds and fish, should have diets formulated in a similar manner to meet the established requirements (Nijboer, 2015b). A veterinary nutritionist should be consulted as required to help tailor diets for animals with a variety of needs (Chandler et al., 2015). In addition, academic support bodies (e.g. Association of Zoos and Aquariums) can provide factsheets on the nutritional care of captive animals (AZA Nutrition Advisory Group, 2020).

Welfare considerations of different types of diet

The type of diet that an owner or animal keeper chooses to feed the individual(s) in their care is crucial to their nutritional welfare. Although commercially prepared diets are still the preferred choice amongst companion animal owners, home-prepared diets (including raw food diets) are becoming increasingly popular (PDSA, 2019). The veterinary team are best placed to advise owners about diet and feeding; evidence-based medicine should be followed and there should be collaboration with the owner to decide upon the best regime for each individual pet (RCVS Knowledge, 2019). If an owner is keen to feed an alternative diet, it is vital to understand why they are motivated to do so and to discuss the advantages and disadvantages, so that the diet selected meets the needs of both the animal and the owner (see also the *BSAVA Guide to Nutrition*).

Commercially manufactured diets

Commercially available pet foods can be categorized by industry standard marketing into the following:

- **Grocery brands** – food that can be bought from the supermarket is fairly well recognized by the general public from large scale mass advertising. Grocery brands rely heavily on public perception of good palatability and appeal to the pet owner
- **Private label brands** – specific-store only brands are becoming increasingly popular in pet superstores; these may be branded to suit different types of owner, with some being marketed in a similar manner to grocery brands whilst others are aimed at a more 'high-end' market
- **Generic pet foods** – these are non-branded foods that can be sold at a very low price point due to low-cost ingredients, manufacturing processes and packaging
- **Speciality brands** – also called premium brands, these foods tend to advertise a higher standard of ingredients and superior manufacturing processes, and are often a higher price point per gram; however, the volume of food that needs to be fed to meet nutritional requirements tends to be less. Veterinary exclusive brands fit within this category
- **Veterinary therapeutic foods** – these should only be provided under veterinary supervision as they usually have a specific purpose. Some of these diets have contraindications (e.g. use in growing animals or use in animals with concurrent medical conditions) and some require a restricted length of feeding time (Crane *et al.*, 2010).

Marketing claims, such as natural, holistic and hypoallergenic, can often be seen on pet food labelling. However, it should be noted that these terms are not protected and definitions may vary (PFMA, 2015a). For example, the European Commission Technical Document on Cosmetic Claims (2017) states "the claim 'hypoallergenic' does not guarantee a complete absence of risk of an allergic reaction and the product should not give the impression that it does". This should be borne in mind when evaluating the appropriateness of a diet for the individual in question.

Manufacturers may use a fixed formula or a closed formula to produce the diet. Fixed formula diets (ingredients and recipe do not routinely change) are more consistent

from batch to batch and are, therefore, preferable to closed formula diets (ingredient composition can vary, as long as the stated nutritional values of the diet are met), especially in animals that are prone to gastrointestinal upset (Barnard *et al.*, 2009; Sanderson, 2013). It should also be noted that manufacturers adhering to high production standards will routinely test the diet throughout the manufacturing process (i.e. from assessing the raw ingredients, to ensuring that the food adheres to the nutritional values required following the cooking process) (Crane *et al.*, 2010). It may be helpful to check the local geographical pet food governing body, as they will have a members list stating which companies adhere to these standards:

- Europe – Fédération Européenne de l'Industrie des Aliments pour Animaux Familiers (FEDIAF) of which there are the following national member organizations:
  - Austria – ÖHTV
  - Belgium – BKVH/CPAF
  - Denmark, Norway and Sweden – NPFA
  - Finland – Lemmikkieläinruokayhdistys
  - France – FACCO
  - Germany – IVH
  - Greece – GPFMA
  - Hungary – HPFA
  - Italy – ASSALCO
  - Netherlands – VKH
  - Poland – Polikarma
  - Portugal–ALIAN
  - Republic of Ireland – PFAI
  - Slovenia – GIZ_PHMZ
  - Spain – ANFAAC
  - Switzerland – VHN
  - United Kingdom – PFMA
- USA – Association of American Feed Control Officials (AAFCO)
- Canada – The Canadian Veterinary Medical Association (CVMA).

Commercially manufactured diets are complete and balanced and, provided that the correct amount is fed, can be a healthy option. However, care should be taken, particularly with dry food, to ensure that it is not fed in excess. Dry food diets tend to have a higher energy content per gram, which increases the risk of overfeeding. Animals should be monitored on a regular basis to ensure that dietary intake and feeding approach is appropriate for the maintenance of a lean body condition and optimal bodyweight. Many manufacturers also produce diets for specific life stages and medical conditions. Feeding a diet formulated for an appropriate life stage or condition ensures that optimal nutrition is delivered to the animal and therefore improves nutritional welfare (Debraekeleer *et al.*, 2010).

Although commercially manufactured diets remain popular amongst owners, the availability of poor quality diets and the recall of some pet food products has contributed to the growing popularity of alternative diets (Freeman *et al.*, 2013; Morelli *et al.*, 2019).

Homemade cooked diets

Homemade cooked diets are becoming increasingly popular with owners (PDSA, 2020) and veterinary professionals need to be able to provide guidance about the advantages and disadvantages of such foods. Owners may get a sense of fulfilment and enrichment from preparing a diet for their pet and may be motivated to do so from a belief that the food will be more 'natural' and 'traditional' (Remillard,

2008). However, it can be costly, time-consuming and less convenient to provide this type of diet. In addition, in the absence of the ability to routinely test the nutritional values of the food, deficiencies or toxicities are more likely to occur (Stockman *et al.*, 2013). If an owner wishes to provide their pet with a homemade diet, then the veterinary team should advise that they consult an appropriately qualified veterinary nutritionist to ensure that only approved recipes and supplements are fed. This is particularly important if the animal is young or in its senior years, when its nutritional requirements differ from that of an adult. For further information, see the *BSAVA Guide to Nutrition*.

Raw diets

Raw diets (also known as raw meat-based diets, 'biologically appropriate raw food' or 'BARF' diets) are becoming increasingly popular with owners (Morelli *et al.*, 2019) and veterinary professionals need to be able to provide guidance about the advantages and disadvantages of such foods.

Veterinary professionals can sometimes feel that it is challenging to have a balanced discussion with owners due to their passion for their selected type of diet (Schlesinger and Joffe, 2011). Owners that have made a decision to feed a raw diet have invariably done so because they believe it to be of benefit to their pet. These owners have often committed a lot of time and energy to researching their chosen diet, but the sources from which they have derived the information may be less than ideal (e.g. internet sites and social media; Morelli *et al.*, 2019). It is important to correct any misconceptions and provide owners with appropriate evidence-based guidance (Davies, 2015).

Proponents of feeding raw meat diets argue that they are more palatable and digestible than dry commercial foods. There is also some emerging evidence for improvement in coat quality and dental benefits; although, raw food diets that contain high quantities of whole or pieces of bone increase the risk of dental and gastrointestinal injury (Frowde *et al.*, 2011; Thompson *et al.*, 2012). Owners may prefer to feed a raw food diet because it is perceived to more closely resemble what dogs would eat in the wild, or because it is more aesthetically interesting than standard kibble style food. In these cases, it may be helpful to discuss alternative enrichment options that can be used with commercial and homemade diets, such as puzzle feeders, scatter feeding or retaining some of the daily ration for training purposes (see Chapters 4 and 6).

One of the main disadvantages associated with raw food diets is the risk of pathogenic infection (van Bree *et al.*, 2018; Davies *et al.*, 2019). A number of pathogens have been identified in both homemade and commercially prepared raw food diets, including:

- *Salmonella* spp. (Weese *et al.*, 2005)
- *Escherichia coli* O157:H7 (Freeman and Michel, 2001)
- *Clostridium* spp. (Weese *et al.*, 2005)
- *Campylobacter jejuni* (Lenz *et al.*, 2009)
- *Toxoplasma gondii* (Taylor *et al.*, 2009)
- *Echinococcus multilocularis* (Antolova *et al.*, 2009).

Thus, it is important that owners consider not only the pet's nutritional welfare but also the potential risk to human health when choosing to feed a raw food diet (e.g. from multiple drug-resistant bacteria). It is essential that adequate precautions are taken to mitigate the risk of infection, including excellent hygiene when handling the food itself and any pet waste.

Inpatients

Due to the risk of pathogen spread to staff and other patients, especially immunocompromised individuals, it is not advised to allow raw feeding of inpatients. Inpatients that are normally fed a raw diet should be isolated where possible, as pathogens can be shed asymptomatically for up to 7 days.

Although there is a growing body of evidence to suggest that raw feeding may be harmful to both pets and owners alike, there is still a lack of large-scale, good quality clinical studies looking at the effects of long-term raw feeding in companion animals (Schlesinger and Joffe, 2011). Many pet owners and some veterinary professionals have anecdotally reported considerable health improvements in animals fed a raw food diet; however, this has not been substantiated in a clinical environment to date. Routine health screening should be undertaken and ideally data collated and published to give the industry a greater understanding of these potential benefits (Freeman *et al.*, 2013).

The American Association of Feed Control Officials (AAFCO) conducts trials to establish whether a food is suitably complete nutritionally for all life stages and to date no raw food diets have been tested in this manner (Davies, 2015). The Pet Food Manufacturers Association (PFMA) (2015a) currently has 11 raw pet food manufacturers listed as members who have to adhere to high quality guidelines and standards; perhaps there may be the opportunity in the future for these companies to undertake clinical studies to confirm the seemingly positive anecdotal evidence for the use of these diets.

If an owner wishes to provide their pet with a raw food diet, then the veterinary team should advise that they consult an appropriately qualified veterinary nutritionist to ensure that only approved recipes and supplements are fed. It should be remembered that dietary requirements can vary greatly depending on the species, breed, age, reproductive status and health of the animal, and that no one diet will provide optimal nutrition. For further information, see the *BSAVA Guide to Nutrition*.

Vegetarian and vegan diets

The number of owners following a vegetarian or vegan lifestyle has increased (Ipsos MORI, 2016), as has interest in feeding pets a vegetarian or plant-based diet, whether this be because owners believe their pet will receive additional health benefits or due to an unwillingness to purchase or handle meat-containing products. There are commercially available vegetarian diets for cats, as well as vegetarian and vegan diets for dogs. However, a study by Kanakubo *et al.* (2015) found that most of the diets assessed were not compliant with labelling regulations and there were concerns regarding the adequacy of essential amino acid content; taurine, in particular, was mentioned due to the obvious risk deficiency poses to cats. If an owner wishes to feed a diet of this type, the PFMA (2015a) advises that a veterinary surgeon or animal nutritionist be consulted to ensure that the diet provided is nutritionally adequate and palatable.

Grain-free diets

Grain-free diets are becoming increasingly popular with pet owners, reflecting a trend within human nutrition of reducing the amount of grain in the diet (NPD Group,

2012). Thus, veterinary professionals need to be able to provide guidance about the advantages and disadvantages of such foods, particularly given that recent studies have questioned the safety of their use.

Owners may state that they wish to feed this type of diet to their pet due to the belief that grains can cause allergies, and that they are an unnecessary filler within pet foods, provide no nutritional value or are a lesser quality ingredient. However, it should be noted that wheat allergies account for only 13% of diet-related allergies and are less common than those associated with dairy proteins or animal proteins found in meat (Mueller *et al.*, 2016). In addition, there is no evidence that the ability of domesticated dogs to digest grain is compromised, and likening them to wolves when comparing grain digestibility has no clinical relevance as they are genetically dissimilar in this regard (Axelsson *et al.*, 2013; Tonoike *et al.*, 2015).

Feeding a diet low in grain content may be beneficial in Irish Setters with familial gluten-sensitive enteropathies (Davies, 2017) and Border Terriers with specific neurological clinical signs (Lowrie *et al.*, 2015); there is evidence that one particular Border Terrier responded well to a gluten-free diet (Lowrie *et al.*, 2016). However, there is more overwhelming evidence that a long-term grain-free diet may be harmful. Golden Retrievers and Labrador Retrievers have been reported to be particularly affected by iatrogenic dilated cardiomyopathy linked to a grain-free diet (US Food and Drug Administration, 2019).

If an owner wishes to provide their pet with a grain-free diet, then the veterinary team should advise that they consult an appropriately qualified veterinary nutritionist to ensure that only approved recipes and supplements are fed. This is particularly important if the animal is young or in its senior years, when its nutritional requirements differ from that of an adult. For further information, see the *BSAVA Guide to Nutrition*.

Welfare considerations of different feeding methods

All species of animals are heterotrophic meaning that they must consume either plant or animal matter to obtain nutrients for life. There are various basic methods for acquiring food; some animals may use one feeding strategy, whilst others may use a combination (Saladin, 2020):

- Browsing – feeding from trees and shrubs
- Burrowing – eating through either wood or soil and sediment
- Filter feeding – straining water to consume small organisms such as plankton
- Grazing – feeding from the land (usually grasses, but can include algae and other water surface plants; see below)
- Foraging for nectar, pollen and seeds – feeding from trees, shrubs and flowers. This is also an essential environmental function for pollination and seed dispersal
- Predation – hunting and consumption of other animals
- Suspension and deposit feeding – consumption of organic matter that settles on the floor of an aquatic environment
- Scavenging – consumption of dead animals or organic matter
- Symbiosis – surviving by living off another animal.

It can be difficult to emulate fully these feeding methods in captive environments. The constituents of the diet may be replicated to a certain extent, but the method in which the animals are fed takes very little time compared with how long their non-captive counterparts take to graze or hunt, which can give rise to the exhibition of negative behavioural traits (Mason *et al.*, 2007).

There are many species-specific considerations. For example, feeding browse to grazing animals (such as giraffes and elephants; Figure 5.1) is highly recommended as it allows them to forage (Clubb and Mason, 2003); rich environments that allow goal-directed and problem-solving behaviour are preferred to 'easier' feeding set-ups (Siegford, 2013). In the case of larger psittacine birds, it is important to consider the method of feeding, particularly if they need to be able to hold and easily manipulate food with their claws (Nijboer, 2015b). Feeding carcasses to scavengers and other carnivores has historically been a worry for zoological establishments due to the fear of visitor complaints. However, it has been shown that exhibition visitors accept this type of feeding and will, in some instances, stay longer to watch animals exhibiting rarely seen natural behaviour (Gaengler and Clum, 2015; Roth *et al.*, 2017).

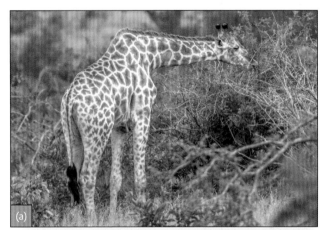

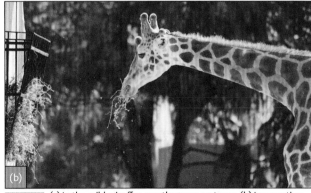

5.1 (a) In the wild, giraffes mostly graze on trees. (b) In a captive environment, presenting browse at height simulates the natural feeding environment.

Five Freedoms

One of the Five Freedoms (see Chapter 2) states than an animal should have freedom from hunger and thirst. However, the veterinary (or captive animal care) team should not be satisfied with just fulfilling this requirement; they should strive to help an animal into a positive mental state through nutrition ▶

(Wolfensohn *et al.*, 2018). Feeding is a core activity and, therefore, if diet and feeding methods are managed to a high standard, the animal will have an overall better quality of life. This is particularly important in a zoological environment, as there is evidence to suggest that animals given more control over the type of food and the manner in which they consume it have an overall increased welfare state (Boissy *et al.*, 2007).

The method by which an animal is fed can also be used to assist an owner or animal care team to control nutrient intake:

- Free choice (*ad libitum*) feeding – this method of feeding allows an animal to consume as much food as it wishes to consume. It is generally advised in lactating animals to allow for adequate caloric consumption for milk production
- Food-restricted feeding – this method of feeding restricts the volume of food fed and may be useful in obese animals as part of a weight management programme. Bodyweight and other condition indicators should be regularly monitored and recorded
- Time-restricted feeding – this method of feeding allows an animal to only eat at certain times of day. It can be useful in training dogs not to free feed, which can help with toilet training puppies; however, it may also encourage feeding beyond the point of satiation (Prendergast, 2010).

Multi-animal households or exhibits pose additional challenges. For most species, it is generally advised to use a separate bowl or other receptacle for each animal. If food aggression is a problem, then feeding animals in entirely different spaces may be helpful (International Cat Care, 2018). Using puzzle-type feeders (Figure 5.2) can assist in redirecting aggressive behaviour into problem-solving and task-oriented behaviour; most species will also find this enriching and rewarding as it better emulates the time it would take for an animal to feed in a natural environment (Rosa *et al.*, 2003; Bryant and Kother, 2014; International Cat Care, 2019). Other enrichment strategies may include scatter feeding and hiding or burying food (see Chapter 4).

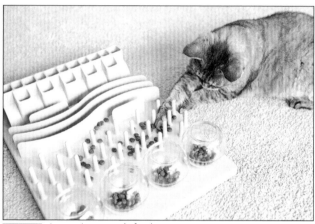

5.2 A cat using a puzzle feeder.
(Veera/Shutterstock.com)

Case example 1: Grazing animals

One of the ways in which animal welfare can be defined is through assessment of whether animals live in a 'natural' environment and have the ability to perform natural behaviours (Phillips, 2010). Grazing behaviour is a type of feeding strategy involving the regular consumption of self-found food and is considered essential for a wide variety of domesticated and wild animal species.

When foraging, an animal has to both search for and harvest its food in a process described as the alternation of movement between feeding stations and 'bite-sets/grazing time' within feeding stations. Foraging behaviour is affected by climatic, topographic and predatory constraints. Forage characteristics of habitats also influence the spatial distribution of herbivores, their diet (intake, choice) and their impact on the environment (Roguet *et al.*, 1998). Grazing animals have feeding preferences, on both a species and individual level which, together with aversions, appear to form early in life (possibly even during gestation) through post-ingestive feedback (Sharpe and Kenny, 2019). The grazing process involves decision-making on a number of levels, with feeding choices based on bite and choice of vegetation, feeding site/patch and home range/territory (Sharpe and Kenny, 2019). Such decisions are based on the optimal foraging theory, which predicts whether an individual will reduce or cease to forage when the reward is outweighed by the perceived predation risk (Webster *et al.*, 2018). Food intake depends on the presentation of the food, the previous experience of the animal with a given food, and to what extent other competing motivations affect the behaviour of the animal (Nielsen *et al.*, 2016). Other constraints include environmental factors and the limits of cognitive abilities, such as memory and discrimination (Roguet *et al.*, 1998). When provided with a number of experimental food patches that are equal in quality, an animal in a safe or preferred environment will exploit a food patch more thoroughly and leave less food behind than an animal in a risky or less preferred environment (Troxell-Smith *et al.*, 2017).

When considering the problems that can arise as a result of insufficient grazing opportunities, it is important to consider two main ecological characteristics of animal species in relation to their feeding and foraging behaviour: body size and primary dietary component (plant or animal). Body size is an evolutionarily selected adaptation which, together with consideration of dietary preference, must be taken into account when designing feeding regimes (Young, 2003). The body size of an animal is inversely proportional to its metabolic rate; thus there is a requirement for small animals to feed frequently on nutrient-dense food that is rapidly available. Conversely, large animals have a slower metabolic rate and can survive on low-quality food whose nutrients can be extracted slowly (Young, 2003). As a consequence, small animals are usually much more active than large animals.

Rabbits

Feeding an appropriate diet to a rabbit is probably the single most important factor in maintaining its health. Rabbits are herbivores and have a complex digestive system involving hindgut fermentation adapted to digest a high-fibre

Case example 1: Grazing animals *continued*

diet consisting mainly of grass. The gastrointestinal tract makes up 10–20% of a rabbit's bodyweight. Gut transit time is rapid and involves the separation of food into digestible and indigestible components within the colon. Indigestible fibre plays an important role in stimulating normal motility of the gut but has no nutritional value and is quickly eliminated from the digestive tract as hard faecal pellets. Digestible components of the diet are moved from the colon to the caecum for fermentation, the products of which include volatile fatty acids (VFAs) and bacteria, which form the rabbit's predominant source of energy and protein, respectively. Around 3–8 hours postprandially, soft, mucus-covered caecotrophs are expelled and ingested, remaining in the stomach for up to 6 hours. Caecotrophy enables the absorption of nutrients and bacterial fermentation products (amino acids, VFAs and vitamins B and K), and the digestion of previously undigested food, thus enhancing nutrient extraction from the diet. VFAs are responsible for 40% of a rabbit's calorie requirement and also facilitate control of pathogenic organisms by helping to maintain the normal pH (6–7) in the caecum.

To maintain gut motility, dental health and caecotrophy, rabbits require a high-fibre, low-carbohydrate diet, consisting predominantly of grass and hay. To meet these requirements, wild rabbits spend an average of 70% of their time grazing and have a dietary intake of approximately 20–25% crude fibre, 15% crude protein and 2–3% fat through consumption of grass alone. In contrast, pet rabbits have limited or no opportunity to graze, exercise or engage in social behaviour, resulting in compromised welfare (Rooney *et al.*, 2014).

The optimal diet for a rabbit should consist of 85% unlimited fresh grass or hay, 10% leafy greens, vegetables and herbs, and 5% good quality commercial pelleted food (Rabbit Welfare Association & Fund, 2020). Unlimited access to clean, fresh water should be provided to meet their daily water requirement of 10% bodyweight. Whilst fresh grass is preferable, good quality hay is a suitable substitute and provides rabbits with a good source of fibre (at least 20%), moderate source of protein (12–15%) and trace minerals. It is also low in fat, starch and sugar. The interaction between ingesta and the occlusal surfaces of teeth during mastication leads to abrasive wear (Winkler *et al.*, 2019). Hay and grass are most effective at achieving repeated tooth-to-tooth contact and promoting dental health due to their silica content and the presence, and abrasive action, of phytoliths. Rabbits receiving a sufficient quantity of hay or fresh forage are at lower risk of fur chewing and subsequent trichobezoar formation.

A hay-based diet promotes increased water intake and the production of higher volumes of less concentrated urine, resulting in a prophylactic effect against urolith formation (Clauss, 2012). The most appropriate type of hay varies according to the age of the rabbit (Figure 5.3). In addition to unlimited grass and hay, leafy greens, vegetables and herbs are important nutritional components and should comprise 10% of a rabbit's diet (Figure 5.4).

Commercially produced concentrate diets ensure nutrient requirements are fulfilled in rabbits consuming insufficient amounts of forage, or where the quality of these items is questionable. Convenience is a major appeal of this type of food to owners, but it should only constitute up to 5% of a rabbit's diet. Concentrate diets are available in a mixed or pellet form. Mixed diets are cereal-based and resemble muesli. The brightly coloured appearance and variation in ingredients make them visually appealing to owners; however, this promotes selective feeding. Rabbits usually favour components such as grains and pulses, which are high in starch, low in fibre and low in calcium, resulting in the consumption of a diet low in essential nutrients and high in protein, fat and carbohydrate (Harcourt-Brown, 1996).

The consumption of mixed diets has been linked to a reduction in hay and water intake, faecal output and caecotroph ingestion, as well as the development of life-threatening dental, digestive and urinary tract disease in rabbits. In contrast, pellet-style diets are grass-based, with ingredients processed into uniform pellets, thus providing a consistent ration and preventing selective feeding. High-quality extruded pellets are considered the optimal choice when selecting a commercially produced rabbit diet. These incorporate long fibre particles and are more palatable and digestible than standard pellet diets. The heated extrusion process improves starch digestibility and reduces carbohydrate overload of the hindgut. Commercial diets with crude fibre levels of more than 18%, indigestible fibre levels of more than 12.5% and protein levels around 15% are recommended.

When selecting an appropriate diet, it is essential to consider the specific energy and nutrient requirements of rabbits at different life stages (Figure 5.5) and in relation to breed, condition and lifestyle. Rabbits absorb calcium at a level directly related to that offered in their food. Maintaining an appropriate dietary calcium content of approximately 1.0%, dietary phosphorus content of approximately 0.4–0.8% and a calcium:phosphorus ratio of between 1.5:1 and 2:1 is vital (PFMA, 2015b).

Approximate age	Type of hay	Justification
7 weeks to 7 months	Unlimited alfalfa hay	Provides the high caloric and calcium content necessary for development and weight gain in young rabbits
7 months to 1 year	Gradually introduce grass hay such as timothy and decrease alfalfa	High in fibre. Coarse varieties provide an abrasive diet and promote dental health
1 year to 5 years	Unlimited timothy, oat or grass hays	Contains lower calcium and high fibre
6 years and up	Continue adult diet if weight is maintained. Feed alfalfa hay if weight loss is a concern (as long as calcium levels are normal)	Alfalfa has a high caloric content and so is good for promoting weight gain, yet it has a high calcium content

5.3 The most appropriate type of hay according to the age of the rabbit.

Case example 1: Grazing animals *continued*

Food item	Considerations when feeding	Herbivores				Omnivores			
		Rabbits	Guinea pigs	Chinchillas	Degus	Gerbils	Hamsters	Mice	Rats
Alliums (including leeks, onions, chives, shallots and garlic)	Contain toxic components that may damage red blood cells and provoke haemolytic anaemia accompanied by the formation of Heinz bodies in erythrocytes of animals	X	X	X	X	X	X	X	X
Asparagus	Contains oxalate, phosphorous and vitamin C	–	✓	X	–	–	✓	✓	✓
Aubergine	Contain alkaloids (solanine), too much of which can cause inflammation	–	✓	X	–	–	✓	✓	✓
Avocado		X	X	X	X	X	X	X	X
Beetroot (raw) and beetroot tops	Contains a small amount of calcium and phosphorus	✓	✓	X	X	✓	✓	✓	✓
Banana	High in potassium and sugar	X	X	X	X	✓	✓	✓	✓
Bok choy		✓	✓	✓	✓	✓	✓	✓	✓
Bread, toast and sugar-free crackers (dry)		X	X	X	X	✓	✓	✓	✓
Breakfast cereal	Should be low sugar or sugar-free varieties	X	X	X	X	✓	✓	✓	✓
Broccoli (raw)	Contains vitamin C and high amounts of vitamin A	✓	✓	✓	✓	✓	✓	✓	✓
Butternut squash	More palatable when cooked	✓	✓	X	✓	✓	✓	✓	✓
Cabbage (green)	Contains high amounts of vitamin C but large intake can cause gas and bloating	✓	✓	✓	✓	✓	✓	✓	✓
Cabbage (red)	Contains high amounts of vitamin C, and a hint of calcium	✓	✓	✓	✓	–	–	–	–
Carrot and carrot tops	Contain oxalate and high amounts of vitamin A and sugar	✓	✓	✓	✓	–	✓	✓	✓
Cauliflower leaves and stalks	Contains high amounts of vitamin C but large intake can cause gas and bloating	✓	✓	X	✓	–	✓	✓	✓
Celery		✓	✓	✓	✓	–	✓	✓	✓
Chard		✓	✓	✓	✓	–	✓	–	–
Chicory		✓	✓	✓	✓	–	✓	✓	✓
Chickpeas	Can be fed roasted, sprouted, canned or boiled. Supplementation found to promote weight gain in guinea pigs	–	✓	–	–	✓	✓	✓	✓
Chickweed	Has white flowers, not to be confused with scarlet pimpernel which is poisonous	✓	–	–	–	–	–	–	–
Chocolate or cocoa	Unsuitable for all small mammals	X	X	X	X	X	X	X	X
Courgette		✓	✓	X	–	–	✓	✓	✓
Corn	Contains vitamin C but is also high in starch. Whole corn should not be fed to rabbits or guinea pigs due to risk of fatal blockages; ground corn may be fed as part of commercial pellets	X	X	X	✓	–	✓	–	–

5.4 A guide to fresh food items that are safe or unsafe to feed to small mammals. Please note this list is not exhaustive. Appropriate research and identification of potential foodstuffs should be undertaken. ✓ = can be offered daily; ✓ = can be offered sometimes/as an occasional treat; X = should never be fed; – = no information available. (continues) ▶

Case example 1: Grazing animals *continued*

Food item	Considerations when feeding	Herbivores				Omnivores			
		Rabbits	Guinea pigs	Chinchillas	Degus	Gerbils	Hamsters	Mice	Rats
Cucumber	Can provide a source of fluid intake in hot weather	✓	✓	X	✓	–	✓	✓	✓
Dairy products and eggs	Low fat varieties	X	X	X	X	–	✓ (scrambled, cooked egg)	✓ (scrambled, cooked egg)	✓ (cottage cheese, cooked egg)
Dandelion leaves		✓	✓	✓	✓	–	–	–	–
Dock	Only the young leaves should be fed, not after it goes to seed	✓	✓	–	–	–	–	–	–
Fruit (citrus)		X	X	X	X	X	X	X	X
Fruit (crunchy) such as apples (without seeds) and pears	Apple seeds are toxic to a number of small mammal species and should not be fed	✓	✓	✓	✓	–	✓	✓	✓
Fruit (dried)	Dried fruit such as raisins, cranberries and bananas are very high in sugar and should therefore be fed only as a treat at a frequency of one piece per week	X	X	✓	X	–	✓	✓	✓
Grains (cooked)		–	–	–	–	–	–	✓	–
Green beans	Contain vitamin C, and can be fed in a raw state. However, be cautious as they also contain calcium and phosphorus	✓	✓	✓	✓	✓	✓	✓	✓
Herbs (dried)		✓	✓	✓	✓	–	✓	–	–
Herbs (fresh) including basil, sage, parsley, mint and coriander		✓	✓	✓	✓	✓	✓	✓	✓
Insect food (live)	Live insects provide mental stimulation, encourage activity and enable expression of natural behaviours	X	X	X	X	–	–	✓	✓
Kale		✓	✓	✓	–	–	✓	✓	✓
Meat products (cooked)		X	X	X	X	✓	✓	✓	✓
Nuts	Should be unsalted variety	X	X	X	X	–	✓ (never almonds)	✓ (never peanuts)	–
Parsnip		✓	✓	–	–	–	–	–	–
Pasta (cooked)		X	X	X	X	–	✓	✓	✓
Peas	Contain phosphorus, calcium and vitamin C	–	✓	X	✓	–	✓	✓	✓
Peppers (bell)	Contain high amounts of vitamin C. Also contain alkaloids (solanine), too much of which can cause inflammation	–	✓ (red)	–	✓	–	✓	✓	✓
Potato (cooked)	Contain alkaloids (solanine), too much of which can cause inflammation. Also high in carbohydrates and starch. Potato leaves can be poisonous to some small mammals and should not be fed	X	X	X	X	–	✓	✓	✓
Pumpkin		✓ (raw)	–	✓	✓	–	–	–	–

5.4 (continued) A guide to fresh food items that are safe or unsafe to feed to small mammals. Please note this list is not exhaustive. Appropriate research and identification of potential foodstuffs should be undertaken. ✓ = can be offered daily; ✓ = can be offered sometimes/as an occasional treat; X = should never be fed; – = no information available (continues) ▶

Case example 1: Grazing animals *continued*

Food item	Considerations when feeding	Herbivores				Omnivores			
		Rabbits	Guinea pigs	Chinchillas	Degus	Gerbils	Hamsters	Mice	Rats
Radicchio		✓	✓	✓	✓	–	–	–	–
Radishes		✓	✓	✓	✓	–	–	✓	✓
Raspberry		✓	✓	X	X	–	✓	–	–
Rhubarb and rhubarb leaves		X	X	X	X	X	X	X	X
Seeds		X	X	X	X	✓	✓	✓	✓
Strawberry		✓	✓	X	X	✓	✓	✓	✓
Spinach	Contains high oxalate levels	✓	✓	✓	✓	✓	✓	✓	✓
Soya yogurt		X	X	X	X	✓	✓	✓	✓
Sprouts	Contain phosphorus and oxalic acid. Large intake can cause gas and bloating	✓	✓	✓	✓	✓	✓	✓	✓
Sweet potato		X	X	X	✓	–	✓	–	X
Tomatoes	Contain alkaloids (solanine), too much of which can cause inflammation. Tomato leaves are poisonous to a number of small mammal species and should be avoided	✓	✓	–	✓	X	X	X	X
Turnips and turnip greens	Low phosphorus:calcium ratio. Contain some vitamin C	✓	✓	–	–	–	–	–	–
Watercress	Contain high amounts of vitamin C. Watch for liver flukes if sourced from streams	✓	✓	–	–	–	–	–	–

5.4 (continued) A guide to fresh food items that are safe or unsafe to feed to small mammals. Please note this list is not exhaustive. Appropriate research and identification of potential foodstuffs should be undertaken. ✓ = can be offered daily; ✓ = can be offered sometimes/as an occasional treat; **X** = should never be fed; – = no information available.

Life stage	Energy requirement	Total protein (%)	Digestible protein (%)	Fat (%)	Fibre (%)	Digestible carbohydrates (NFE, %)	Total digestible nutrients (%)
Maintenance	100 kcal ME x bodyweight (kg) $^{0.75}$	12	9	1.5–2	14–20	40–45	50–60
Growth	A multiple of 1.9 to 2.1 [a]	16	12	2–4	14–16	45–50	60–70
Gestation	A multiple of 1.35 to 2.0 [a]	15	11	2–3	14–16	45–50	55–65
Lactation (with litter of 7–8)	A multiple of 3.0 [a]	17	13	2.5–3.5	12–14	45–50	65–75

5.5 Specific energy and nutrient requirements of rabbits at different life stages in relation to total diet. ME = metabolizable energy; NFE = nitrogen-free extract; [a] = in relation to maintenance value.
(FEDIAF, 2013; Mayer, 2015)

Small mammals

Given their high metabolic rate, it is natural for many small mammals to feed almost continuously. The nutritional requirements of small mammals vary across species and life stage (Figure 5.6). As with rabbits, the diet of most species should contain a variety of fresh food items (see Figure 5.4) and only a small percentage of commercially produced concentrate food. Foraging is an essential feeding practice and behavioural need for a range of animals, including myomorphs, hystricomorphs and sciuromorphs. Many of these species are highly exploratory and have adapted to working for their food; therefore, captive animals unable to replicate this natural feeding behaviour are at an increased risk of developing mental and physical health problems and behavioural stereotypies. These include barbering, over-grooming, excessive chewing (cage bars or other materials), aggression and circling. Whilst small mammals have their own species-specific behaviours and needs, most do better in a complicated space, created with multilevel caging or the use of cage furniture to simulate an environment similar to that of their wild counterparts. Structural items that are safe to gnaw should also be provided. Similar methods of feeding to those previously described for rabbits can help to encourage natural foraging behaviours, whilst promoting exercise and reducing the risk of obesity.

▶

Case example 1: Grazing animals *continued*

Generic nutritional requirements	Species-specific nutritional requirements and dietary-related considerations	
Herbivores		
• Hindgut fermenters • Consume a grass- and plant-based diet • Require high levels of dietary fibre and therefore need plenty of good quality fresh hay and/or grass on a daily basis • Provision of fresh herbs or leafy green vegetables offer dietary variety and behavioural enrichment • Alongside grass, hay and fresh food, a portion of species-specific commercial pelleted pet food ensures that nutrient requirements are fulfilled • Have open-rooted teeth and therefore require an abrasive diet	Guinea pigs	• Require vitamin C supplementation – have a minimum dietary requirement of 10 mg/kg/day (30 mg/kg/day in pregnancy) • Some forms of vitamin C supplementation are unstable and oxidize readily. Commercial diets containing stabilized forms should be fed and appropriate storage conditions should be maintained in accordance with manufacturer's guidance once opened • High vitamin A requirement • High dietary calcium can lead to urinary tract disease and should be avoided
	Chinchillas	• Natural diet includes the consumption of tough and fibrous vegetation, low in energy content. This requires high dietary fibre intake and prolonged mastication for the extraction of nutrients • Recommended diet consists of a good quality grass hay and a small amount of commercially produced chinchilla pellets. Sole feeding of commercial pellets should be avoided • Fruit and small amounts of greens offer suitable treats but sugar-rich foods should be avoided • Any dietary change should be conducted gradually and with close monitoring of faecal output
	Degus	• Natural diet includes grass, leaves, herbs, seeds, fruits, fresh cattle/horse droppings and crops • Captive animals should be fed grass hay alongside commercial chinchilla pellets and occasional amounts of fresh greens
Omnivores		
• Consume a plant- and animal-based diet • In their natural habitat, omnivores also eat grass, seeds, grains and insects • Small amounts of fresh fruit and vegetables should be provided • Alongside fresh food, a portion of species-specific commercial pelleted pet food ensures that nutrient requirements are fulfilled	Gerbils	• Coprophagic • Natural diet includes coarse grasses, roots, seeds and occasional invertebrates • Captive animals can be fed a commercial pelleted rodent diet with added fruit, vegetables and hay • Gerbils will eat sunflower seeds to the exclusion of other foods. These are high in cholesterol and low in amino acids, vitamins and minerals, particularly calcium, contributing to obesity and musculoskeletal disorders
	Hamsters	• Coprophagic • Hoard food; care should be taken when feeding meat and fresh food. Old food should be removed regularly • Fluid requirement of 10 ml/100 g BW • Begin eating solid food at 7–10 days old • Energy requirement (kcal/day) = $110 \times BW^{0.75}$ • Protein requirements range from 16% (maintenance) to 20% (reproduction) • Carbohydrate and fat requirements are a 60–65% and 5–7%, respectively
	Mice and rats	• Opportunistic and are prone to obesity if fed a high-sugar or high-calorie diet • To avoid dietary imbalances, a commercial, pelleted rodent diet should be fed, supplemented with a wide variety of fresh food in moderation • Excessive supplementation can result in dietary imbalance, obesity or gastrointestinal upset
Carnivores		
• Consume mainly or exclusively an animal-based diet • Alongside fresh food, a portion of species-specific commercial pelleted pet food ensures that nutrient requirements are fulfilled	Ferrets	• Require a good quality high-protein diet • Fat content can vary from 9–28% but ferrets are prone to obesity so food intake should be closely monitored and a high-calorie diet avoided • Have a short gut and fast gut transit time; carbohydrate and fibre intake should be low • A natural diet of whole carcasses and dry commercial pelleted food is recommended for the prevention of dental disease

5.6 Nutritional requirements and dietary considerations for small mammals. BW = bodyweight.

Case example 1: Grazing animals *continued*

Reptiles

Meeting the physical, mental and behavioural demands of reptiles is reliant on the provision of an optimal environment, diet and, if relevant, compatible cage mates (Pasmans *et al.*, 2017). In contrast to endotherms, ectotherms are characterized by low metabolic rates, low energy requirements, and low food intakes (Lagarde *et al.*, 2003). Reptiles consume a variety of food types and utilize a range feeding strategies; feeding behaviours vary according to diet, which can itself be complex. Given the highly specific nutritional requirements required by some reptilian species, replicating the natural diet for captive animals can be particularly challenging (Pasmans *et al.*, 2017). Many primarily herbivorous reptiles such as tortoises, green iguanas and uromastyx have adapted to live in arid/semi-arid areas where climatic conditions can be harsh and food scarce, necessitating lengthy periods of foraging over large distances. Optimizing foraging efficiency is further complicated as their food resource often consists of fibrous plant materials, considered to be of poor nutrient value (Lagarde *et al.*, 2003). Captive reptiles are often presented with excessive amounts of easily accessible food which, given their low metabolism and relative inactivity, results in malnourishment, boredom, frustration and other health and behavioural problems.

Birds

In comparison to their captive counterparts, wild birds are surrounded by unpredictable stimuli to which they have adapted to respond and, therefore, are able to exert a certain degree of control over their environment. It has been suggested that birds working for food in the presence of identical free food (contra-freeloading) exert control over aspects of their environment and that non-food-deprived birds prefer variable to constant reinforcement.

Chickens and parrots are two examples of birds that would naturally graze in the wild and spend a significant amount of time searching for food. In captivity, insufficient provision of foraging opportunities results in frustration, boredom and the exhibition of a variety of undesirable and stereotypical behaviours, including psychogenic pterotillomania (feather plucking) and mutilation. It is surmised that feather pecking stems from redirected foraging motivation and therefore the provision of forages to birds is most likely to decrease feather-pecking behaviour (Dixon *et al.*, 2010). However, this behavioural problem can also be associated with other management factors, such as social isolation and lack of environmental stimuli, as well as medical conditions. A full history should be obtained to ascertain the cause. Figure 5.7 details the nutritional requirements and dietary considerations for chickens and parrots.

Zoological species

A wide range of wild animal species dedicate a significant amount of time to foraging. Not only does this prompt activity, it also promotes the animal's expression of cognitive skills, such as problem-solving, as well as exploratory behaviour and fine-tuned motor skills (Bennett *et al.*, 2014). The controlled diets and provisioned feeding experienced by many captive animals contrast radically with the ever-changing foraging and decision-making processes of daily life by their wild counterparts.

Feeding regimes are just one of the factors found to influence the display of abnormal stereotypical behaviours in captive wild animals, such as repetitive pacing, swaying, head-bobbing, bar-biting, self-mutilation, over-grooming or excessive licking. The provision of rich, naturalistic enclosures with a variety of stimuli, unpredictable feeding schedules, and extractive foraging opportunities, together with chances for exploration, social interaction and housing, are likely to contribute to positive affective states in animals and have the potential to decrease the performance of abnormal behaviours (Wolfensohn *et al.*, 2018).

Horses

Horses are selective grazers; fibre should constitute at least 50% of the diet, and in many cases up to 100%, with grass as the principal constituent. Whilst at pasture, horses spend approximately 70% of their time (around 17 hours per day) grazing and demonstrate a range of foraging behaviours, including locomotion, selection, manipulation and ingestion of food. At times of increased grass quality and quantity, horses can eat up to 4% of their bodyweight per day; however, a maximum of 1.5–2% bodyweight is recommended (British Horse Society, 2019).

Stabled horses and those with limited access to pasture are maintained in conditions very different from those in which they evolved, often being provided with a single low-forage diet, straw bed and concentrate rations. This undesirable type of management is linked to a variety of health problems and the exhibition of stereotypical and redirected behaviour patterns, including crib biting, weaving, windsucking and pawing (Goodwin *et al.*, 2002; Thorne *et al.*, 2005). For horses with restricted or no access to pasture, the provision of a multiple forage diet, together with foraging enrichment and the promotion of more natural feeding behaviours can help to improve health and welfare.

Medical problems

Lack of, or inadequate, forage (quantity or quality) has been identified as a contributory factor to a number of medical problems. Owner education about optimal feeding regimes is therefore essential. Nutrition is recognized as vital and regardless of the reason for an animal's presentation at the clinic, all aspects of the diet should be assessed for every animal at every veterinary visit.

Case example 1: Grazing animals *continued*

	General dietary considerations	Suitable additions to a commercial pellet diet [a,b]	Foods to avoid [a]	Age and life stage of bird	Oils/fats	Protein	Fibre	Ash
Chickens	• The provision of a complete commercial diet, formulated for the appropriate age and life stage, should constitute 90% of the daily dietary intake and ensures that basic dietary requirements are met • Other food items can be offered as treats and for environmental enrichment but these should be kept to a minimum (no more than 10% of daily dietary intake) • It is illegal to feed kitchen scraps unless the household is 100% vegan, but vegetables straight from the garden are permitted • Using feed-balls or hiding favoured treats encourages natural feeding behaviours	Fresh food including: • Cabbage • Cauliflower leaves • Spinach • Dandelions • Pasta • Hardboiled egg • Corn-on-the-cob • Invertebrates including mealworms • Fruit such as apples and strawberries are suitable to be fed only as occasional treats	• 'Junk food' – anything processed and high in salt, fat or sugar • Avocado • Chocolate or cocoa • Products containing caffeine or alcohol	Chick (6 weeks to 8 weeks)	3.5%	18.0%	4.5%	6.0%
				Growers (9 weeks to 20 weeks)	3.5%	16.0%	4.5%	5.5%
				Layers (21 weeks to 7 weeks)	2.7%	16.0%	5.5%	12.5%
				End of lay (72 weeks onwards)	4.0%	16.0%	4.0%	14.0%
Parrots [c]	• Wild parrots eat a variety of foodstuffs depending on location, species, availability and time of year; attempting to replicate this in captivity can be challenging • The mainstay of a pet bird's diet (approximately 80% of the food consumed) should be a premium commercial pellet supplemented with fresh food • Pelleted and extruded foods provide balanced nutrition; however, these diets alone do not provide sufficient physical or mental stimulation • Traditional mixed, un-supplemented seed-based diets are often deficient in essential amino acids, vitamins and minerals, high in fat and carbohydrate and promote selective feeding • One of the most important dietary minerals is calcium. To utilize this, birds require vitamin D3, which is activated by ultraviolet (UV)B light. The calcium:phosporus ratio should be maintained around 2:1 • Fresh water should always be available and preferably placed away from the food source to encourage exercise and prevent contamination • 'Feeding time' for wild parrots is usually very social. When tempting a captive bird on to pellets, or when introducing a novel food item, it can be useful to do so at the same time as the owner is eating • Some parrots are specialist feeders and require appropriate diets including grain, fruit and nectar-based	Fresh food including: • Soaked pulses • Leafy green vegetables • Seeds and nuts should make up only 10% of the entire diet but are good training aids and occasional treats Whole wheat pasta and cooked whole grains including brown rice can be suitable in moderation. Offering whole food items such as corn-on-the-cob with the husk still on, wrapping favoured food items in paper or making use of foraging toys will encourage birds to forage for food. It is important to be aware of the energy density of supplemented food	• Dairy produce • 'Junk food' – anything processed and high in salt, fat or sugar • Avocado • Meat • Chocolate or cocoa • Peanuts • Tapioca • Products containing onion, garlic, caffeine or alcohol	Juvenile	–	20%	–	–
				Pubertal	–	20%	–	–
				Maturity	2.0–4.0%	10–15%	–	–

5.7 Nutritional requirements and dietary considerations for chickens and parrots. – = data cannot be specified. [a] Please note this list is not exhaustive: appropriate research and identification of potential foodstuff should be undertaken. [b] Any food source offered should be fit for human consumption and preferably organic. [c] The information in this table does not apply equally across all parrot species: the reader is urged to research the individual needs of species they work with. See the BSAVA Manual of Psittacine Birds for more information.
(Jones and Dodd, 2012; Davies, 2016)

Case example 1: Grazing animals *continued*

Dental disease

Small mammals with open-rooted teeth, such as rabbits, guinea pigs and chinchillas, are at an increased risk of developing dental disease if fed high quantities of processed soft food and an insufficiently fibrous, abrasive and plant-based diet. Whilst the occlusion of these animals may be sound, without sufficiently vigorous or lengthy chewing, the teeth will overgrow, preventing normal prehension and mastication of food and closure of the mouth (Legendre, 2002). It is therefore essential that the main constituent (at least 70–85%) of their diet is naturally abrasive, good quality grass, with the remainder comprising a variety of greens. Whilst hay is considered by many owners to be a suitable substitute for grass, studies suggest that access to natural grazing and vitamin D from sunlight may promote more effective dental wear than unlimited access to hay (Müller *et al.*, 2015; Norman and Wills, 2016).

Obesity

Obesity is a multifactorial condition, with several risk factors contributing to weight gain in different species. For grazing species, some of the main contributory factors include access to, and type of grazing, together with a relative lack of physical activity. The provision of commercial food in a bowl enables easy and rapid consumption, leaving much of the animal's time unoccupied. This can lead to undesirable behaviours, including gnawing and food aggression. Animals provided with a natural high-fibre diet that takes several hours to search for and graze on are better able to develop and exhibit natural foraging behaviours and benefit from increased activity and stimulation.

Gastrointestinal stasis

Insufficient consumption of dietary fibre in rabbits and hystricomorph rodents reduces gut motility, increasing the risk of gastrointestinal stasis. In captive animals, a lack of exercise and limited opportunity to exhibit natural species-specific behaviours, such as grazing, further contributes to gut hypomotility. Other contributory factors include pain, anorexia, dehydration, environmental stressors and dental disease (often a secondary factor due to the consumption of an incorrect diet).

Gastrointestinal stasis is one of the most serious conditions seen in rabbits and requires prompt action by the owner and treatment by the veterinary healthcare team. Anorexic animals should be examined as soon as possible following reduction or cess ation of food intake. Supportive care is critical with stress reduction and the provision of warmth, pain relief, fluid therapy and nutritional support considered important first aid measures (Johnson, 2019). The key principles of treatment in cases of gastrointestinal stasis include rehydration of the patient and stomach contents, alleviation of pain, provision of nutrition and treatment of any underlying disorders. Re-establishing gut motility is reliant on the ingestion of fibrous food; therefore, free-choice hay and water together with a variety of greens should be offered. Pharmacological treatment generally involves analgesia and prokinetic therapy with or without the administration of antacids. Treatment alone is insufficient and identification of the underlying cause is essential to prevent recurrence.

Equine gastric ulcer syndrome

Equine gastric ulcer syndrome (EGUS) is a general term used to describe erosive and ulcerative diseases of the stomach in horses. More recently, equine squamous gastric disease (ESGD) and equine glandular gastric disease (EGGD) have been proposed as terms that more specifically describe the affected anatomical region (Sykes *et al.*, 2015). The prevalence of gastric ulceration in horses varies with breed, use and level of training, as well as between ESGD and EGGD.Horses continually secrete gastric acid and prolonged exposure of the proximal stomach to a low pH environment has been identified as the primary cause of EGUS (Reese and Andrews, 2009). Normal grazing behaviour stimulates the production of saliva, which helps to buffer the naturally acidic stomach contents, resulting in a pH ≥4 for a large portion of the day. Pasture turnout is considered to reduce the risk of EGUS, although evidence to support this is conflicting. Similarly, free access to fibrous feed or frequent forage feeding is widely considered to reduce the risk of gastric ulceration, although strong evidence supporting this position is also lacking, and the impact of forage feeding in the absence of other risk factor reduction might not be as great as previously believed (Sykes *et al.*, 2015).

Whilst large-scale epidemiological studies are lacking in relation to EGGD, nutrition-related risk factors for the development of ESGD appear to include:

* Fasting and intermittent starvation
* Increased time between forage feeding (>6 hours between meals)
* Feeding grain at 1% bodyweight to stabled and non-exercising horses, 1 hour before hay is fed
* Starch intake exceeding 2 g/kg bodyweight per day
* The provision of straw as the only forage
* Intermittent access to water.

The primary goals of treatment and management are pain relief, healing and the prevention of secondary complications (Reese and Andrews, 2009). Pharmacological treatment indicated in the management of both ESGD and EGGD focuses on suppressing gastric acid secretion and increasing stomach pH (Sykes *et al.*, 2015).

▶

Case example 1: Grazing animals *continued*

Environmental, dietary and nutritional management have traditionally been identified as playing an important role in EGUS; however, strong evidence supporting certain nutritional recommendations is lacking, particularly in relation to the role of diet in EGGD. The following recommendations in relation to nutritional management have been proposed by Sykes *et al.* (2015) and are primarily based on risk factors identified for ESGD:

- Continuous access to good quality grass pasture is considered ideal. Free choice or frequent feedings (4–6 meals per day) of hay (minimum of 1.5 kg (dry matter; DM)/100 kg bodyweight per day) might be a suitable replacement
- Overweight animals at risk of EGUS should receive a minimum amount of high-quality forage (1.5 kg (DM)/100 kg bodyweight per day); the forage should be mature and have a low energy content
- Straw can be fed at <0.25 kg (DM)/100 kg bodyweight per day, but should not be the only forage provided
- Grain and concentrate food should be fed as sparingly as possible:
  - Feeding more than 1–2 kg of sweet feed per meal can result in the excessive production of VFAs and should be avoided
  - Grains such as barley and oats can be substituted to decrease fermentation to VFAs
  - The diet should not exceed 2 g/kg bodyweight of starch intake per day or more than 1 g/kg bodyweight of starch per meal
  - Concentrate meals should not be fed <6 hours apart
- Water should be provided continuously
- Vegetable oils such as corn oil might help to reduce the risk of EGGD.

Foraging enrichment

Normal behaviour must be considered not only in terms of what is natural for a particular species, but also whether the range and context are appropriate. For example, in the wild, food is seasonal and randomly distributed and its availability cannot be guaranteed. In contrast, the feeding schedules for captive animals, including pets, may be stricter and foraging is often simpler. Less time and effort is required by the animal to search for and manipulate food, thus negatively affecting their natural foraging behaviour, resulting in frustration and boredom (Charmoy *et al.*, 2015).

The relationship between inadequate foraging opportunities and the exhibition of stereotypical and redirected behaviour patterns has been well documented in many species (Goodwin *et al.*, 2002; Thorne *et al.*, 2005; Schepers *et al.*, 2009; Malmkvist *et al.*, 2013). Foraging enrichment is therefore considered one of the most effective strategies to improve animal welfare and reduce such behaviours (van Zeeland *et al.*, 2013).

Extending foraging time through dietary enrichment and modifications to the feeding method can help to increase activity levels and promote more naturalistic behaviour (Hosey, 2005). Providing a variety of enrichment also creates a healthier environment and caters for individual preference (Rooney and Sleeman, 1998). When considering environmental adaptation or use of resources to promote foraging opportunities, it is important to introduce these slowly and under observation, particularly when multiple animals are present. Materials and dietary choices must be safe, non-toxic and appropriate to the age, life stage, physiology and species of animal. A number of dietary-related enrichment examples are given in Figure 5.8. See Chapter 4 for more information on feeding enrichment.

Non-device-based foraging enrichments

- Rather than placing food/meals in one location, it can be scattered, smeared, frozen or hidden to encourage animals to forage, hunt and manipulate their food
- Suspension of food from hanging points within the enclosure (such as the furniture, roof or sides) is unpredictable in movement, providing stimulation for animals
- Implementing unpredictable feeding schedules
- Providing food items that take a longer period of time to consume
- Alternating the frequency and scheduling of feeding
- Providing carcass feeding to carnivores
- Variation in the diet and provision of novel food items
- Use of a multiple level platform
- Providing a suitable substrate to enable foraging and digging
- Changes in food size or texture (e.g. diced or whole food, frozen or juice) to alter foraging and feeding patterns
- Providing live food. In the UK, the feeding of live vertebrate prey is illegal

Device-based foraging enrichments

- Providing gnawing surfaces and opportunities for activity
- Use of puzzle feeders and limited access food hoppers
- Use of scent-infused sacks
- Placing food inside hollow toys, balls, cardboard boxes or tubes pierced with holes
- Hiding food in cardboard boxes or tubes filled with straw, hay or other species-appropriate material
- Hiding food in deep substrate such as straw, hay, shredded paper, wood shavings, blankets, wood chip or another species-appropriate material

5.8 Examples of foraging-related enrichment strategies that can be adapted and implemented for different species of animal. (Adapted from Jennings and Prescott, 2009)

Clinical diseases related to poor nutritional welfare

Malnutrition is a serious condition that occurs when an individual's diet does not contain the correct amount of nutrients (National Health Service, 2020). The term does not just apply to animals that are not receiving enough nutrients – it can also be used to indicate that an animal is being given too many nutrients; in the UK more animals are now suffering with malnutrition because of obesity than are suffering with emaciation (PDSA, 2019).

Obesity

At the most recent estimation, veterinary professionals considered 51% of dogs, 44% of cats and 29% of small mammals to be either overweight or obese (PFMA, 2019b). Animals may become obese as a result of a variety of reasons (Jones, 2019):

- Higher than necessary calorie intake
- Incorrect diet
- Too many or inappropriate treats and table scraps
- Lack of sufficient and appropriate exercise
- Enclosure/environment
- Neutering
- Genetics.

Veterinary professionals are acutely aware of the massive detrimental impact obesity has on the welfare of their patients (Marshall et al., 2010). Overweight dogs have an overall lifespan that is 2 years shorter than that of a dog of a healthy weight (Marshall et al., 2010) and although cats do not appear to have a reduced lifespan due to obesity, there is evidence that their quality of life is impacted as owners of overweight animals spend 36% more on diagnostic procedures than owners of healthy cats (Banfield Pet Hospital, 2019). Unsurprisingly, the small animal and exotic pet populations reflect the same trend in increasing obesity (PFMA, 2018), and the health problems encountered in dogs and cats can also be seen in rabbits (Carroll et al., 1999), rodents (Buettner et al., 2007), reptiles (Frye, 1984) and birds (Schoemaker et al., 1999).

Unfortunately, this pattern also appears to be reflected in the captive animal population. Certain reptile species gain weight in captivity because of an inappropriate diet coupled with a natural propensity to store fat (Donoghue, 2006; Rawski and Jozefiak, 2014). Obesity has also been documented in smaller primates such as lemurs (Schwitzer and Kaumanns, 2001) and marmosets (Power et al., 2013), as well as larger species such as chimpanzees (Videan et al., 2007); the latter having been proven to have similar health problem to humans, including obesity-related hypertension (Ely et al., 2013).

The problem of obesity can seem overwhelming, but with discussion and education it has been proven that over 50% of owners who agree with the obesity assessment of the veterinary team will take steps to reduce the weight of their pet (Cairns-Haylor and Fordyce, 2017). These conversations can be difficult but veterinary staff should remember that their duty of care is to the animal and that nutritional welfare is a priority. It is important to feed an appropriate diet when putting an animal on a weight loss programme; whether that be a diet that has been specifically formulated for weight reduction or a recipe that has been formulated by a certified animal nutritionist, as restricted intake of food not manufactured for weight loss can put animals at risk of nutrient deficiencies (Gaylord et al., 2018). The veterinary care team and owner/keeper should work together to ensure that the animals in their care are healthy and fed an appropriate diet.

Underweight animals and weight loss

Underweight animals present a management challenge for the veterinary care team and, with the increasingly aging pet population (Wallis et al., 2018), geriatric weight loss is an area of senior care to consider. Animals (particularly cats) over the age of 11 lose body condition rapidly over time (Gross et al., 2010). Anorexia is common and can be due to a number of age-related conditions, including decline in taste and smell perception, dental disease, physical debilitation, and chronic disease and the drugs associated with its management (Gross et al., 2010). Diet recipes and formulations should be reassessed for patients over 11 years of age (Laflamme, 1997).

It is important to remember that cachexia, anorexia and hyporexia can be associated with various chronic diseases; the disease causing the clinical signs should be treated as the priority and the appropriate diet chosen according to the diagnosis (Gagne and Wakshlag, 2015). Cachexia associated with cancer, in particular, is associated with weight loss, reduced nutritional intake and inflammation. In these cases, cachexia is made worse by the side effects from surgery and associated treatments, such as radiotherapy and chemotherapy, which can cause inappetence, anorexia, nausea, vomiting and diarrhoea, and thus contribute to further weight loss (Hand et al., 2011).

Although there are very few documented cases, refeeding syndrome is a particular concern in cats; it can be fatal in starved or severely malnourished individuals, as the weakened cardiovascular system cannot cope with the reintroduction of fluid and electrolytes if enteral or parenteral nutrition is used without caution (Weinsier and Krumdieck, 1981; Brenner et al., 2011; DeAvilla and Leech, 2016). The degree of malnutrition sustained by an individual may increase the risk of developing refeeding syndrome, but it has also been noted in patients who have had only a brief period of starvation (Chan, 2015). It is known to occur in small ruminants that have received parenteral nutrition (Luethy et al., 2020) and reptiles (Boyer and Scott, 2019), and there has been one documented incidence of refeeding syndrome in a group of dogs (Silvis et al., 1980). Recovery from refeeding syndrome can be achieved and seeking specialist nutritional knowledge is recommended as very specific feeding protocols have to be utilized (Armitage-Chan et al., 2006).

Other nutrition-related diseases

Malnutrition can also refer to an inappropriate diet that leads to health problems, other than those that are specifically weight-related; when formulating a diet for any species, care should be taken to ensure that it meets the needs of the animal. For example, although dental wear is common in nearly all mammals, especially as they age, captive big cats (Hope and Deem, 2006), bears (Kitchener, 2004) and great apes (Lowenstine et al., 2015) appear to have a greater incidence of dental disease than their wild counterparts. Thus, care should be taken to ensure that the items they are fed avoid ingredients known to increase the risk of dental disease and that the feeding methods implemented promote good dental health.

For carnivores and omnivores this can be achieved by providing different food stuffs in the diet that mimic the variety encountered in the natural environment (e.g. a whole carcass, including hair, organs and rumen, rather than select cuts of meat). Fresh and soft bones help to keep the teeth clean and less susceptible to disease (hard bones and ice enrichment should be avoided due to the risk of tooth fracture) (Briggs and Scheels, 2005). Providing a variety of items allows an animal suffering from dental disease to select the foods that are less difficult for them to consume, thereby reducing the risk of associated weight loss. This experience also provides enrichment as the individual has autonomy over which items to consume (Krebs et al., 2018).

Malnutrition in reptiles arising from an improper diet, as well as poor husbandry and feeding management, can lead to a multitude of diseases, including metabolic bone disorder, hypo- and hypervitaminosis A, hypovitaminosis B1, biotin and iodine deficiency, and hypovitaminosis E (Donoghue and McKeown, 1999; Wilkinson, 2015). Animals fed vertebrate prey should be given animals that have been fed a complete and nutritious diet. In addition, the method of thawing the prey items should ensure minimal water loss, as carnivorous species rely on their food for the majority of their water intake (Nijboer, 2015a).

There has been a lack of progression of nutritional understanding for ectotherms, but it is vital to ensure that they are exposed to ultraviolet (UV) light in order to maintain homeostasis and stimulate circadian rhythms to allow for vitamin D synthesis and calcium metabolism. Provision of thermal gradients in the environment allows an individual to adjust their body temperature as they would in the wild, which is vital for metabolism, and these environmental requirements continually change with season, age and reproductive status (Barten and Simpson, 2019).

Case example 2: Welfare compromises that can be caused in wild species by habituation through food

The intentional and unintentional feeding of wild animal species by human beings is a worldwide phenomenon that occurs for a variety of reasons. Whilst often motivated by good intentions, the appropriateness of this practice is controversial and is often a source of human–wildlife conflict (Orams, 2002; Dubois and Fraser, 2013).

What is habituation?

Habituation is defined as a reduction in response as a result of repeated exposure to a stimulus. Through this adaptive learning process, the stimulus elicits a change in behaviour in the absence of any training (Thompson, 2015).

Human disturbance is driving the decline of many species, both directly and indirectly (Samia et al., 2015). Wild and non-domesticated animals often perceive humans as predators and are generally human averse, avoiding people where possible and responding to human encounters by fleeing and retreating to cover (Knight, 2009). As such, sightings of these animals are often unpredictable and brief.

Over time, some species may become more tolerant of the presence of humans, but the extent to which they do is largely driven by the type of environment in which they live and by their body size (Samia et al., 2015). Free-ranging and captive wild animals with habituation and regular exposure to humans lose their fear of them, no longer viewing them as a threat and may allow closer contact. While this provides people with an incredible opportunity to view wildlife, habituation can be dangerous for both animals and humans (Orams, 2002; Nyhus, 2016).

Why and how is food habituation used in wild animal species?

Evidence suggests that animals and humans habituate on a variety of behavioural and physiological responses to repeated presentations of food cues (Epstein et al., 2009). In wild species this process, known as provisioning, offsets the human-aversive behaviour through the provision of food, exploiting their appetite and attraction to food, and acting as a form of bribery (Knight, 2009). Habituating animals to tolerate the presence of humans is often a slow process. The use of food can expedite the familiarization process in provisioned animals, resulting in their positive attraction to humans, whom they associate with food (Knight, 2009).

Four broad categories have been proposed by Dubois and Fraser (2013) to describe the main reasons for feeding wild animal species:

- Tourism
- Research
- Opportunistic
- Management.

Tourism

Ecotourism, in which travellers visit natural and often threatened environments to support conservation efforts and boost local economies, has become increasingly popular over recent years and often includes an element of wildlife tourism. This involves encounters with non-domesticated, wild animals either in their natural environment (on land or at sea; Figure 5.9) or in captivity, and entails attractions at fixed sites, tours, experiences available in association with tourist accommodation or unguided encounters by independent travellers (Higginbottom, 2004). Given the difficulty associated with locating and detecting free-ranging terrestrial and aquatic-based wild animals, habituation is considered a possible solution and has been described by Woodford et al. (2002) as a 'taming process'.

▶

Case example 2: Welfare compromises that can be caused in wild species by habituation through food *continued*

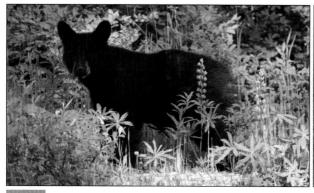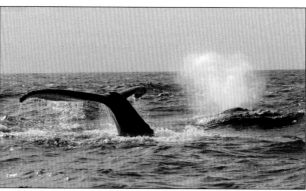

5.9 Encounters with wild animals in their natural environment are a popular aspect of ecotourism.

Over time, the relationship between the animal and food-giver develops with animals becoming more active solicitors rather than passive recipients of food. Animals may begin to exhibit begging behaviour and, longer term, may demonstrate human-centred aggression and violence (Knight, 2009). A reduction in their fearfulness and antipredator responses increases their vulnerability and predation risk.

Captive wildlife tourism is made possible due to zoos, wildlife parks, animal sanctuaries and aquaria. The behaviour of animals, particularly mammals, within these environments is often modified using standard operant conditioning and classical conditioning techniques through which food can be used as a type of positive reinforcement (Young and Cipreste, 2004; Miller and King, 2013).

Figures 5.10 and 5.11 detail the advantages and disadvantages of this form of habituation for free-ranging and captive wild animals, respectively.

Advantages
• Localizes the animals thus minimizing search time and enabling a more efficient form of wildlife viewing • Accelerates habituation, expediting the process of familiarization • Increased public awareness of wildlife and subsequent support for conservation • Benefits to human beings include: • Entertainment • Ability to observe/photograph wild animals • Educational purposes • Helping to counteract human actions perceived to have a negative effect on wild animals such as habitat destruction

Disadvantages
• Denies animals the opportunity to conceal themselves • Promotes the consumption of an inadequate and unsuitable diet • Habitation leads to secondary changes in the pattern of foraging. Provisioning results in primary changes in the process of food acquisition • Animals become positively attracted to humans, whom they associate with food; some animals may become docile, others aggressive/violent to humans • Animals may pose a nuisance to local residents • Animal attacks on humans increase the likelihood of animal culling • Potential for intra- and inter-species aggression • Increases animals' vulnerability to poaching, acting as a facilitator to the illegal pet trade • Contact with humans may spread disease • Increased chances of animals sustaining injury through close proximity to vehicles (see Figure 5.14) • Marine wildlife is at further risk of injury through contact with fishing gear and the ingestion of plastic and other non-edible items discarded by human beings

5.10 Advantages and disadvantages of the use of food provisioning for free-ranging wild animals.

Advantages
• Helps to avoid the need for immobilization via chemical or physical restraint • Improved safety of staff • Enhanced social management and opportunity through training techniques that increase affiliative behaviours and decrease aggression • Helps to improve staff attitudes to animals under their care • Improved psychological wellbeing through desensitization techniques that directly address fear and discomfort • Creates learning opportunities for animals which can be a form of enrichment • Increased public awareness of wildlife and subsequent support for conservation

Disadvantages
• Depending on the choice of food used, obesity or dental disease

5.11 Advantages and disadvantages of the use of food provisioning for captive wild animals.

▶

Case example 2: Welfare compromises that can be caused in wild species by habituation through food *continued*

Research

Safeguarding animal welfare and refining animal husbandry are essential factors to consider in research and management, both from an ethical standpoint and for the scientific integrity of the results (Boleij *et al.*, 2012). Animals recruited to research laboratories often undergo a period of acclimatization, which includes habituation, desensitization and training for procedures and husbandry tasks that will be involved in experimental use. Positive reinforcement training methods, such as the provision of food cues, are frequently used to reward desired behaviour in laboratory animals and are considered a valuable tool for their humane care and use.

In scientific studies, provisioning may also be used in an attempt to tame or habituate free-ranging animals, so they can be studied more closely and answer ecological questions when food is not a limiting factor (Dubois and Fraser, 2013). Natural or novel foods may be provided directly (by hand) or indirectly (at feeding stations). Dubois and Fraser (2013) recommend that these studies avoid permanent food conditioning, are conducted over short periods of time, involve small sample sizes and are overseen by research ethical committees.

The use of these techniques is associated with the acceleration of acclimation, helping to turn a potentially negative experience into a more predictable and positive one (Schapiro and Everitt, 2006). A reduction in stress level also results in more positive interactions with humans and increased responsiveness to training. Species groups that respond particularly well to positive reinforcement training techniques in the laboratory include pigs, dogs and non-human primates (Schapiro and Everitt, 2006).

Figure 5.12 details the advantages and disadvantages of food provisioning in research.

Advantages
• Facilitates data collection that is of optimal quality and might otherwise be impossible to collect without more invasive means
• Reduced opportunities for injury to animals and staff during procedures
• Potentially less stressful for the animal
• Provides a form of enrichment through greater mental stimulation and control
• Useful as part of a formal socialization programme, as part of animals' acclimatization and early phases of training
• More satisfactory human–animal interaction resulting in improved animal wellbeing

Disadvantages
• Animals in their own habitat may demonstrate aggressive altercations and/or food competition
• Care must be taken not to provide items that are high in 'empty' calories which could result in increased bodyweight and associated health-related problems
• Risk of dietary imbalances
• Difficulties have been reported in young animals if they are poorly socialized with humans as they become stressed and will not take food (Prescott and Buchanan-Smith, 2007)

5.12 Advantages and disadvantages of the use of food provisioning in research.

Opportunistic

A variety of anthropogenic and other food sources are attractive to wild animal species. These may be obtained by opportunistic feeding via pet food, rubbish bins, compost, landfill sites, gardens and directly from humans. The feeding of wild birds in residential gardens, parks and other public spaces is one of the most common and socially accepted forms of opportunistic feeding in Western culture (Dubois and Fraser, 2013). Wildlife living in and around urban areas, such as foxes and badgers, will access gardens, backyards and open spaces to exploit chances for opportunistic feeding. Repeated interaction with humans or pets, especially when being intentionally fed, is likely to lead to habituation of these animals (Figure 5.13).

In their natural environment, wild animals adapt to fluctuations in the availability of food and seasonal variation of their diet. Opportunistic feeding by the human population provides an artificial abundance of food and withdrawal of this food source can lead to habituated and highly food-conditioned animals becoming stressed and aggressive. Over time, animals can become a nuisance or public safety risk (Figure 5.14), with the public response involving the use of non-lethal or lethal methods of population control. The modification of human behaviour to prevent intentional and unintentional feeding can help to prevent human–wildlife conflict; feeding wildlife in public locations is generally discouraged and occasionally prohibited.

Figure 5.15 details the advantages and disadvantages of opportunistic food provisioning.

Management

The use of management or 'supplemental' feeding of wild animals to achieve conservation objectives and promote animal welfare is well documented and performed under many contexts. Such a food resource can benefit both individuals and wider populations of wildlife. Length of programme, size of the species population and choice of food provision are all factors considered influential to the effects and outcome of this feeding method (Milner *et al.*, 2014). Murray *et al.* (2016) recommend adopting the following feeding practices:

- Provide food that is nutritionally appropriate for the target species
- Make food available at lower densities for short periods at unpredictable times and places to prevent aggression
- Avoid feeding during times of migration, pulses of new recruits and epidemics

Figure 5.16 details the advantages and disadvantages of the use of management food provisioning.

▶

Case example 2: Welfare compromises that can be caused in wild species by habituation through food *continued*

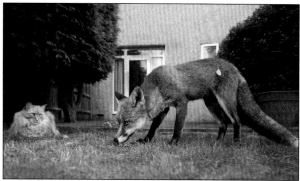

| 5.13 | Intentional feeding together with repeated interaction with people or pets is likely to lead to habituation of wild animals.
(Giedriius/Shutterstock.com)

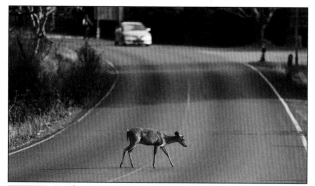

| 5.14 | Food provisioning can increase the risk of animals sustaining injury through close proximity to vehicles.
(Janejira Sriharaj/Shutterstock.com)

Advantages

- Improved survival and breeding rates
- Increased public awareness of wildlife and subsequent support for conservation
- Benefits to human beings include:
  - Pleasure from wildlife contact and a connection with nature
  - Gaining the trust of animals
  - Educational purposes
  - Entertainment
  - Gaining a sense of usefulness and kindness
  - Ability to observe/photograph wildlife
  - Helping to counteract human actions perceived to have a negative effect on wild animals such as habitat destruction

Disadvantages

- Facilitates the spread of disease
- Promotes the provision of inadequate and imbalanced nutrition
- Increased risk of window strikes by birds
- Interferes with the seasonal variations in food availability
- Food can attract rodents and other wildlife
- Increased risk of predation to wildlife
- Irregular cleaning of bird feeders can lead to fungal or bacterial infections
- Increased risk of aggression and injury towards people
- Potential damage to property

| 5.15 | Advantages and disadvantages of the use of opportunistic feeding.

Advantages

- Improved individual or population performance, including improved body condition and reduced winter mass loss
- Diverts animals away from certain areas and food types, thus protecting crops, forestry and natural habitats
- Facilitates the recovery or re-establishment of endangered species
- Reduces human–wildlife conflict

Disadvantages

- Increases the risk of pathogen transmission resulting in the promotion of disease and infection
- Risk of dietary imbalances

| 5.16 | Advantages and disadvantages of the use of management feeding.

References and further reading

American Animal Hospital Association (2003) *The Path to High-Quality Care: Practical Tips for Improving Compliance*. American Animal Hospital Association, Lakewood, Colorado

Antolova D, Reiterova K, Miterpakova M *et al.* (2009) The first finding of *Echinococcus multilocularis* in dogs in Slovakia: an emerging risk for spreading of infection. *Zoonoses and Public Health* **56**, 53–58

Armitage-Chan E, O'Toole T and Chan D (2006) Management of prolonged food deprivation, hypothermia, and refeeding syndrome in a cat. *Journal of Veterinary Emergency and Critical Care* **16**, S34–S41

Axelsson E, Ratnakumar A, Arendt M-J *et al.* (2013) The genomic signature of dog domestication reveals adaptation to a starch-rich diet. *Nature* **495**, 360–364

AZA Nutrition Advisory Group (2017) *Body Condition Scoring Resource Center.* Available from: nagonline.net/3877/body-condition-scoring

AZA Nutrition Advisory Group (2020) *Factsheets.* Available from: nagonline.net/tag/factsheet

Banfield Pet Hospital (2019) *State of Pet Health 2019 Report.* Available from: www.banfield.com/state-of-pet-health

Barnard DE, Lewis SM, Teter BB and Thigpen JE (2009) Open- and Closed-Formula Laboratory Animal Diets and Their Importance to Research. *Journal of the American Association for Laboratory Animal Science* **48**, 709–713

Barten S and Simpson S (2019) Lizards. In: *Mader's Reptile and Amphibian Medicine and Surgery, 3rd edn*, ed. S Divers and S Stahl, pp. 152–161.e1. Elsevier Saunders, Philadelphia

Becvarova I, Prochazka D, Chandler ML and Meyer H (2016) Nutrition Education in European Veterinary Schools: Are European Veterinary Graduates Competent in Nutrition? *Journal of Veterinary Medical Education* **43**, 349–358

Bennett AJ, Perkins CM, Harty NM *et al.* (2014) Assessment of foraging devices as a model for decision-making in nonhuman primate environmental enrichment. *Journal of the American Association for Laboratory Animal Science* **53**, 452–463

Bissell HA, Sullivan K, Kendrick E and Maslanka M (2019) Assessing the nutritional welfare and status of animals. *13th Zoo and Wildlife Nutrition Foundation/AZA Nutrition Advisory Group Conference on Zoo and Wildlife Nutrition, St. Louis, MO, Sept 29–Oct 2, 2019*

Bloomsmith MA (2014) *Training animals*. Available from: www.nc3rs.org.uk

Boissy A, Manteuffel G, Jensen MB *et al.* (2007) Assessment of positive emotions in animals to improve their welfare. *Physiology & Behavior* **92**, 375–397

Boleij H, Salomons AR, van Sprundel M *et al.* (2012) Not all mice are equal: welfare implications of behavioural habituation profiles in four 129 mouse substrains. *PLoS ONE* **7**, 1–8

Boyer T and Scott P (2019) Nutritional Therapy. In: *Mader's Reptile and Amphibian Medicine and Surgery, 3rd edn*, ed. S Divers and S Stahl, pp. 1173–1176.e1. Elsevier Saunders, Philadelphia

Brenner K, KuKanich KS and Smee NM (2011) Refeeding syndrome in a cat with hepatic lipidosis. *Journal of Feline Medicine and Surgery* **13**, 614–617

Briggs BM and Scheels DDS (2005) Selection of proper feeds to assist in the dental management of carnivores. *Paper presented at the 6th Conference of the AZA Nutrition Advisory Group on Zoo and Wildlife Nutrition, Omaha, NE*

British Horse Society (2019) *Pasture Management*. Available from: www.bhs.org.uk/advice-and-information

British Veterinary Association (2020) *BVA, BVNA, BVZS and BEVA policy position on obesity in dogs, cats, horses, donkeys and rabbits*. Available from: www.bva.co.uk

Bryant Z and Kother G (2014) Environmental enrichment with simple puzzle feeders increases feeding time in fly river turtles (*Carettochelys insculpta*). *The Herpetological Bulletin* **130**, 3–5

Buettner R, Schölmerich J and Bollheimer LC (2007) High-fat diets: modeling the metabolic disorders of human obesity in rodents. *Obesity* **15**, 798–808

Cairns-Haylor T and Fordyce P (2017) Mapping discussion of canine obesity between veterinary surgeons and dog owners: A provisional study. *Veterinary Record* **180**, 149

Carroll JF, Summers RL, Dzielak DJ *et al.* (1999) Diastolic compliance is reduced in obese rabbits. *Hypertension* **33**, 811–815

Chan DL (2015) Refeeding syndrome in small animals In: *Nutritional Management of Hospitalized Small Animals*, ed. DL Chan, pp. 159–164. Wiley-Blackwell, Hoboken

Chandler M, German AJ and Woods G (2020) *BSAVA Guide to Nutrition*. Available from: www.bsavalibrary.com

Chandler M, Haro CV and Weeth L (2015) Benefits of a veterinary small animal nutritionist in practice. *Vet Times* **December 04, 2015**

Charmoy K, Sullivan T and Miller LJ (2015) Impact of different forms of environmental enrichment on foraging and activity levels in gorillas (*Gorilla gorilla gorilla*). *Animal Behavior and Cognition* **2**, 233–240

Clauss M (2012) Clinical Technique: Feeding Hay to Rabbits and Rodents. *Journal of Exotic Pet Medicine* **21**, 80–86

Clubb R and Mason G (2003) *A Review of the Welfare of Zoo Elephants in Europe*. University of Oxford, Oxford

Cooper B, Mullineaux E and Turner L (2020) *BSAVA Textbook of Veterinary Nursing, 6th edn*. BSAVA Publications, Gloucester

Crane SW, Moser EA, Cowell CS *et al.* (2010) Commercial Pet Foods. In: *Small Animal Clinical Nutrition, 5th edn*, ed. MS Hand and LD Lewis, pp. 157–190. Mark Morris Institute, Topeka

Davies G (2016) Chicken Nutrition. *The Veterinary Nurse* **7**, 273–277

Davies M (2015) Evidence-based nutrition: raw diets. *Veterinary Times* **VT45.46**

Davies M (2017) Cereals and grains found in dog food – a health benefit or risk? *Veterinary Times* **VT47.37**

Davies RH, Lawes JR and Wales AD (2019) Raw diets for dogs and cats: a review, with particular reference to microbiological hazards. *Journal of Small Animal Practice* **60**, 329–339

Dawkins MS (2004) Using behaviour to assess animal welfare. *Animal Welfare* **13**, S3–S8

DeAvilla MD and Leech EB (2016) Hypoglycemia associated with refeeding syndrome in a cat. *Journal of Veterinary Emergency and Critical Care* **26**, 798–803

Debraekeleer J, Gross KL and Zicker SC (2010) Introduction to Feeding Normal Dogs. In: *Small Animal Clinical Nutrition, 5th edn*, ed. MS Hand and LD Lewis, pp. 251–255. Mark Morris Institute, Topeka

Dixon LM, Duncan IJH and Mason GJ (2010) The effects of four types of enrichment on feather-pecking behaviour in laying hens housed in barren environments. *Animal Welfare* **19**, 429–435

Donoghue S (2006) Nutrition. In: *Reptile Medicine and Surgery, 2nd edn*, ed. S Divers and D Mader, pp. 251–298. Elsevier Saunders, St. Louis, USA

Donoghue S and McKeown S (1999) Nutrition of Captive Reptiles. *Veterinary Clinics of North America: Exotic Animal Practice* **2**, 69–91

Dubois S and Fraser D (2013) A Framework to Evaluate Wildlife Feeding in Research, Wildlife Management, Tourism and Recreation. *Animals* **3**, 978–994

Ely JJ, Zavaskis T and Lammey ML (2013) Hypertension Increases With Aging and Obesity in Chimpanzees (*Pan troglodytes*). *Zoo Biology* **32**, 79–87

Epstein LH, Temple JL, Roemmich JN *et al.* (2009) Habituation as a determinant of human food intake. *Psychological Review* **116**, 384–407

European Commission (2017) *Technical document on cosmetic claims*. Available from: ec.europa.eu/growth/sectors/cosmetics_en

Fédération Européenne de l'Industrie des Aliments pour Animaux Familiers (2013) *Nutritional Guidelines for Feeding Pet Rabbits*. Available from: www.fediaf.org

Freeman L, Becvarova I, Cave N *et al.* (2011) WSAVA Nutritional Assessment Guidelines. *Journal of Small Animal Practice* **52**, 385–396

Freeman LM and Michel KE (2001) Evaluation of raw food diets. *Journal of the American Veterinary Medical Association* **218**, 705–709. Erratum in: *Journal of the American Veterinary Medical Association* **218**, 1716

Freeman LM, Chandler ML, Hamper BA and Weeth LP (2013) Current knowledge about the risks and benefits of raw meat-based diets for dogs and cats. *Journal of the American Veterinary Medical Association* **243**, 1549–1558

Frowde PE, Battersby IA, Whitley NT *et al.* (2011) Oesophageal disease in 33 cats. *Journal of Feline Medicine and Surgery* **13**, 564–596

Frye FL (1984) Nutritional disorders in reptiles. In: *Diseases of Amphibians and Reptiles*, ed. GL Hoff, FL Frye and ER Jacobson, pp. 633–660. Springer, Boston, MA

Gaengler H and Clum N (2015) Investigating the impact of large carcass feeding on the behavior of captive Andean condors (*Vultur gryphus*) and its perception by zoo visitors. *Zoo Biology* **34**, 118–129

Gagne JW and Wakshlag JJ (2015) Pathophysiology and clinical approach to malnutrition in dogs and cats. In: *Nutritional Management of Hospitalized Small Animals*, ed. DL Chan, pp. 117–127. Wiley-Blackwell, Hoboken

Gaylord L, Remillard R and Saker K (2018) Risk of nutritional deficiencies for dogs on a weight loss plan. *Journal of Small Animal Practice* **59**, 695–703

Goodwin D, Davidson HPB and Harris P (2002) Foraging enrichment for stabled horses: effects on behaviour and selection. *Equine Veterinary Journal* **34**, 686–691

Gross S, Jewell DE, Yamka KL *et al.* (2010) Macronutrients. In: *Small Animal Clinical Nutrition, 5th edn*, ed. MS Hand and LD Lewis, pp. 49–105. Mark Morris Institute, Topeka

Hand MS, Zicker SC and Novotny B (2011) *Small Animal Clinical Nutrition Quick Consult*. Mark Morris Institute, Topeka

Harcourt-Brown FM (1996) Calcium deficiency, diet and dental disease in pet rabbits. *Veterinary Record* **139**, 567–571

Harcourt-Brown N and Chitty J (2005) *BSAVA Manual of Psittacine Birds, 2nd edn*. BSAVA Publications, Gloucester

Higginbottom K (2004) Wildlife Tourism: An Introduction. In: *Wildlife Tourism: Impacts, Management and Planning*. Common Ground Publishing, Victoria, Australia

Hope K and Deem SL (2006) Retrospective study of morbidity and mortality of captive jaguars (*Panthera onca*) in North America: 1982–2002. *Zoo Biology* **25**, 501–512

Hosey GR (2005) How does the zoo environment affect the behaviour of captive primates? *Applied Animal Behaviour Science* **90**, 107–129

International Cat Care (2018) Aggression between cats. Available from: icatcare.org/advice/aggression-between-cats

International Cat Care (2019) *Puzzle feeders*. Available from: icatcare.org/advice/puzzle-feeders

Ipsos MORI (2016) *Vegan Society Poll*. Available from: www.ipsos.com/ipsos-mori/en-uk

Jennings M and Prescott MJ (2009) Refinements in husbandry, care and common procedures for non-human primates. *Laboratory Animals* **43**, S1:2–S1:47

Johnson DH (2019) Gastrointestinal Stasis Syndrome in Small Herbivores. *91st Western Veterinary Conference, Las Vegas, NV, 17–20 February 2019*

Jones C (2019) Dog obesity: a community study. *VN Times* **19.10**

Jones R and Dodd C (2012) Birds: biology and husbandry. In: *BSAVA Manual of Exotic Pet and Wildlife Nursing*, ed. M Varga, R Lumbis and L Gott, pp. 58–79. BSAVA Publications, Gloucester

Kanakubo K, Fascetti AJ and Larsen JA (2015) Assessment of protein and amino acid concentrations and labeling adequacy of commercial vegetarian diets formulated for dogs and cats. *Journal of the American Veterinary Medical Association* **247**, 385–392

Kipperman B, Morris P and Rollin B (2018) Ethical dilemmas encountered by small animal veterinarians: Characterisation, responses, consequences and beliefs regarding euthanasia. *Veterinary Record* **182**, 548

Kitchener A (2004) The problems of old bears in zoos. *International Zoo News* **51**, 282–293

Knight J (2009) Making wildlife viewable: habituation and attraction. *Society & Animals* **17**, 167–184

Krebs BL, Marrin D, Phelps A, Krol L and Watters JV (2018) Managing aged animals in zoos to promote positive welfare: A review and future directions. *Animals* **8**, 116

Laflamme D (1997) Nutritional Management. *Veterinary Clinics of North America: Small Animal Practice* **27**, 1561–1577

Lagarde F, Bonnet X, Corbin J *et al.* (2003) Foraging behaviour and diet of an ectothermic herbivore: *Testudo horsfieldi*. *Ecography* **26**, 236–242

Legendre LFJ (2002) Malocclusions in guinea pigs, chinchillas and rabbits. *Canadian Veterinary Journal* **43**, 385–390

Lenz J, Joffe D, Kauffman M *et al.* (2009) Perceptions, practices, and consequences associated with foodborne pathogens and the feeding of raw meat to dogs. *Canadian Veterinary Journal* **50**, 637–643

Lowenstine LJ, McManamon R and Terio KA (2015) Comparative pathology of aging great apes: Bonobos, chimpanzees, gorillas, and orangutans. *Veterinary Pathology* **53**, 250–276

Lowrie M, Garden OA, Hadjivassiliou M *et al.* (2015) The Clinical and Serological Effect of a Gluten-Free Diet in Border Terriers with Epileptoid Cramping Syndrome. *Journal of Veterinary Internal Medicine* **29**, 1564–1568

Lowrie M, Hadjivassiliou M, Sanders DS and Garden OA (2016) A presumptive case of gluten sensitivity in a border terrier: a multisystem disorder? *Veterinary Record* **179**, 573

Luethy D, Stefanovski D and Sweeney R (2020) Refeeding syndrome in small ruminants receiving parenteral nutrition. *Journal of Veterinary Internal Medicine* **34**, 1674–1679

Malmkvist J, Palme R, Svendsen PM *et al.* (2013) Additional foraging elements reduce abnormal behaviour – fur-chewing and stereotypic behaviour – in farmed mink (*Neovison vison*). *Applied Animal Behaviour Science* **149**, 77–86

Marshall WG, Hazelwinkel HAW, Mullen D *et al.* (2010) The effect of weight loss on lameness in obese dogs with osteoarthritis. *Veterinary Research Communications* **34**, 241–253

Mason G, Clubb R, Latham N and Vickery S (2007) Why and how should we use environmental enrichment to tackle stereotypic behaviour? *Applied Animal Behaviour Science* **102**, 163–188

Mason GJ (2010) Species differences in responses to captivity: stress, welfare and the comparative method. *Trends in Ecology and Evolution* **25**, 713–721

Mayer J (2015) Nutrient requirements of rabbits. In: *MSD Veterinary Manual.* Available from: www.msdvetmanual.com

McGreevy PD, Thomson PC, Pride C *et al.* (2005) Prevalence of obesity in dogs examined by Australian veterinary practices and the risk factors involved. *Veterinary Record* **156**, 695–701

Miller R and King CE (2013) Husbandry training, using positive reinforcement techniques, for Marabou stork *Leptoptilos crumeniferus* at Edinburgh Zoo. *International Zoo Yearbook* **47**, 1–10

Milner JM, van Beest F, Schmidt KT *et al.* (2014) To feed or not to feed? Evidence of the intended and unintended effects of feeding wild ungulates. *Journal of Wildlife Management* **78**, 1322–1334

Morelli G, Bastianello S, Catellani P and Ricci R (2019) Raw meat-based diets for dogs: survey of owners' motivations, attitudes and practices. *BMC Veterinary Research* **15**, 74

Mueller RS, Oliry T and Prélaud P (2016) Critically appraised topic on adverse food reactions of companion animals (2): common food allergen sources in dogs and cats. *BMC Veterinary Research* **12**, 9

Müller J, Clauss M, Codron D *et al.* (2015) Tooth length and incisal wear and growth in guinea pigs (*Cavia porcellus*) fed diets of different abrasiveness. *Journal of Animal Physiology and Animal Nutrition* **99**, 591–604

Murray MH, Becker DJ, Hall RJ *et al.* (2016) Wildlife health and supplemental feeding: A review and management recommendations. *Biological Conservation* **204**, 163–174

National Health Service (2020) *Overview: Malnutrition.* Available from: www.nhs.uk/conditions/malnutrition

Nielsen BL, de Jong IC and De Vries TJ (2016) The use of feeding behaviour in the assessment of animal welfare. In: *Nutrition and the Welfare of Farm Animals*, ed. C Phillips, pp. 59–84. Springer, Cham

Nijboer J (2015a) Nutrition in Reptiles. In: *MSD Veterinary Manual.* Available from: www.msdvetmanual.com

Nijboer J (2015b) Overview of Nutrition: Exotic and Zoo Animals. In: *MSD Veterinary Manual.* Available from: www.msdvetmanual.com

Nijboer J, Fidgett A, Clauss M *et al.* (2011) Course of action. *EAZA Zooquaria* **5**, 26–27

Norman R and Wills AP (2016) An investigation into the relationship between owner knowledge, diet, and dental disease in guinea pigs (*Cavia porcellus*). *Animals* **6**, 1–9

NPD Group (2012) *Is Gluten-Free Eating a Trend Worth Noting?* Available from: www.npdgroup.co.uk

Nyhus PJ (2016) Human-wildlife conflict and coexistence. *The Annual Review of Environment and Resources* **41**, 143–171

Orams MB (2002) Feeding wildlife as a tourism attraction: a review of issues and impacts. *Tourism Management* **23**, 281–293

Pasmans F, Bogaerts S, Braeckman J *et al.* (2017) Future of keeping pet reptiles and amphibians: towards integrating animal welfare, human health and environmental sustainability. *Veterinary Record* **181**, 450

People's Dispensary for Sick Animals (2019) *PDSA Animal Wellbeing (PAW) Report 2019.* Available from: www.pdsa.org.uk

People's Dispensary for Sick Animals (2020) *PDSA Animal Wellbeing (PAW) Report 2020.* Available from: www.pdsa.org.uk

Pet Food Manufacturers Association (2015a) *PFMA Fact Sheets.* Available from: www.pfma.org.uk/fact-sheets

Pet Food Manufacturers Association (2015b) *Rabbits – Nutritional Requirements.* Available from: www.pfma.org.uk

Pet Food Manufacturers Association (2018) *PFMA Annual Report 2018.* Available from: www.pfma.org.uk/annual-reports

Pet Food Manufacturers Association (2019a) *PFMA Annual Report 2019.* Available from: www.pfma.org.uk/annual-reports

Pet Food Manufacturers Association (2019b) *PFMA Obesity Report 2019.* Available from: www.pfma.org.uk/pet-obesity-reports

Phillips C (2010) Definitions and concepts of animal welfare. In: *The Welfare of Animals; the Silent Majority*, ed. C Phillips, pp. 1–11. Springer, Queensland

Phillips-Donaldson D (2015) *Has grain-free pet food surpassed trend status?* Available from: www.petfoodindustry.com

Power ML, Ross CN, Schulkin J, Ziegler TE and Tardif SD (2013) Metabolic consequences of the early onset of obesity in common marmoset monkeys. *Obesity* **21**, E592–E598

Prendergast H (2010) Nutritional requirements and feeding of growing puppies and kittens. In: *Small Animal Pediatrics*, ed. ME Peterson and MA Kutzler, pp. 58–66. Elsevier Saunders, St Louis, USA

Prescott MJ and Buchanan-Smith HM (2007) Training laboratory-housed non-human primates, part 1: a UK survey. *Animal Welfare* **16**, 21–36

Pyke GH (2019a) Foraging: A fundamental activity for all life. In: *Encyclopedia of Animal Behavior, 2nd edn*, ed. MD Breed and J Moore, pp. 75–79. Elsevier, Philadelphia

Pyke GH (2019b) Optimal Foraging Theory: An Introduction. In: *Encyclopedia of Animal Behavior, 2nd edn*, ed. MD Breed and J Moore, pp. 111–117. Elsevier, Philadelphia

Rabbit Welfare Association & Fund (2020) *Rabbit Diet.* Available from: rabbitwelfare.co.uk

Rawski M and Jozefiak D (2014) Body condition scoring and obesity in captive African Side-Neck Turtles (*Pelomedusidae*). *Annals of Animal Science* **14**, 573–584

Reese RE and Andrews FM (2009) Nutrition and dietary management of equine gastric ulcer syndrome. *Veterinary Clinics of North America: Equine Practice* **25**, 79–92

Remillard RL (2008) Homemade diets: attributes, pitfalls, and a call for action. *Topics in Companion Animal Medicine* **23**, 137–142

Roguet C, Dumont B, Prache S *et al.* (1998) Selection and use of feeding sites and feeding stations by herbivores: A review. *Annales de Zootechnie* **47**, 225–244

Rolph NC, Noble PJM and German AJ (2014) How often do primary care veterinarians record the overweight status of dogs? *Journal of Nutritional Science* **3**, e58

Rooney MB and Sleeman J (1998) Effects of selected behavioral enrichment devices on behavior of Western Lowland Gorillas (*Gorilla gorilla gorilla*). *Journal of Applied Animal Welfare Science* **1**, 339–351

Rooney NJ, Blackwell EJ, Mullan SM *et al.* (2014) The current state of welfare, housing and husbandry of the English pet rabbit population. *BMC Research Notes* **7**, 1–13

Rosa C, Vitale A and Puopolo M (2003) The puzzle-feeder as feeding enrichment for common marmosets (*Callithrix jacchus*): a pilot study. *Laboratory Animals* **37**, 100–107

Roth EK, Visscher NC and Ha RR (2017) Food for thought: assessing visitor comfort and attitudes toward carcass feeding at the ABQ BioPark Zoo. *Anthrozoös* **30**, 227–235

Royal College of Veterinary Surgeon's Knowledge and Sense About Science (2019) *Evidence-Based Veterinary Medicine Matters: Our Commitment to the Future.* Available from: knowledge.rcvs.org.uk

Saladin KS (2020) *Feeding Strategies.* Available from: www.biologyreference.com

Samia DSM, Nakagawa S, Nomura F *et al.* (2015) Increased tolerance to humans among disturbed wildlife. *Nature Communications* **6**, 1–8

Sanderson SL (2013) Dog and Cat Foods. In: *MSD Veterinary Manual.* Available from: www.msdvetmanual.com

Schapiro SJ and Everitt JI (2006) Preparation of animals for use in the laboratory: Issues and challenges for the Institutional Animal Care and Use Committee (IACUC). *ILAR Journal* **47**, 370–375

Schepers F, Koene, P and Beerda B (2009) Welfare assessment in pet rabbits. *Animal Welfare* **18**, 477–485

Schlesinger DP and Joffe DJ (2011) Raw food diets in companion animals: a critical review. *Canadian Veterinary Journal* **52**, 50–54

Schoemaker NJ, Lumeij JT, Dorrestein GM and Beynen AC (1999) Nutrition-related problems in pet birds. *Tijdschrift Voor Diergeneeskunde* **124**, 39–43

Schwitzer C and Kaumanns W (2001) Body weights of ruffed lemurs (*Varecia variegata*) in European zoos with reference to the problem of obesity. *Zoo Biology* **20**, 261–269

Sharpe P and Kenny LB (2019) Grazing behavior, feed intake, and feed choices. In: *Horse Pasture Management*, ed. P Sharpe, pp. 121–139. Academic Press, London

Siegford JM (2013) Multidisciplinary approaches and assessment techniques to better understand and enhance zoo nonhuman animal welfare. *Journal of Applied Animal Welfare Science* **16**, 300–318

Silvis SE, DiBartolomeo AG and Aaker HM (1980) Hypophosphatemia and neurological changes secondary to oral caloric intake: a variant of hyperalimentation syndrome. *The American Journal of Gastroenterology* **73**, 215–222

Stockman J, Fascetti AJ, Kass PH and Larsen JA (2013) Evaluation of recipes of home-prepared maintenance diets for dogs. *Journal of the American Veterinary Medical Association* **242**, 1500–1505. Erratum in: *Journal of the American Veterinary Medical Association* **245**, 177

Sykes BW, Hewetson M, Hepburn RJ *et al.* (2015). European College of Equine Internal Medicine Consensus Statement–Equine Gastric Ulcer Syndrome in Adult Horses. *Journal of Veterinary Internal Medicine* **29**, 1288–1299

Taylor MB, Geiger DA, Saker KE *et al.* (2009) Diffuse osteopenia and myelopathy in a puppy fed a diet composed of an organic premix and raw ground beef. *Journal of the American Veterinary Medical Association* **234**, 1041–1048

Thompson HC, Cortes Y, Gannon K *et al.* (2012) Esophageal foreign bodies in dogs: 34 cases (2004–2009). *Journal of Veterinary Emergency and Critical Care* **22**, 253–261

Thompson RF (2015) Habituation. In: *International Encyclopedia of the Social & Behavioural Sciences, 2nd edn*, ed. JD Wright, pp. 480–483. Elsevier, Amsterdam

Thorne JB, Goodwin D, Kennedy MJ *et al.* (2005) Foraging enrichment for individually housed horses: Practicality and effects on behaviour. *Applied Animal Behaviour Science* **94**, 149–164

Tonoike A, Hori Y, Inoue-Murayama M *et al.* (2015) Copy number variations in the amylase gene (AMY2B) in Japanese native dog breeds. *Animal Genetics* **46**, 580–583

Troxell-Smith SM, Whelan CJ, Magle SB *et al.* (2017) Zoo foraging ecology: development and assessment of a welfare tool for captive animals. *Animal Welfare* **26**, 265–275

US Food & Drug Administration (2019) *FDA Investigation into Potential Link between Certain Diets and Canine Dilated Cardiomyopathy.* Available from: www.fda.gov/animal-veterinary

van Bree FPJ, Bokken GCAM, Mineur R *et al.* (2018) Zoonotic bacteria and parasites found in raw meat-based diets for cats and dogs. *Veterinary Record* **182**, 50

van Zeeland YRA, Schoemaker NJ, Ravesteijn MM *et al.* (2013) Efficacy of foraging enrichments to increase foraging time in Grey parrots (*Psittacus erithacus erithacus*). *Applied Animal Behaviour Science* **149**, 87–102

Videan EN, Fritz J and Murphy J (2007) Development of guidelines for assessing obesity in captive chimpanzees (*Pan troglodytes*). *Zoo Biology* **26**, 93–104

Wallis LJ, Szabó D, Erdélyi-Belle B and Kubinyi E (2018) Demographic Change Across the Lifespan of Pet Dogs and Their Impact on Health Status. *Frontiers in Veterinary Science* **5**, 200

Warwick C, Arena P, Lindley S *et al.* (2013) Assessing reptile welfare using behavioural criteria. *In Practice* **35**, 123–131

Webster C, Massaro M, Michael DR *et al.* (2018) Native reptiles alter their foraging in the presence of the olfactory cues of invasive mammalian predators. *Royal Society of Open Science* **5**, 1–10

Weese JS, Rousseau J and Arroyo L (2005) Bacteriological evaluation of commercial canine and feline raw diets. *Canadian Veterinary Journal* **46**, 513–516

Weinsier RL and Krumdieck CL (1981) Death resulting from overzealous total parenteral nutrition: the refeeding syndrome revisited. *The American Journal of Clinical Nutrition* **34**, 393–399

Wilkinson SL (2015) Reptile wellness management. *Veterinary Clinics of North America: Exotic Animal Practice* **18**, 281–304

Winkler DE, Schulz-Kornas E, Kaiser TM *et al.* (2019) Forage silica and water content control dental surface texture in guinea pigs and provide implications for dietary reconstruction. *Proceedings of the National Academy of Sciences* **116**, 1325–1330

Wolfensohn S, Shotton J, Bowley H *et al.* (2018) Assessment of welfare in zoo animals: Towards optimum quality of life. *Animals* **8**, 110

Woodford MH, Butynski TM and Karesh WB (2002) Habituating the great apes: the disease risks. *Oryx* **36**, 153–160

WSAVA, Global Nutrition Committee (2022) *Global Nutrition Toolkit.* Available from: wsava.org/wp-content/uploads/2021/04/WSAVA-Global-Nutrition-Toolkit-English.pdf

Young RJ (2003) Food and foraging enrichment. In: *Environmental Enrichment for Captive Animals*, ed. RJ Young, pp. 85–106. Blackwell Publishing, Oxford

Young RJ and Cipreste CF (2004) Applying animal learning theory: training captive animals to comply with veterinary and husbandry procedures. *Animal Welfare* **13**, 225–232

Useful websites

AZA Nutrition Advisory Group
nagonline.net

Pet Food Manufacturers' Association
www.pfma.org.uk

WSAVA Global Nutrition Guidelines
wsava.org/global-guidelines/global-nutrition-guidelines/

Chapter 6

Welfare-focused animal training

Jim Mackie and Chirag Patel

Introduction

This chapter will look at a contemporary approach to training and its role in the care and welfare of captive and companion animals. The goal is to use the latest scientific evidence and ethical grounding to provide a chapter of fundamental knowledge and everyday practical tips. Case studies and training plans are provided throughout, and the reader is encouraged to modify these for their own use. Training that focuses on the principles of operant conditioning (see Chapter 3) while providing the learner with choice and control is considered a gold standard by the authors. Most importantly, this chapter aims to help readers to improve the lives and welfare of the animals in their care.

Animal training and the integrated approach

Animals have been trained by humans for millennia in various forms, but until recently training was not reliant on scientific principles; instead, techniques were handed down anecdotally from generation to generation. From raptors to elephants, dolphins to horses, animals were trained for human needs, often using coercive techniques with little consideration for animal welfare or the emotional state of the individual. The first use of Skinner's modern, evidence-based techniques in a zoological collection was with marine mammals in 1958 but it was not until much later, in the 1990s, that they became a commonly applied facet of zoo animal management. Similarly, in the companion animal world, it is generally agreed that operant conditioning became prevalent following the publication of Karen Pryor's *Don't Shoot the Dog!* in the 1980s (Pryor, 1999). The perception of animal training has come a long way in a short time, and it is now an essential part of companion and domestic animal care, zoo animal behaviour management and behaviour-based husbandry.

Zoological collections as models for welfare-focused training

Zoological collections and zookeepers have embraced the concept of animal training for improved welfare, especially in medical care. All over the world, zoo animals are trained for an incredible variety of ▶

Zoological collections as models for welfare-focused training *continued*

behaviours in many contexts and across all taxonomic groups. In many ways, zoological collections are setting the standard for training for improved welfare and these experiences and skills are increasing all the time.

This chapter draws on the author's [JM] experience in zoological settings to provide examples of behaviours that can be achieved through training and ways these can be used to improve animal welfare. The underlying principles for training zoo animals and domestic species are the same; the reader is encouraged to adapt the protocols provided in case examples throughout the chapter for use in their day-to-day interactions with any species.

Definitions

What is learning?
A change in behaviour as a result of experience.

Why use the word change?
The term change is preferred when referring to the acquisition of a new behaviour, as learning does not always involve acquiring something but does always involve change (Chance, 1998).

What is behaviour?
Anything an animal or person does that can be measured (see below and Chapter 3 for further definition) (Skinner, 1938; Moore, 2011).

What is experience?
Defined as events that occur in the animal's environment or surroundings (Chance, 1998).

Behaviour

Behaviour is anything an animal does when interacting with its environment. This includes overt behaviours observable by others, such as moving to a water source, as well as internal processes, such as thinking. Similarly, 'environment' refers to internal (e.g. hormonal and other biochemical changes) and external (e.g. food availability) factors that influence behaviour. Eating, drinking, exercising, playing, socializing and participating in veterinary care all involve behaviour. Behaviour is discussed at length in Chapter 3.

BSAVA Manual of Practical Veterinary Welfare. Edited by Matthew Rendle and Jo Hinde-Megarity. ©BSAVA 2022

Training

Simply put, training is teaching, where teaching can be considered as arranging or creating circumstances that change the way other individuals feel and behave. Training is an applied technology derived from the field of behaviour analysis, which is a natural science studying environmental variables and their influence on behaviour. Most behaviour animals engage in is influenced by their environment – training is the tool by which such behaviour can be managed.

Often trainers or teachers worry that the animal will not learn, but learning is not optional – it is a function of biology. Caregivers should bear in mind that they are teachers and every interaction with an animal is a potential learning experience, whether it is part of a formal training scenario or not. *The important thing to consider is not whether, but what, an animal is learning.*

Routine cleaning

Even routine cleaning of an enclosure or tank is a potential learning experience and caregivers should approach it as teachers. Rather than expecting the animals to actively avoid us so we can work without disturbance, we should use practical applications of behaviour science, such as enclosure modification or non-coercive training methods. This way we are not creating an aversive association with us, but rather teaching the animals which behaviours will result in them gaining reinforcers.

Reasons for training animals

Animals are actively trained for a variety of reasons, including ease of medical care, improved husbandry, enrichment and behaviour modification. In zoological collections, training may also be useful for demonstrations, public interaction, safe working, and to support conservation, research and education. These reasons fit into two broad categories (Ramirez, 1999):

- Primary reasons: these benefit the individual being trained directly
- Secondary reasons: these benefit other animals, humans and the wider environment.

The focus for any animal training programme should be to provide a net welfare benefit to the animal (Department for Environment, Food and Rural Affairs, 2012). Welfare benefits associated with using trained behaviour include providing alternatives to traditional animal management techniques, such as box training for transportation instead of manual restraint (see Chapter 7), hand injection instead of darting and target training instead of herding. Where training occurs for secondary reasons, there must also be a welfare benefit to the individual animal.

Integration of training

Behaviour and learning occurr throughout all areas of animal care and welfare, and training should be considered a vital part of any holistic approach to animal management.

Case example 1: Muzzle training – dog

Muzzle training of dogs is performed for secondary reasons – to prevent injury to other people or animals. However, training a dog to accept a muzzle may also have net welfare benefits; for example, it may mean they are able to engage in enriched experiences, such as walking, that would be unsafe without a muzzle. The programme outlined below is suitable for dogs that have had negative associations with a muzzle, or where no previous associations with the muzzle have been made.

Principles

- Find a suitable reinforcement for the dog. Food and attention are more practical than toys, as they are useable with a muzzle. Treats such as cheese, sausage and chicken, cut into small pieces (0.5 cm), work for most dogs.
- Contexts where a muzzle is indicated must be avoided until the programme is finalized.
- Proceed to the next step only if the dog shows no signs of stress when offered food.
- When signs of stress are observed (e.g. licking the nose, yawning or pulling away), training must be taken back to the previous step.

Sequence

1. Put the muzzle on the floor when the dog is not in the room. Let the dog enter the room and feed them treats when they are in the vicinity of the muzzle (within about 1 metre).
2. Repeat step 1, but with the treats scattered on the floor up to and around the muzzle.
3. Hold the muzzle in one hand, parallel to your body. Feed treats with the other hand. The muzzle should be kept still in this phase.
4. Extend the hand holding the muzzle by flexing the elbow. Keep the muzzle fixed in this position. Feed treats with the other hand. If the dog shows no signs of stress, try feeding the treats closer and closer to the muzzle.
5. Feed treats from the muzzle. Start by putting treats on the brim and then progressively moving them further towards the closed end of the muzzle.
6. Once the dog will willingly put their face in the muzzle, do it up for a few seconds, then remove it and offer another treat in the muzzle without doing it up.
7. Repeat step 6 but gradually increase the time with the muzzle on.
8. When the dog is comfortable with the muzzle resting on their face, the strap can be done up and the muzzle left on for a short time.
9. The time wearing the muzzle can be gradually increased in non-threatening circumstances.

Care must be exercised to watch the dog for overheating since panting is restricted when a muzzle is worn. To minimize the impact of this, a basket-style muzzle should be used, rather than a close-fitting nylon muzzle (see Chapter 4).

A research project at the Zoological Society of London (ZSL) required two zoo-housed dogs to wear GPS tracking technology attached to their collars (Figure 6.1). The data collected helped conservation scientists in the field interpret corresponding data from collars attached to wild dogs. Although useful field data was being collected, the wild dogs could not be observed all the time, so information was missing. CCTV cameras at the zoo provided 24/7 observation: this allowed identification of missing behaviours, which were then matched to data from wild individuals. This helped support conservation plans in the wild. Despite the obvious benefits overall, training for research is not a primary reason to train an animal as it does not provide a net welfare benefit to the individual. Welfare provision was ensured by utilizing the enclosure modifications needed to train the dogs to allow for regular weighing, hand injections and voluntary transportation.

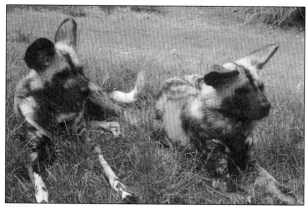

6.1 Arican wild dogs at ZSL London Zoo with GPS monitoring collars attached via trained behaviour.
(Courtesy of Luke Harvey)

Animal training is the technology that allows veterinary professionals and other carers to ethically manage the behaviour of animals they interact with. As such, training should be given the same importance as providing nutrition and veterinary care and it should not be considered an optional extra.

"Just as one would never consider developing an animal care program without a veterinary component, a nutritional component, a social component, and an environmental component; nobody should consider caring for an animal without a behavioral management component (training*) integrated into the program" (Ramirez, 1999).

*The word 'training' has been added by the authors and does not appear in the original quote.

Fundamentals of animal training

Trainers must understand the fundamentals of teaching and learning in order to train ethically and effectively. This chapter provides a foundation, and the authors recommend readers study further when implementing specific training protocols. The *BSAVA Manual of Canine and Feline Behavioural Medicine* provides in-depth practical advice. The author [JM] also recommends *Zoo Animal Learning and Training* (Melfi *et al.*, 2019), and *Animal Training: Successful Animal Management Through Positive Reinforcement* (Ramirez, 1999).

Communication

The various ways in which we interact with animals during training sessions determine whether the training will be successful. Animal training involves a two-way flow of information reliant on feedback from the animal and the correct interpretation of that feedback by the trainer. Training is sometimes likened to a 'dance' or a 'conversation' – these terms emphasize that both parties are equal participants.

Communication requires the trainer to:

- Know what is required of the animal – both the end goal and each approximation (see 'Approximation', below)

- Communicate clearly to the animal with visual and verbal stimuli – all verbal communication must have meaning to the animal. Extraneous dialogue should be restricted
- Adopt the correct body language
- Listen, watch and adapt to the animal – respond to feedback
- Evaluate and record each session and communicate progress between trainers.

Techniques

There are five recognized techniques for training new behaviours. They are subdivided into two categories – antecedent and consequent techniques:

- **Antecedent techniques** are reliant on a prompt to evoke behaviour:
  - **Luring** – using a desirable stimulus to guide an animal to a position or to perform a particular behaviour
  - **Baiting** – using a desirable stimulus to encourage an animal to a particular location
  - **Physical manipulation or moulding** – physically moving the animal into the desired position
- **Consequent techniques** are reliant on the outcome of the behaviour:
  - **Capturing** – waiting until the animal performs the desired behaviour and reinforcing at that moment
  - **Shaping** (through successive approximations) – reinforcing the learner for exhibiting closer and closer approximations to the desired behaviour.

Each of these techniques is used frequently in both zoo and companion animal training but certain considerations need to be taken into account. When using prompts, these need to be faded out as quickly as possible to prevent the stimulus becoming the cue itself, but not so fast as to confuse the animal and lose the behaviour. Generally, training will utilize more than one technique at a time. In zoological collections, physical moulding is normally discouraged as it is unlikely that the animal will have sufficient trust in the trainer to feel comfortable with the tactile nature of this technique.

Approximation

The technical definition of shaping by successive approximations is: "Gradually modifying some property of responding by differentially reinforcing successive approximations to a goal behaviour" (Association of Zoos & Aquariums (AZA) and American Association of Zoo Keepers (AAZK), 2016).

Prior to beginning training a new behaviour with an animal, the trainer should prepare a training plan. This requires a clearly defined target behaviour, for example, 'male western lowland gorilla – chest presentation for auscultation'. The behaviour can be broken down into a series of 'approximations' (i.e. small steps to the end goal. It is important not to be too prescriptive or detailed in the) training plan as one of the key elements of training is to respond to behavioural feedback from the animal. If the plan is too precise, it can reduce the potential for adjustment during and between sessions. In the example of the gorilla, a simple training plan may look as follows:

- Background – the individual is trained for the following foundation behaviours (see 'Foundation behaviours', below): calm behaviour, shifting, stationing and targeting (touch with the right index finger). A member of the veterinary team will need to perform the actual examination so they will need to be included in the training plan after the target behaviour has been trained.
1. Separate the individual according to the existing husbandry routine.
2. Begin by reinforcing calm behaviour at the training location.
3. Use existing targeting behaviour to extend the arm upwards.
4. Reinforce any chest contact with the mesh.
5. When he has touched the mesh with his chest a few times, place the behaviour under stimulus control by phasing out the target and inserting the cue word 'chest'.
6. When he is presenting his chest to the mesh on cue, increase the duration of the behaviour.
7. Add allowance of physical contact with chest behaviour using a hand touch.
8. Test response to stethoscope and reinforce recognition of the novel stimuli.
9. Replace hand with stethoscope.
10. Attempt auscultation examination and transfer behaviour to the veterinary team.

There is plenty of scope in this plan for evaluation and adjustment. If the targeting behaviour does not elicit the correct response, the trainer could use a food lure or the behaviour could be captured.

Pre-planned approximations are subject to change according to the results of individual training sessions. For example, if the trainer presents the stethoscope during the session, but the animal reacts in a negative way by moving away from the training station, the trainer should reassess and return to a previous approximation – return to station, touch a target or offer eye contact. This process is called relaxing criteria; the criteria can be increased after the animal is in a calm state or can be reserved for a future session. The trainer should then focus on making the stethoscope a desirable stimulus, perhaps using the classical conditioning technique of pairing the undesired stimulus (stethoscope) with a desired stimulus (favoured food items).

One essential component of animal training is knowing when to move on to the next approximation. It is very easy to be too fast or too slow, both of which can have a detrimental impact on progress. Moving too fast risks the animal becoming overwhelmed by the intensity of the training and refusing to participate; moving too slow risks teaching an animal one part of the training so well it refuses to move to the next step. The author [JM] has made both of these mistakes with the aforementioned results. Those that work with a range of species will have to learn how fast to move from one approximation to the next with each species, though the training principles are no different when working with dogs, cats, exotic pets or zoo animals. Some of this learning will always be through experience, but knowing the general rules and principles provides a good head start and minimizes the likelihood of making too many mistakes.

Foundation behaviours

It is a good idea with any training to begin with simple foundation behaviours. These can be different depending on the institution but are always a series of basic behaviours. They are primarily designed to provide the building blocks to achieve other, more invasive, behaviours such as presentation for hand injections. The author [JM] uses the following foundation behaviours:

1. **Calm behaviour** (Figure 6.2a) – establishing calm behaviour and ensuring there is a good human–animal bond is an important first step in any training programme. This can be achieved by reinforcing any calm behaviour in the presence of the caregiver. The calm behaviour must be observable and measurable. For example, it could be maintaining eye contact with the trainer for a few seconds before receiving reinforcement. It may be as simple as taking food from the trainer's hand without moving away directly after receiving reinforcement or continuing to eat food placed on the ground while the trainer moves around the training area. All of these behaviours can be observed and described to other caregivers.
2. **Targeting** (Figure 6.2b) – teaching an animal recognition of a novel object and asking them to touch it with a body part. This can be as simple as asking the animal to touch their nose to a ball on the end of a stick. Learning to touch the target means they can be moved from one place to another by following the object or can be asked to stay in one location.
3. **Stationing** (Figure 6.2c) – teaching an animal to remain in one location for a prolonged duration. The trainer should look to reinforce calm behaviours. This behaviour can be very useful for weighing animals. Training them to step on to a mat or board can facilitate other behaviours, such as those useful for conscious radiography.
4. **Shifting** – essentially, this is teaching the animal to move from one location to another, for example, from an outside paddock to an inside den. The antecedent stimulus for this behaviour can be an audio cue, such as a human voice or the sound of a shaker, and results in a desired outcome (such as a favoured food item) after the behaviour is completed.
5. **Audio recall** (Figure 6.2d) – this is the action of fast movement from one location to another, within a short time frame, following the sound of a stimulus such as a whistle or bell. This fast response behaviour can be

used in emergencies to move an animal to a safe area, or it can be used to call an animal towards a training station.

6. **Transportation** (Figure 6.2e) – teaching transportation proactively, before it is necessary, is helpful in reducing the stress associated with moving animals. For small animals, transport training is likely to involve training the individual to enter a crate and remain calm while the door is closed for increasingly prolonged periods of time (see Chapter 7). For larger animals, a trailer or container is more likely to be used.

The first foundation behaviour described above is calm behaviour/trust, which includes eye contact. This behaviour is particularly useful when the animal has previously mastered a behaviour but is not performing it when cued.

Waiting for a few seconds, then reinforcing eye contact or a calm behaviour at station gives the animal the opportunity to receive reinforcement, encouraging continued participation. This is called the least reinforcing scenario (LRS) (AZA/AAZK, 2016).

In modern zoological institutions, animal caregivers are often encouraged to teach these foundation behaviours as a proactive behaviour management measure. If the animal knows these simple behaviours it can make more invasive procedures, such as blood sampling or hand injections, much easier to train (see 'Training to facilitate clinical care', below). Similarly, teaching these foundation behaviours to companion animals minimizes the stress of a visit to the veterinary practice. In addition, positive reinforcement training gives animals coping skills in their captive environment (Melfi *et al.*, 2019).

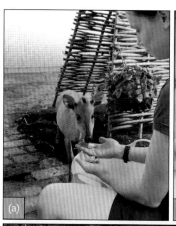
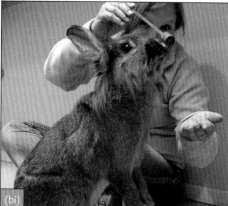
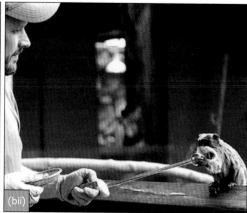
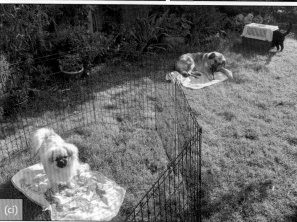
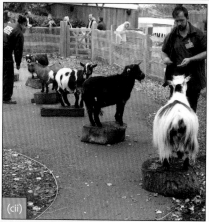
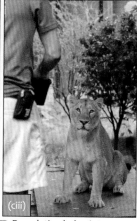
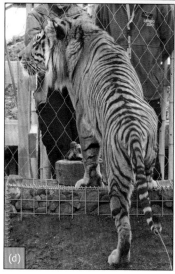
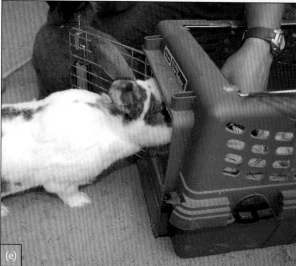

6.2 Foundation behaviours. (a) This keeper is reinforcing a red forest duiker for displaying calm behaviour. (bi) This rabbit has been trained to touch a target with the end of its nose. (bii) This emperor tamarin has been taught to touch a target with its hand. The principles of stationing are the same for (ci) dogs and cats as for (cii) pygmy goats. (ciii) This Asiatic lion is being stationed following an enriched feeding event. (d) This Sumatran tiger is receiving a food reinforcer following a recall behaviour. (e) This rabbit is being trained to travel in a pet carrier.

(a, bii, cii, courtesy of the Zoological Society of London; bi, e, courtesy of Barbara Heidenreich; d, courtesy of Darren Martin)

Dogs

Case example 3: Sit and stay exercises – dog

Sit and stay exercises are designed to teach a dog to focus attention on a person for direction in order to receive behavioural cues. Trust and acceptance of hand feeding are essential steps in the training process.

Principles

- Small food treats are used for positive reinforcement.
- In some cases, a headcollar and lead may be useful.
- Begin practising in a familiar area with minimal distractions. As the dog learns the task at hand, vary the location. Finally, add distractions.
- Initially, plan several short sessions over the course of the day. As you progress, sessions may vary from 5 to 15 minutes.

Stage 1: Reward attention

1. Stand directly in front of the dog.
2. Show the treat to the dog, ask the dog to 'sit', give them the treat.*
3. Show the treat to the dog, say 'sit and stay', count to 2, reward with the treat.*
4. Repeat, randomly varying the count from 1 to 10 during each session.*

   *Reward the dog if they sit quietly and look directly at you. During initial lessons, the treat may be used to lure attention.

- Throughout the lesson, speaking to the dog might help them to relax.
- The dog should remain in the 'sit' position until they are released with a verbal cue such as 'OK'.

Stage 2: Reward relaxed attention

During the initial sessions, the dog may be excited about earning treats. They may bark or offer other behaviours they have learned.

- Try to ignore any barking or pawing. Wait quietly; withhold the reward until they offer the 'sit' as instructed.
- With repetition, the dog will begin to understand that the only way to earn a treat is to sit calmly and watch you. A subtle relaxation of the dog's body posture may be noticed – reward these postures.

Stage 3: Add distance and distractions

Once the dog can consistently sit–stay and quietly watch you for 10 seconds, you are ready to ask them to stay as you move away.

1. Stand directly in front of the dog.
2. Ask them to 'sit and stay' while you take a step away and return. Give a treat.*
3. Repeat the sequence, randomly varying the distance. Return to the dog and reward with the treat.*
4. As you progress, add some distractions such as clapping your hands, knocking on the floor or bouncing a ball.
5. Finally, walk to the door, and then knock on the door. After each event, return to the dog and give a treat.*
6. Alternate randomly between challenging tasks and simple ones.
7. Always end your lesson on a positive note. Pick an easy task, such as a series of 1-second 'sits'.

   *Reward the dog if they sit quietly and look directly at you.

Stage 4: Add challenging distractions

Sit–stay exercises can be used to manage many problem behaviours, including jumping up on guests and running after bicycles. The dog's reaction to these triggers can be reduced, but the process must be gradual.

Begin a lesson far enough away from the trigger that the dog is able to sit and stay. A lead and/or headcollar should be used for control, but this should not be a struggle. Use very high-value rewards.

Example: Sit–stay to control jumping up on guests (this exercise should not be attempted until the dog has mastered the sit–stay while a family member walks to the door, opens and closes the door, and then returns to the dog).

1. When the guest enters the house, the dog should be restrained by lead (and headcollar) several feet from the door, out of the path of the visitor.
2. The dog should sit and stay to earn high-value treats.
3. Keep the dog's attention, rewarding quiet behaviour, while the guest settles.
4. Maintain the sit–stay for several minutes. Do not release the stay until the dog has relaxed and is not attempting to look towards the guest.
5. Once the dog is calm, they may be released to greet the visitor.
6. The guest should pet the dog only if it sits quietly.

Case example 4: Stationing – dog

The 'place' command, a form of stationing, is an effective tool for managing behaviours like excessive barking. Although barking can be interrupted, it will likely resume if the trigger remains. It can be very helpful to give the dog an acceptable alternative behaviour.

Place

It is necessary to establish a suitable place. This can be a dog bed or mat that is near the owner's main sitting area but away from the main window.

Stage 1

Begin training in the absence of any offending stimulus.
1. Ask the dog to 'stay'.
2. Go to the place and put a treat on it.
3. Release the dog with 'OK'.
4. As the dog approaches the treat, say 'mat' or 'bed', as appropriate.
5. Follow along, ask the dog to 'sit' and give a second treat.
6. Repeat, varying the starting distance.

Stage 2

Put the treat on the spot when the dog is not watching. Ask them to 'mat' or 'bed'; follow along, ask them to 'sit' and give a second treat.

Stage 3

When the dog begins to bark, for instance at a person passing by, attract their attention to interrupt the bark then send them to the chosen place. Reward.
1. Use a down–stay or sit–stay command to keep the dog in place; food titbits may be used to reward this quiet behaviour.
2. Alternatively, fasten a lead and bring the dog to an area of the house where they will not encounter the stimulus.

Tips

- If the home is very large, more than one 'place' may need to be set up.
- This method is less appropriate if there are several dogs present, young children in the home, or if the dog displays insecurity around food.
- In multi-dog households, it is possible to train one dog at a time while the others are confined elsewhere.
  - Rather than leaving the treat on the floor, hold the treat in your hand.
  - Show the treat.
  - Encourage the dog to follow you as you both walk to the 'place'. Ask the dog to 'sit' and reward.
  - Repeat until the dog begins to trot ahead towards its 'place', anticipating the treat. The moment the dog moves ahead, give the command 'mat' or 'bed', meet the dog at the 'place' and give the treat.

Case example 5: Recall training – dog

Teaching a dog to come back when called when it is off the lead is helpful for its safety and the peace of mind of the owner.

Stage 1: Introduce attention and cue

1. Stand close to the dog – just a few steps away. Allow it to sniff and explore while you hold the lead loosely.
2. Attract the dog's attention: squeak a toy, rattle a treat bag, make an odd sound.
3. The moment the dog looks towards the sound, give the command to 'come'.
4. Immediately reward with a high-value treat or toy.
5. Release the dog to sniff and explore.

   Repeat this sequence several times per session, varying the value of rewards.

Stage 2: Increase distance

1. When the dog has responded briskly and reliably for 2–3 sessions at close range, increase the distance between you and the dog.
2. The sequence should be the same: attract attention first, then call, then reward. At this point, the reward should be of moderate value.
3. For the next few sessions, vary the distance randomly. Sometimes call from a few steps away, sometimes from the end of a long line. Again: attention first, command, then the dog receives a reward.

Case example 5: Recall training – dog *continued*

Stage 3: Distractions

1. Add some distractions – a new toy in the area or a friend walking by.
2. Get the dog's attention.
3. Once the dog looks towards you, say 'come'. This time, a high-value reward should be used. Be careful not to use the 'come' command before you have the dog's attention.

Stage 4: Off-lead in a safe area

1. If you have a fenced training area, or if there is no risk of the dog running off into traffic or inadvertently injuring someone, then the same sequence may be followed off-lead.
2. Remove the lead, call from a short distance away, and give a high-value reward.
3. This time, as you reward, clip the lead on. Reward again, then unclip the lead and let the dog go and play.

Stage 5: New location

When the dog is performing reliably, take them to a new location, attach a long lead and start at the beginning.

Stage 6: Active recall

1. Encourage the dog to run (e.g. throw a toy).
2. While the dog is active and engaged, use a distraction such as a whistle or bell, then call and reward with a very high-value treat.
3. Let the dog go back to play.

Tips

- Use a long lead until performance is optimal.
- Conduct initial sessions in a quiet area.
- Consistently rewarding the dog whenever it returns will help to keep recall strong. High-value treats should be used initially and may be largely replaced by verbal praise and physical affection after recall is established.
- Fussing a bit with the collar as the reward is given will prepare the dog for times when it is off-lead and has to be restrained.
- Avoid repeating commands. If the dog is not paying attention, it is not associating anything with the sound of the command and the existing recall could become extinct.
- If the dog is removed from the play area immediately after obeying a recall command and being placed on a lead, it is being inadvertently punished for good behaviour.

Cats

Domestic cats are far less frequently trained than their canine counterparts. Even relatively simple procedures such as crate training or recall are not often attempted. Owners remark that their cat is not food motivated or that they are not responsive to training. This is most likely due to motivating operations, natural history or past experiences.

It may be worth attempting to train in the evening when the cat is most active, or trying tactile reinforcement rather than food in the initial stages of training. A preference test to determine which food item creates the highest motivation could be undertaken. There will almost certainly be something that each cat will find worth behaving for – in the authors' experience roast chicken never fails!

Case example 6: Audio recall – cat

A simple whistle recall is one of the first things dog owners teach their pets. It can also be very useful with cats that are allowed to range freely. Many cat owners will have spent time wondering where their cat has got to, and more often than not it will be within range of a whistle.

Recall training is used frequently for various cat species in zoological collections and can be applied to domestic animals; the steps below outline one approach. The audio device can be a whistle, a shaker, a doorbell – basically anything that can be sounded outside and can be heard at a fairly long distance. Note that this procedure is designed to call the cat back to the sound of the cue, to a set location such as the back door of the house.

1. Baiting. Place a very high-value food item on a place mat or other clearly marked station with the cat far enough away that it has to move towards it.
2. Observing the behaviour. Allow the cat to approach the food and eat. Repeat this action several times until the cat is moving towards the station at pace as soon as the food is placed there.
3. Inserting the cue. When the cat is moving towards the food insert the audio cue by sounding it just before the cat finds the food reinforcement. If it is sounded too far before or after eating, the connection with the sound will not occur. Repeat this 5–8 times.

Case example 6: Audio recall – cat *continued*

4. Phasing out the bait. This time do not add food to the station, just use the audio cue. When the cat moves towards the station, be ready to reinforce with food as quickly as possible. Repeat this several times to be sure the cat has made the connection between the sound and the behaviour of running to the station.
5. Testing the cue. Sound the cue when the cat is not visible. The cat should stop whatever it is doing and run towards the station for food.
6. Testing with a distraction. The cat should respond to the cue even it is doing something highly engaging, such as interacting with another cat. Test the response to the cue by giving it something else, such as a favourite toy, before sounding the cue.

Case example 7: Crate training – cat

There are several ways to crate train a cat. Shaping, luring, baiting and capturing are all appropriate. The following plan uses baiting and luring as the primary methods. It is worth noting that, unless you are training a kitten with no previous experiences of transportation, there is a good chance a transport crate will elicit a fear response. A period of habituation and counter-conditioning may be necessary before the training plan below can be used. Habituation may include leaving the crate in the garden with no expectation for the cat to interact with it at all. Over time the cat will realize there is no need to expend energy in being fearful of it. Counter-conditioning could mean leaving some high-value foods near the crat and then inside it. It may be necessary to remove the door for this part of the process, or even take the top half of the box away. All these methods have worked for the author [JM] when retraining a cat that has encountered aversive experiences during a visit to the veterinary surgery. The cat clearly connected those experiences with the crate and was sensitized to it.

1. Place a small piece of food inside the crate, allow the cat to enter and eat the food.
2. While the cat is inside the crate, offer more food through the side of the crate.
3. Offer the food lure only through the side of the crate (Figure 6.3a).
4. Replace the food lure with a finger tap on the side of the crate (Figure 6.3b). As the cat enters, replace the finger with the food reinforcer.

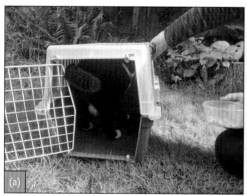
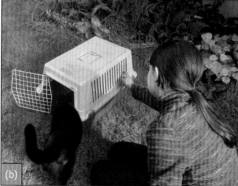

6.3 (a) A food lure is being used to prompt the cat to enter the crate. (b) The food lure is phased out and replaced with a finger tap.

5. Use the finger tap to cue the cat inside the crate. As it enters, present the food at the front of the crate (Figure 6.3c). Repeat this action several times to build duration. This step can be placed under stimulus control by inserting the cue 'turn around'.
6. Desensitize the cat to the door closing – this should be done outside the crate. Station the cat just outside the crate and repeatedly open and close the door, offering reinforcement for each repetition. After a few repetitions, insert the cue 'closing door'.
7. With the cat stationed inside the crate, offer the cue 'closing door'. Slowly close the door and continue to offer food, always being aware of feedback from the cat. If it stops taking food, stop closing the door and if it moves towards the door, open it. Removing the stimulus the cat does not like is important at this stage but should quickly be replaced with the door opening only when the cat is showing calm behaviour by taking food.

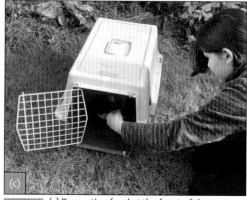

6.3 (c) Presenting food at the front of the crate encourages the cat to turn around. The food lure is then faded and replaced with the verbal cue 'turn around'.

▶

Case example 7: Crate training – cat *continued*

8. Once the cat accepts the door closing fully, build duration in the crate by offering several reinforcers through the door (Figure 6.3d).
9. Use a second person to lift the box while continuing to offer reinforcement.
10. Test the complete behaviour. Cue the cat into the box and ask it to turn around before slowly closing the door. Reinforce through the door. Lift the box and walk around before placing the box back on the ground, then reinforce. Open the door and reinforce the cat for staying inside. Cue leaving the crate with a finger tap on the floor and reinforce (Figure 6.3e).

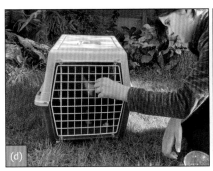
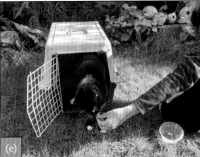

6.3 (d) Slowing the rate of reinforcement teaches the cat to sit in the crate for longer periods. (e) The cat is reinforced upon leaving the crate, having demonstrated the complete behaviour of entering and sitting calmly with the door shut.

The later stages of the process can include taking the box to the car for a drive. Any additional steps should be done with sensitivity, testing the response to stimuli such as the sound of the engine and the movement of the vehicle.

Small mammals

The physical nature and relative lack of risk associated with handling small mammals often results in manual restraint being viewed as an acceptable method of management. Case example 8 outlines a training protocol based on classical conditioning that has historically been recommended to make procedures such as handling less aversive for the animal. Nowadays, this philosophy is being challenged. Training should start by building a shared reinforcement history between the owner and animal with simple foundation behaviours such as targeting and crate training. The reinforcement history results in an improved human–animal bond, which means handling and restraint can be taught in a voluntary way. Case example 9 outlines a similar training protocol that makes use of operant conditioning and encourages voluntary engagement from the animal.

Training can and should be part of the small mammal caregiver's toolkit. One useful resource for rabbit and guinea pig training is Animal Training Fundamentals (see 'Useful websites', below), which provides a series of videos to demonstrate how to start training small mammals.

Case example 8: Establishment of calm behaviour and trust in a rabbit

The protocol below represents an effort to implement welfare-focused training when teaching a rabbit to accept handling, but it does not incorporate operant conditioning or consider the animal's agency. The general framework could be adapted by incorporating other techniques, in order to give the animal greater control and agency, which would greatly improve its welfare potential. Below the protocol, some steps that could be taken to improve it are provided. It should be borne in mind that whenever we are teaching animals new behaviours, both types of learning (classical and operant) will be at play (see Chapter 3).

Principles

- Associate a cue word with being lifted, so the rabbit is not surprised when picked up.
- Make the association pleasant enough that the rabbit and owner might mutually enjoy handling.

Stage 1: Reward acceptance of stroking

1. If the rabbit has displayed fear aggression in the past, then stroking should initially be done with a soft baby brush on a piece of dowel, so that the rabbit cannot bite the person. Otherwise, start with the hand.
2. Provide a few mouthfuls of the rabbit's favourite treat, such as fresh herbs.
3. Whilst it is eating, gently stroke the rabbit along the head, gradually along the back and around the chest, all the time softly saying the rabbit's name and the cue word (e.g. 'Thumper, lift').
   - Only continue while the rabbit is eating, and only gradually move to areas where it is less comfortable being touched.
4. Once the rabbit is relaxed being stroked whilst eating, move on to stage 2.

Case example 8: Establishment of calm behaviour and trust in a rabbit *continued*

Stage 2: Introduce lifting and restraint

1. Whilst the rabbit is eating, lift the hindquarters a few centimetres and put them back down again.
2. Follow this up by pushing your fingers gently between the front legs whilst offering the food.
3. When the rabbit is consistently relaxed with this, it is possible to begin picking the rabbit up.
   - It is important to support the hindquarters and the chest area. Fingers should be placed through the front legs so that the rabbit's weight is supported along the forearm and it cannot leap out of the hand. All rabbits should be handled securely but gently with two hands.

Improvements

Target behaviour could be used to call the rabbit – allowing it to interact on its terms with reinforcement of any interaction. A verbal cue could be added when the rabbit comes to the target, which then acts as a recall signal. Once the rabbit is approaching when called with either a target or voice recall, a combination of food reinforcers and physical contact (if the animal is expressing calm behaviours) can be used to develop a shared reinforcement history that will enhance the human–animal bond.

The target should then be used to ask the rabbit to hop into the trainer's lap; again a combination of food and tactile reinforcement should be used to reinforce the behaviour of staying in the lap for a prolonged duration. Using the method described above, pair desired stimuli with the small steps of being lifted, moving at a slow pace to ensure the handling is pleasant for both participants.

Ultimately, with training as an integrated component of an owner's (or veterinary practitioner's) husbandry techniques, asking the rabbit, or any other small mammal species, to hop into a crate or on to a lap replaces the majority of times when manual handling is actually required. Even simple procedures such as nail clipping can be achieved by a combination of recall, targeting on to a lap and then pairing food and tactile reinforcers with the equipment and sensations associated with the procedure.

Case example 9: Operant conditioning to facilitate handling of guinea pigs

At Copenhagen Zoo, the education team care for a number of animals that frequently participate in education sessions with groups of school children. Historically, these animals were handled and managed without the use of operant conditioning, as is typical with most domestic animals used for education in zoological collections. Copenhagen Zoo's training coordinator, Annette Pedersen, worked with the care staff to integrate trained behaviour into the programme in order to ensure voluntary participation in the sessions with children. They also used training to facilitate routine husbandry and medical care with a range of species, including chickens, rabbits and guinea pigs.

The first priority was to replace manual restraint handling with a voluntary operant behaviour. This was achieved by teaching each individual guinea pig to walk on to a tray (Figure 6.4) where it would receive reinforcement. Then each animal was taught to be lifted up in a canvas cloth. Once comfortable with this process, the guinea pig was moved from the tray to someone's lap where food reinforcement continued to be offered.

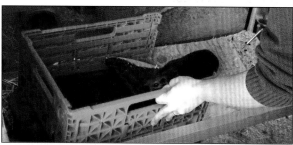

6.4 This guinea pig is learning to walk on to a tray containing a canvas cloth. Teaching the behaviour of walking into a crate affords the animal more agency than manually picking it up.
(Courtesy of Annette Pedersen)

This process can be described using the four-term contingency (see 'Four-term contingency', below):

- Antecedent: tray is lowered into enclosure
- Behaviour: guinea pig walks on to tray
- Consequence: food reinforcer is given to the guinea pig.

This behaviour was subsequently used in education sessions where the guinea pig would be moved from one child's lap to another, giving each child the opportunity to have a close contact experience with the animal. If a guinea pig refused to walk on to the tray for a session, the trainer moved to the next guinea pig, ensuring that each animal had the ability to choose whether or not to participate in the session.

The behaviour of choosing to leave the enclosure for reinforcement was also used to complete simple husbandry procedures (Figure 6.5). These behaviours were not trained separately but were possible due to the reinforcement history of human–animal contact.

Case example 9: Operant conditioning to facilitate handling of guinea pigs *continued*

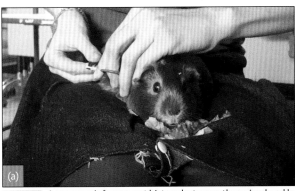
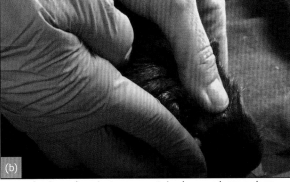

6.5 A strong reinforcement history between the animal and human makes it much easier to carry out simple procedures such as (a) nail trimming and (b) applying eye ointment without causing undue stress.
(Courtesy of Annette Pedersen)

Zoological species

Case example 10: Zoo animal transport

In the author's [JM] experience, one frequently asked question from zookeepers and veterinary surgeons (veterinarians) is 'How can we train an animal to travel for 10 hours to another zoo?' The answer is simple: we cannot. What we can do is make sure the transportation vessel has a history of positive reinforcement. This way we are giving the animal the power to cope with a potentially stressful situation. Anecdotally, these coping skills are evidenced by a return to normal feeding patterns and social interaction behaviours following voluntary transfer to another zoological collection. Further research into the transportation of animals in and between zoological collections is ongoing.

The value of a positive association with transportation methods should also be highlighted to all owners. It is important that dogs are allowed time to get used to travelling in cars with crates or seat belt harnesses. Cats and rabbits can be desensitized to their carriers by having them as a normal part of their home/enclosure, whilst birds and other exotic species can also be trained using positive reinforcement methods so that they are more accepting of, and less stressed by, travelling.

Four-term contingency

For a complete functional overview when considering behaviours and training, the environmental influences that occur before (antecedents) and after (postcedents) the behaviour must be noted. The four-term contingency allows consideration of all the important components required to assess and understand behaviour and design a training plan to change or teach new behaviours. The elements of the four-term contingency are: motivating operations (MOs), antecedents (A), behaviour (B) and consequences (C). Behaviour is defined briefly above and in detail in Chapter 3; each of the other elements is covered briefly below, including how they relate to each other and how to make use of this model.

Case example 11: Four-term contingency evaluation of a cat scratch

If a veterinary surgeon states that a cat scratched them, this tells us that scratching occurred but, because this only focuses on part of the behaviour (B), we do not know when this occurred or why it occurred. The full picture might be that when the veterinary surgeon touched the cat's abscess (A), the cat scratched (B), which resulted in the veterinary surgeon moving their hand away from the abscess (C). This provides much more information and allows us to study the scratching behaviour and form a hypothesis as to why it could have occurred. In moving their hand away, the veterinary surgeon negatively reinforced the behaviour of scratching, and the cat will be more likely to scratch in similar situations in the future (see Chapter 3).

Motivating operations

Motivating operations are environmental variables that alter the reinforcing or punishing effectiveness of subsequent stimuli. Motivating operations can be used to ensure an animal is prepared to offer or perform behaviours on cue for a chosen reinforcer. The principles of reinforcement and punishment are discussed in Chapter 3.

In the case of zoo animals, training reinforcers are primarily food-based, with a few animals, for example Malayan tapirs, responding well to tactile and play-based reinforcers. Reinforcers for companion animals are more likely to be verbal, tactile or play-based, though food reinforcers are still common. Increasingly, the feeling of control as a primary reinforcer has been considered an important aspect of zoo animal training, and this should be incorporated into companion animal training wherever possible. It is important to frequently reassess the strength of reinforcers, and to understand that no single reinforcer will be effective in every context.

When food is the primary reinforcer, there are several techniques that can be used to build the necessary motivation required to elicit behaviour. These methods must be carefully evaluated to ensure individual animal welfare and are dependent on species-specific ethology. One method

Case example 12: Ring-tailed lemurs – crate training

A group of ring-tailed lemurs was trained to enter a transport crate, using small pieces of sweet potato used as a food reinforcer. Initially, food was used to lure the animal into the crate. After a few repetitions, the food lure was phased out and replaced with a visual cue (a finger tap on the mesh of the crate). Once the animal was trained to fully enter the crate on cue, with the doors open, the use of control came into play. Firstly, the trainer started to move the doors with the animal stationed outside the crate. Each time the door moved it was preceded by a verbal cue: 'door opening'. The trainer waited to see visual recognition of the door moving – this recognition was then reinforced with food. Once the trainer was sure the animal understood the link between the door moving and food being offered, and the animal remained calm and focused on the trainer, not the door, training could continue inside the crate.

With the animal fully inside the crate, the trainer offered the verbal cue 'door closing' and started to close the door very slowly. If the animal looked at the door, the trainer stopped closing the door but continued to offer food for remaining inside and showing calm behaviour. To begin with, the trainer would allow the animal to leave and would fully open the door if the animal moved towards it, ensuring the animal felt control over the stimulus. However, very quickly the trainer would use the action of opening the door to reinforce calm behaviour, rather than to reinforce moving towards the door. This was actually negative reinforcement: using the removal of the undesired stimulus (the door) to reinforce the behaviour of remaining calm in the crate. This was combined with feeding, which meant positive reinforcement quickly replaced negative. Food was offered outside the crate and then the animal cued back inside to repeat the process. Gradually, criteria were raised, with the end result being an animal that was comfortable inside the crate and felt in control at all times during the training process, as if their eyes or body language were in charge of the movement of the door.

A similar protocol can be used with any species required to enter a carrier or crate for travel. The principles remain the same, for example, for cat carriers (see Case example 7, above), raptor transport boxes and horse trailers.

involves removing a highly desired food item from an animal's daily allowance and only offering it during training sessions. This creates a relative deficit, strengthening the reinforcing value of the item. Thus, whilst the animal has access to all other food items in its daily budget, at any time the animal is called for training it should leave those food items and participate in training with enthusiasm to earn its favourite food. Owners will often have a good idea of their animals' favourite foods; for example, a pet iguana may be fed mostly vegetables but have a clear preference for the fruit that makes up a small part of its daily ration. For a zoo animal, such as an emperor tamarin, keepers may offer a variety of food items and let the animal choose a favourite. However, it is more difficult to train a Philippine crocodile, for example, using food as they generally feed once or twice a week. In this instance, it may be necessary to use all the food allowance for that day to facilitate trained behaviour. In all cases, it is not suitable to rely on hunger to motivate animals as this can lead to aggression towards trainers/owners and conflict with conspecifics.

Antecedents

In behavioural science, there are two types of antecedent – distant and direct. Direct antecedents are what immediately precedes a behaviour occurring; in animal training this is often a visual stimulus (for example, a target) or verbal stimulus (a cue word such as 'sit'). Distant antecedents concern the ethology of a species. When training an animal, the first thing you must do is find out as much as you can about its natural history: What is the animal physically and mentally capable of? What challenges is it adapted to overcome in a natural environment? What are its feeding strategies and social interactions? Coupling these facts with knowledge of the individual history of the animal provides important information for planning a programme.

Antecedent arrangement: Antecedent arrangement is the term used for any modification or alteration of an animal's habitat to help make it easier for them to perform a desired behaviour and harder to perform an undesired

behaviour, and it has a huge impact on the potential success of a training plan.

This applies to all behaviour modifications, training or otherwise. For example, a polar bear at Yorkshire Wildlife Park required daily topical treatment on the pads of its feet. Keepers installed a soft absorbent mat on the floor across the width of a passage between two areas of the exhibit. The pad was soaked with the medicated liquid and the bear would walk across it twice a day during routine husbandry. This antecedent arrangement made the behaviour of walking across the mat easier to achieve without the need to train any new behaviours.

For zoo animals, most medical training occurs in protected contact conditions, where a protective barrier is necessary for human health and safety. The barrier also provides a sense of security to the animal so, even with animals where daily husbandry occurs in 'free contact' conditions that are not dangerous to the caregiver, it is often advisable to train in protected contact.

Antecedent arrangement is one of the most important components of zoo animal training. It can fundamentally change the way an animal approaches a training situation from being challenging to easy, it applies to all taxonomic groups and is often simple to install. For example, changing the location of training with callitrichids (New World monkeys) from the forest floor to a balcony replicates the natural behaviour of occupying mid-canopy rainforest, giving the animals a greater sense of control over the environment and interactions with people. When training crocodiles to enter a crate for blood sampling, half submerging the crate in water allows them to quickly learn to follow a target and swim into the crate to receive reinforcement. This is a simple adjustment from placing the crate on land, where crocodiles will struggle.

With large carnivores, a simple antecedent is placing a heavy object, such as a log, in a lateral position adjacent to the barrier. This teaches the animal to adopt a sternal position, which is necessary for hand injections. The addition of a 'letter box' aperture enables the trainer or veterinary surgeon to safely access the tail, which is the optimal way to take blood samples in wild cat species.

Antecedent arrangements are commonly employed in companion animal training. For example, parrots can be quite territorial and, thus, their cage may not be the best place to start a training session – providing a play stand from which training sessions can be run is a simple form of antecedent arrangement. Case example 3 states sit–stay training should begin in a familiar area with minimal distractions; the home will be a much easier environment for a dog to learn in than a busy park that provides ample opportunity for undesirable behaviours.

All of these techniques can be extrapolated for use with other species and should be an important part of any care plan. For example, evaluating the animal's current level of training should be considered when discussing an upcoming elective procedure, in order to help the owner to understand how to implement changes that can help the process go more smoothly (i.e. training a dog or cat to be comfortable giving their paw and having their leg held can help with intravenous access). It is vital that these discussions take place as early as possible, so that the animal and the owner have enough time to implement these training requests correctly and without rushing.

Consequences

Simply put, consequences are the stimuli that follow a behaviour and determine whether the behaviour is likely to increase or continue (reinforcement) or decrease (punishment). The science of behaviour change (i.e. operant conditioning) uses the operant quadrant to demonstrate how consequences affect future probable behaviour:

* Positive reinforcement – adding an appetitive stimulus
* Postivie punishment – adding an aversive stimulus
* Negative reinforcement – removing an aversive stimulus
* Negative punishment – removing an appetitive stimulus.

It is very important to state here that the language used should be interpreted without the existing connotations certain words carry. Positive does not mean good, negative does not mean bad; they mean adding and removing, respectively. Similarly, punishment does not have the same meaning in operant conditioning as it does in common parlance. Punishment simply reduces a behaviour while reinforcement increases it. It is extremely important to remember this when using the associated terminology. It is very easy to assume that all negative reinforcement is bad training and all positive reinforcement is good training, but this is incorrect. However, there is evidence to show that the use of punishment when training animals can lead to undesired side effects such as generalized fear, apathy and aggression (see Chapter 3).

The context and welfare of the individual animal should be considered at all times when deciding on training methods. There are many examples in the zoological collection environment where removing a stimulus necessarily precedes, or accompanies, positive reinforcement. For example, when beginning to train large herds of ungulates to move to an indoor area, food can be offered far away from the dens. When the animals start to eat, the trainer moves away. This process is repeated with the food closer to the dens and each time the trainer leaves this negatively reinforces the action of eating. Eventually, the food is offered inside the dens and the behaviour is placed under stimulus control using, for example, the sound of a bell. However, it should be noted that in some cases, it is hard to build enough trust between the human caregiver and the animal to allow positive reinforcement to occur.

Case example 13: Flamingos at Copenhagen Zoo

Copenhagen Zoo has a flock of 65 flamingos and limited staff resources, so it was decided that the flamingos would be trained to enter indoor housing using negative reinforcement. The keeper would slowly walk towards the flock and when it began to move away from him, he would move backwards, reinforcing the behaviour of movement towards the indoor house by removing the aversive stimulus (himself). If the flamingos stopped, he would move forwards again and repeat the process until they were fully inside the house. This process was repeated with the addition of gentle hand clapping. In a very short time, the entire flock learned to move inside the house just from the sound of the hand clap without any movement from the keeper at all. When they were inside they had access to food reinforcers, pairing negative with positive reinforcement. It is important that this process is completed very quickly and by experts who can recognize when the behaviour of the birds is calm and relaxed. If the birds are at all stressed they will not learn the behaviour correctly.

Training to facilitate clinical care

Desensitization

Many veterinary practices are now encouraging owners to bring their dogs to the surgery prior to a procedure to habituate them to the surroundings. In some cases, dogs may have developed an aversion to the veterinary practice and require some desensitization to attempt to reduce the aversive behavioural response. Firstly, it is important to be able to observe and measure a behaviour before trying to reduce it. Practitioners often refer to stress, but this is an overused word which needs to be defined and described.

Case example 14: Desensitization – fearful German Shepherd Dog x Golden Retriever

When Rosie, a German Shepherd Dog x Golden Retriever, arrived at the veterinary surgery she exhibited fearful behaviours including licking, tucking her tail between legs, cowering and flight movement away from staff. Additionally, she would not accept appetitive stimuli, such as food or physical contact, and would not engage in any behaviours associated with calmness, such as sniffing the ground or interacting with the environment in other ways. She would express calm behaviours and take food reinforcers when inside the car. ▶

Case example 14: Desensitization – fearful German Shepherd Dog x Golden Retriever *continued*

The observable behaviours were modified using a simple behaviour plan and offering appetitive stimuli of preferred food items and physical contact. Throughout the process, the observable behaviours were measured – if the dog expressed any behaviours associated with fear, the process was slowed down. As long as the dog expressed behaviours associated with calmness, the process moved to the next step.

1. Drive to the veterinary surgery and stay in the car park, offer appetitive stimulus while the dog is inside the car with the door closed.
2. Park at the surgery and open the car boot, offer stimulus while the dog remains calm in the boot.
3. Park at the surgery and offer stimulus while a veterinary receptionist stands adjacent to the boot.
4. Allow the receptionist to offer stimulus and while the dog is in the car.
5. With the dog in the car park, offer stimulus then ask the receptionist to do the same.
6. When the dog is engaging with the environment of the car park, switch the role of the receptionist to a veterinary surgeon or veterinary nurse.
7. Repeat the process in the waiting area and then in the consultation room itself.
8. When the dog is fully comfortable and expressing calm behaviours in each location and with more than one veterinary surgeon or nurse, the process can move to training for simple medical procedures such as auscultation.

Scale training

A simple starting point for any medical care programme is teaching the animal to sit on scales (Figure 6.6). Depending on the species and individual history, this can be as simple as presenting the device on or near the normal training area, or it may require considerable acclimatization and training. A fear response shown by the animal can usually be challenged by antecedent arrangement (Figure 6.6a) or counter-conditioning.

Scale training more than one animal

Training multiple animals in any scenario always presents a challenge, generally due to competition for high-value resources such as food. Good planning, antecedent arrangement and teaching foundation behaviours such as stationing and shifting are essential facets for successful group training. The first question a trainer must answer before starting is: should I separate or station? Most zoo animal training involves shifting and isolation, and placing

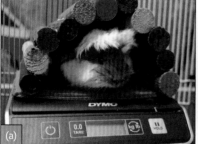 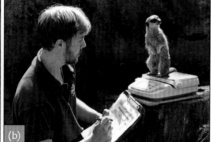 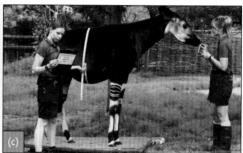

6.6 Scale training uses stationing behaviour to facilitate weighing an animal. (a) This guinea pig is being weighed under a familiar shelter, an example of antecedent arrangement to train new behaviours. (b) The scales for this meerkat have been placed on a raised surface, which makes it easier to train one individual at a time. (c) This okapi is demonstrating both stationing and targeting behaviours, allowing it to be weighed and measured.
(a, Courtesy of Barbara Heidenreich; b, c, Courtesy of the Zoological Society of London)

Case example 15: Scale training a green-winged macaw

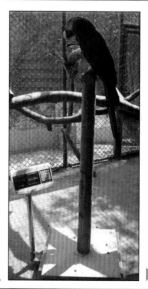

Ruby, a green-winged macaw (*Ara chloropterus*) with no previous training experience, was trained to step on to an elevated perch in the first week of a quarantine period following import to ZSL London Zoo (Figure 6.7). The training programme outlining the foundation behaviours and small approximations towards this behaviour was:

1. Motivating operations – walnuts were chosen as a primary reinforcer and removed from the diet.
2. Desensitization to the scales – platform scales were placed in the corridor outside the den to allow the bird to visually acclimatize to the novel stimulus.
3. Shifting and recall through name recognition – walnuts were offered in feed stations in the inside den and outside flight and the name 'Ruby' was inserted while the bird moved between stations.
4. Hand feeding to develop trust between the animal and trainer – walnuts were offered to Ruby by hand, first in protected contact (to give Ruby a sense of security and control), then in free contact.

6.7 The custom-made T perch that helped Ruby to sit on the scales is an example of antecedent arrangement. ▶

Case example 15: Scale training a green-winged macaw *continued*

5. Walnuts were used as a lure to move Ruby from one branch to another and then the food lure was phased out and replaced with a finger tap as a visual cue.
6. The scales, now with a custom-made high T perch, were placed in the outside flight while Ruby was locked inside. Ruby was allowed access to the scales and given time to acclimatize to them. When it was clear the scales elicited no fear response, training recommenced.
7. The foundation behaviours of hand feeding and cued movement using audio recall and the finger tap stimulus were used to encourage Ruby on to the high perch.

Ruby was successfully weighed less than 1 week after import from another UK collection with no previous training experience. Further behaviours trained during the 28-day quarantine period were crate training for transfer to the exhibit and presentation for microchip reading.

---

a physical barrier between each conspecific is guaranteed to prevent conflict over resources. However, physical separation is sometimes not possible, for example in large aviaries, and it can pose different problems. Social animals may be reliant on conspecifics for a feeling of control and reassurance; a highly intelligent carnivore or primate could become aggressive towards conspecifics when reintroduced following a training session, especially if that training session is with a subordinate animal. Whether separating or stationing is used, it is imperative that each individual animal receives reinforcement of equal value throughout the process, either directly from the trainer or via enriched feeding or another high-value activity.

Scale training in protected contact

There are many examples of animals being weighed without physical contact in zoological collections. The most effective way to enable this is through antecedent arrangement. Weigh boards, with blocks positioned to encourage an animal to stand, sit or lie correctly, mean that the trainer only needs to have the trust of the animal in order to gain a correct weight. Similarly, primates can be weighed with hanging scales.

Case example 16: Scale training three primate species in one exhibit

Keepers responsible for a walk-through exhibit housing multiple emperor tamarins (*Saguinus imperator*), a single golden-headed lion tamarin (*Leontopithecus chrysomelas*) and multiple coppery titi monkeys (*Callicebus cupreus*) needed to be able to weigh all the animals with a minimal impact on welfare. Each species was taught a different audio recall which enabled the group of dominant emperor tamarins to be called to one station for weighing, the single golden-headed lion tamarin to be called to another station and placed in a box, and the subordinate coppery titi monkeys to be called to a third location to be target trained. The species could then be rotated through each location allowing all three to be weighed in succession. Discriminative stimuli and food reinforcers were chosen carefully; for example, the titi monkeys received walnuts, which the emperor tamarins did not like, reducing the likelihood of resource conflict.

▶

Case example 16: Scale training three primate species in one exhibit *continued*

The training plan was:

1. Preference test each species (and individuals) for primary reinforcers.
2. Motivating operations – remove primary reinforcer from the diet for 3 days.
3. Using food luring, teach a different sound to each species.
4. Target train each species with a discriminative stimulus – e.g. bamboo stick for the titi monkey, lollipop target for the emperor tamarin.
5. Create a custom-made scale perch or block for each species and station and train them to it.
6. Use target and station training to reinforce individuals of the same species for allowing conspecifics to be weighed.
7. Switch location of species using recall behaviour.

Induction of anaesthesia

Induction of anaesthesia in zoo animals varies according to species and enclosure provision, and traditional methods normally include some element of manual restraint for gas induction or hand injection, or darting with a blow pipe or gun. These methods are still used and are important skills for any zoo veterinary surgeon or veterinary nurse to have but significant progress has been made and there is an increasing desire to apply voluntary trained behaviour to achieve the same end goal. Hand injection has replaced darting as the go-to method for anaesthesia induction in larger mammal species, with many zoological collections routinely training large carnivores, great apes and hoofstock for hand injection.

There are significant benefits to adopting training for hand injection in place of darting or manual restraint for induction. Firstly, the time to recumbency is quicker when achieved through trained behaviour, which suggests a reduction in hormones such as adrenaline. Secondly, the dose required to achieve full induction is significantly reduced, which saves money and reduces associated risks. Anecdotally, a 'smoother' recovery from the effects of anaesthesia has been described when hand injection was used in a range of mammalian species including lions, tigers and primates. These benefits influence the welfare of the animal and can help improve anaesthetic safety.

The use of trained behaviour to achieve induction of anaesthesia through hand injection can be extended to a wide variety of mammal species. These injections can be delivered through a protective barrier, in a custom-made crate or in free contact. There are important considerations for each scenario:

- If you intend to inject in free contact, is it safe for trainer, veterinary surgeon and animal?
- If you are injecting an animal via a protective barrier, is the animal going to retreat to a higher location where it may fall when the anaesthetic takes effect?
- Does the crate you have designed allow for access and comfort?

Hand injections in a custom-made enclosed chute

One way to ensure that a hand injection is delivered successfully, and with minimal risk of injury to the animal during the time to recumbency, is to train an animal to enter a custom-made injection crate or chute. The author's [JM] experiences with this method are numerous, although each scenario presents a different experience for the individual and it is more suited to certain species.

Hand injections in free contact or an open chute

This method is used for animals that are not appropriate for chute training or are housed in facilities that make protected contact training impossible, and that are considered safe for human contact following a risk assessment.

Hand injections in protected contact

The majority of hand injections in the zoological collection environment are delivered through a protective barrier. This is primarily for human safety, but it also ensures that the training offers a feeling of control to the animal whose participation is dependent on a reliable recall to the training station. Success is again reliant on motivation and antecedent arrangement, with a particular emphasis on ensuring there is a safe transition to recumbency following the injection.

Case example 17: Hand injection in a crested porcupine

One successful and necessary use of hand injection in a custom-made enclosed chute involved a crested porcupine at ZSL London Zoo and a modified mesh dog cage with a board installed in the middle. This board could be moved to adjust the available cage width depending on the stage of the training.

This individual knew the foundation behaviours of recall and stationing, which were trained in free contact in the large outside area of the exhibit prior to the injection training.

1. The cage was placed inside the enclosure and the animal was allowed to habituate to its presence with no stimuli (such as food) available, in order to ensure that the animal did not experience a dilemma (i.e. I do not trust the cage, but I want the food: what do I do?). This process was followed up with some conditioning by placing food around the cage after observations confirmed there was no fear response to the cage.
2. With the chute set at the greatest width, the porcupine was trained to enter the chute using a food lure of small pieces of nuts.
3. The food lure was phased out and replaced with a shaker audio cue and reinforcement delivered when the animal was fully inside the chute.
4. The animal was trained for increased duration inside the cage.
5. Gradually, the width of the chute was reduced until the right side of the porcupine was pushed up against the mesh.
6. The porcupine was then trained to exit the chute and enter a large transport crate, using the same audio cue (shaker).
7. The sequence of entering the chute, remaining at station for up to a minute and leaving the chute to enter the crate was repeated until it became a chained behaviour.
8. The next stage was to introduce the veterinary surgeon and allow the animal to habituate to their presence. This process also involved some conditioning, with the veterinary surgeon delivering food reinforcers while the animal was inside the chute.
9. The final stage was to apply a small amount of pressure to the board while the veterinary surgeon applied pressure to the right-hand side of the rump of the animal using a dummy syringe. If the animal stopped taking reinforcers from the trainer during this stage, the pressure of the board was relaxed and the veterinary surgeon desisted with the dummy injection.
10. The actual injection was successful with the board held in position but without the need to squeeze the porcupine against the mesh. The porcupine then entered the transport crate where it became recumbent.

Chute training for hand injections has also been successful in ring-tailed lemurs, coppery titi monkeys, servals, gentle lemurs, golden-headed lion tamarins and Asiatic small-clawed otters.

Case example 18: Hand injection in aye-ayes

In the case of the aye-aye, an animal that is naturally cautious and requires a trusting relationship with the caregiver to be successfully managed in captivity, the decision was made to attempt hand injection in free contact. However, a risk assessment concluded that there needed to be some form of barrier to provide safe access for the veterinary surgeon who would be delivering the injection. Aye-ayes are very destructive, so any equipment used during training must be removable or made of metal; in addition, the ability to move and isolate animals from the training area is very useful.

Firstly, each individual was taught the foundation behaviours of hand feeding: building a trusting relationship with the keeper, stationing and shifting between the different areas of the enclosure.

The key to success in this case was good antecedent arrangement. A custom-made station was built that incorporated an open chute, a mesh panel for safe access to inject, and a T-perch with a half coconut shell to place

---

Case example 18: Hand injection in aye-ayes *continued*

reinforcers in and to encourage the aye-ayes into the ideal position for injections. A transport crate was placed in the corner of the den.

During regular training sessions each aye-aye was:

1. Recalled to an enclosed den while the injection station was installed in the training den.
2. Recalled to the training den and allowed to habituate to the equipment.
3. Allowed to interact with the station with a keeper present. Each interaction (visual or tactile) was reinforced.
4. Encouraged using luring to stand on its back legs holding on to the T-perch. The lure was phased out and replaced with a finger tap on the perch.
5. Rewarded for spending an increased duration at the station in the correct position.
6. Encouraged to enter the crate following each repetition of stationing behaviour.
7. Classically conditioned to the keeper touching its right thigh (i.e. food was placed in the coconut shell and whilst the aye-aye took the food the tactile work continued).
8. Habituated to the presence of a second person (e.g. veterinary nurse) in the training area.
9. Acclimated to injection with a dummy needle, with the veterinary surgeon positioned to the animal's right.

The training was completed with several repetitions of stationing, dummy injection and voluntary, cued entry to the transport crate. This training worked more than once with three aye-ayes who had very different histories and personalities, and resulted in a fast and smooth induction to anaesthesia.

Case example 19: Hand injection in African wild dogs

The first successful hand injection training at ZSL London Zoo was completed by the author [JM] in 2013 with three African wild dogs (*Lycaon pictus*). The training programme was specifically requested by the veterinary team to replace darting for delivery of annual vaccinations for leptospirosis. This training took a long time, approximately 6 months, as difficulties with motivation and trust building needed to be overcome. The dogs received large enriched-carcass feeds, the joint consumption of which was considered crucial for the social dynamic of the group, and the training allowance was taken from the same carcasses. Motivation was hard to develop in this scenario as the dogs were intelligent enough to understand that if they waited a few hours they would receive the same food item as they were being offered by the trainer, both in a larger quantity and in a more stimulating way, without having to be in close proximity to a trainer. Various methods to build trust and increase motivation were trialled without resorting to the hunger state. These included offering enrichment to the dogs in the form of scatter feeds while the keeper was present, the use of negative reinforcement (if the dogs looked at or approached the trainer the food would be dropped and the trainer would walk away), name recognition and eye contact (any recognition of the trainer would be reinforced by throwing meat over the barrier). Once the dogs were comfortably taking food from the trainer using tongs for safety, a variety of behaviours were introduced to help keep the sessions interesting. Targeting, stand up and sit behaviours were trained before moving on to any tactile work. To achieve the correct position for injection, sternal recumbency with the rump against the mesh barrier, the environment was modified with a heavy log that the dogs could stand or lie behind. A second person was added to the training, and they began to replicate the injection with a dummy syringe.

Every time you train a new species, or individual for that matter, you learn something new. One prerequisite for invasive procedures such as hand injections in zoo animals is to attempt to recreate exactly the same conditions during training sessions as in the actual event. For example, using the same size of needle and filling the syringe with the same amount of liquid that will be needed on the day itself. In the case of the dogs, it was not enough to fill the syringe with water to replicate the vaccine as their incredible sense of smell meant they knew that the liquid inside the syringe was different to that used in training. This led to an unsuccessful first attempt – the dogs knew something was different on the day and refused to participate. However, even if this was known in advance, the cost of the vaccine prohibited using it as a training tool. Water continued to be used for training but the syringe was covered in a neutral smell, stronger than the aroma of the vaccine, which the dogs habituated to prior to the next attempt.

Despite taking a long time, these techniques were successful. All three dogs were vaccinated by hand injection and it was a key learning experience for the trainers involved.

The vaccinations were administered in protected contact in a large outside exhibit without the need for separation, as this group allowed each animal to approach the training station in turn without competition for food reinforcers. Not relying on hunger to build motivation was a definite plus in this scenario. Unfortunately, it is not possible to hand inject an individual dog for anaesthesia in this way. Firstly, there is a significant risk that the other dogs could injure the conspecific during the process of induction; secondly, there is a human risk in entering a large outside enclosure with a dog even if it seems completely recumbent. For these reasons, all anaesthesia was achieved by separating individuals in to internal dens for darting.

The anaesthetic protocol was improved after the installation of crates in the inside dens in 2017, in response to an export request. A new breeding group, introduced to the exhibit in 2016, had successfully reared 11 pups and the female offspring were to be moved to ZSL Whipsnade Zoo. The crates were installed on the outside of the mesh panels and, following a period of habituation to the new equipment, the training of an audio recall to enter the new training area, and time for the keepers to get to know and station individuals, each dog was encouraged to enter the crate in turn. Once inside, they were taught to lie down and the sliding door, operated by the trainer at the font of the

Alternatives to anaesthesia

Despite significant advances in the use of trained behaviour to improve induction of anaesthesia in zoo animals, it is preferable to avoid anaesthesia where possible. Trained voluntary behaviours, such as presenting body parts for blood sampling, radiography and dental examinations, can provide enough clinical information to negate the need for a full anaesthetic event (Figure 6.8).

Animal behaviour management should focus on proactive and preventive care rather than reactive care. Good nutrition, enrichment and enclosure design form the basis of a preventive regime, and training programmes that focus on foundation behaviours and preventive healthcare will result in the least intrusive management plan. Following this philosophy can often remove the need for other intrusive interventions, such as manual restraint (see 'Avoiding anaesthesia in avian and reptile species', below).

Avoiding anaesthesia in avian and reptile species

Routine training of zoo birds and reptiles is not as prevalent as in mammals, but there is a direct and meaningful benefit to using training techniques, especially to prevent manual restraint and anaesthesia.

Foot health is an ongoing issue in captive birds. Miguel Santos, formerly of Zoomarine in Portugal, modified a wooden box with mirrors to allow close-up examination of the underside of several bird species' feet. This proactive tool, coupled with daily routine station training, facilitates early identification and treatment of potential foot problems. This design was widely disseminated among zoo professionals and sees frequent use as it is appropriate for a range of species.

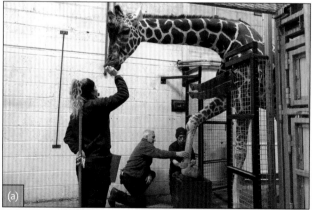

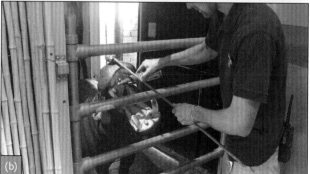

6.8 (a) Trained behaviour allows examination of this giraffe's foot without anaesthesia and facilitates radiography and hoof trimming. (b) This hippopotamus is voluntarily allowing dental care to be carried out using trained targeting behaviour.
(a, Courtesy of Anusia Acus; b, Courtesy of the Zoological Society of London)

Case example 20: Nail clipping in a Sulawesi crested macaque *continued*

4. The animal was conditioned to accept human nail clippers, through visual recognition initially and then tactile.
5. A veterinary surgeon was introduced to the training, who inspected and then trimmed the nail.
6. The process was repeated for the other hand as a proactive measure.

Case example 21: Bumblefoot in a king vulture

At ZSL London Zoo, the author [JM] and bird keeper colleagues trained a king vulture to present its feet at a protective barrier to allow topical treatment of bumblefoot. This behaviour was achieved using the following steps:

1. Target training – teaching the bird to touch a coloured disc target with its beak. Any visual recognition of the target was reinforced with a small piece of meat.
2. The target was held slightly out of reach of the bird, so she reached upwards to touch the target and lifted one foot to maintain balance. This behaviour was captured and reinforced.
3. After just a few repetitions, the bird would present her foot when the target was hung just above her reach. This behaviour could be repeated for either foot depending on whether the target was placed to her right or left.
4. While the foot was presented, conditioning commenced to allow a keeper to touch the underside of each foot.
5. Topical medication was applied to the affected area during the foot presentation behaviour.

The king vulture in this example was a fascinating bird and a wonderful learner. The individual had been labelled as unpredictable and aggressive towards certain keepers, but a simple solution to this was to work with her in a protected contact setting. Teaching audio recall and stationing helped build a good human–animal bond and the cognitive experience of learning was a major motivating factor for the bird. Participation in training sessions could even occur directly after a large feed.

Editor's note [JHM]

The methods detailed here for training zoo animals rely on basic principles that can be applied to any species, including domestic pets – if a tiger can be trained to present for a blood sample to be obtained, it should not be a struggle to trim a pug's nails! Members of the veterinary profession can and should be more proactive in sharing training techniques with owners. Small steps that are simple to teach can reduce stress and fear for animals during consultations. For example, asking a new puppy or kitten owner to practice lifting their pet's tail and holding it over its back can really help with temperature taking.

Acknowledgement

The authors gratefully acknowledge the assistance of Barbara Heidenreich of Animal Training Fundamentals (see 'Useful websites', below), who provided images for use in this chapter as well as invaluable guidance on rabbit training.

References and further reading

Association of Zoos & Aquariums and American Association of Zoo Keepers (2016) *AZA/AAZK Animal Training Terms & Definitions*. Available from: www.aazk.org/wp-content/uploads/AZA-AAZK-Training-Terms-2016.pdf

Chance P (1998) *Learning and Behavior*. Thomson Wadsworth, Belmont

Department for Environment, Food and Rural Affairs (2012) *Secretary of State's Standards of Modern Zoo Practice*. Available from: www.gov.uk

Horwitz DF and Mills DS (2009) *BSAVA Manual of Canine and Feline Behavioural Medicine, 2nd edn*. BSAVA Publications, Gloucester

Melfi VA, Dorey NR and Ward SJ (2019) *Zoo Animal Learning and Training*. Wiley-Blackwell, Hoboken, New Jersey

Moore J (2011) Behaviorism. *The Psychological Record* **61**, 449–463

Pryor K (1999) *Don't Shoot the Dog!: The New Art of Teaching and Training, revised edn*. Bantam Books, New York

Ramirez K (1999) *Animal Training: Successful Animal Management Through Positive Reinforcement*. Shedd Aquarium Society, Chicago, Illinois

Skinner BF (1938) *The Behavior of Organisms*. Appleton-Century, New York City

Useful websites

Animal Training Fundamentals
animaltrainingfundamentals.com

Chapter 7

Optimizing animal welfare in clinical practice

Heather Bacon and Hayley Walters

Introduction

Veterinary professionals aim to optimize the welfare of their patients as part of their ethical duty of care, as well as to ensure improved clinical and surgical outcomes for the animal and help build a good veterinary surgeon (veterinarian)–client–patient relationship. However, the fear and anticipated discomfort that a patient often experiences at, and therefore associates with, the veterinary practice can make handling and treating them difficult and/or dangerous. Distressed patients may have increased circulating levels of stress hormones, which can affect the immune system and hinder recovery from disease or surgery; these patients may also require higher doses of anaesthetic agents or other medications, which could be associated with an increased risk of complications. However, with thoughtful planning of each area of the clinic, an understanding of the animal's perspective, and staff awareness of low-stress handling and restraint methods, a patient's experience of the clinic can be much more positive. If procedures are well planned to minimize the compromise to patient welfare, then patients, owners and staff members will all benefit.

Building the 'welfare bank account'

The first visits to the veterinary clinic are often extremely negative for an animal (e.g. vaccinations, microchipping, neutering); patients learn from these negative experiences and can become sensitized to future visits. Fear of the clinic can result in the animal having to be carried or dragged in, muzzled for examination and forcefully restrained. This is not only unpleasant for the animal but is often cited by owners as a reason for not seeking veterinary attention, and may result in delayed treatment or poor owner compliance with treatment. Often these negative experiences can be mitigated by building the 'welfare bank account' (Fisher, 2015).

To help build the bank account, owners should be advised to bring their pet to the clinic on a regular basis to allow gentle exposure to the staff and environment (weight or development checks provide the ideal opportunity for this type of interaction). Owners can be asked to bring in their animal's favourite treat or toy, to make the experience as rewarding as possible. Staff should be available to 'fuss' the animal, if this is something the pet enjoys, either in the waiting room or outside in the car park. These visits should be encouraged from a young age to help establish a relationship between the veterinary practice and the owner and the patient.

Making a deposit or withdrawal

We can consider an animal's relationship with the veterinary clinic to be like a bank account (Fisher, 2015) (Figure 7.1).

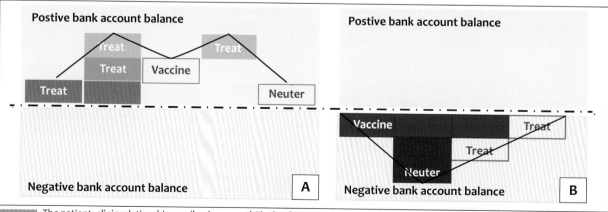

7.1 The patient–clinic relationship as a 'bank account'. The bank account balance is shown by the solid line and the 0 threshold by the dashed line. A indicates how investing in the bank account through positive welfare experiences can mitigate the impact of necessary aversive procedures on the patient–clinic relationship, whilst B indicates that a focus on routine aversive procedures may create a significant deficit within the patient–clinic relationship, which can be difficult to recover.
(© Heather Bacon)

Making a deposit or withdrawal *continued*

Each animal starts its relationship with the clinic with a balance of zero (i.e. neither positive nor negative in terms of its welfare experience). However, each time the animal has an aversive experience we make a 'withdrawal' from that bank account and the more aversive the experience, the larger the withdrawal. If a significant 'debt' is accrued, it can be difficult to enter into positive equity, even with repeated positive experiences. Animals that are constantly 'overdrawn' in their relationship with the clinic are much more likely to experience poor welfare in the clinic and display behaviours that are problematic for the veterinary staff to manage.

However, animals that have built up their 'bank account' through a series of positive experience 'deposits' with the clinic are much more likely to behave positively and to trust the veterinary staff. This means that when a 'withdrawal' or aversive experience is necessary, there is a positive trust balance and the experience is therefore less likely to negatively affect the patient–clinic relationship or result in unwanted or dangerous behaviours.

Pre-visit information for owners

Owners should be given pre-visit advice on how to make their pet's visit to the clinic less stressful when they register or book their appointment. Owners should be advised to allow the animal to toilet before their appointment as it will improve their pet's comfort on the journey and whilst being examined. Large meals should be avoided before appointments in case the animal experiences travel sickness, but small high-value treats (if permitted) should be available to help reassure the pet whilst travelling or waiting to be seen. Owners should be encouraged to bring their pet's own bedding to increase olfactory familiarity. Waiting in the car, rather than the waiting room, should be advised to reduce the time the animal may spend surrounded by potentially frightening smells, sights and sounds.

Advice should also be offered on the ideal cat carrier. The ideal carrier should have a detachable lid, as well as a front door, allowing the animal to stay in the base and be examined, or to walk out if it chooses to. It should be made of a solid material so the base does not flex when the animal stands up, and made of a material that can easily be wiped clean should toileting accidents occur. There should always be a thick towel or blanket in the bottom for the animal to grip on to and burrow into: ideally, this should be a familiar blanket or bedding that offers a reassuring scent.

Smaller animals, such as rabbits and rodents, should be securely housed in draughtproof but ventilated transport boxes and provided with bedding and food. Boxes should have a secure but removable lid, allowing the animals to be observed and examined in the box, but also easily handled when needed. Ectothermic animals should be transported with appropriate life support systems, including temperature gradients, water quality and humidity parameters where possible. Thermal stress may adversely affect the health status and recovery of ectotherms. Large snakes should be transported in a bag with a secure tie.

Wildlife and zoo species seen in the clinic environment will be highly stressed by any human handling or interaction. They should be secured in a small transport box or crate, depending on size. The box should be as small as possible to reduce the opportunity for escape behaviours that could result in injury, such as thrashing, butting or tunnelling (Figure 7.2). The box should be ventilated but secure and kept dark with minimal human interaction. Wildlife species should not wait in the waiting room.

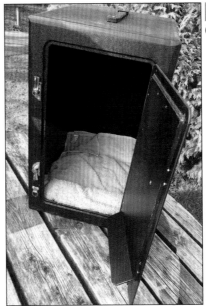

7.2 A raptor transport box. (Courtesy of John Chitty)

Habituation, desensitization and counter-conditioning

Many animals arrive at the veterinary clinic stressed or overexcited from the journey. Habituation, desensitization and counter-conditioning to the transportation carrier and travelling in the car may help to reduce stress and anxiety, allowing for a more pleasant journey and easier handling on arrival at the veterinary practice. This must be done slowly and sensitively, but may be of huge benefit to the animal for future veterinary visits. See Chapters 3 and 6 for further information.

Habituation

Habituation is a form of non-associative learning in which a response to a stimulus decreases after repeated or prolonged presentations of that stimulus. In animals, habituation occurs by exposing the individual to a particular event or feature of the environment so that the animal learns to ignore it or becomes used to it, as there are no consequences to the event or feature. Most species can be habituated to voluntarily spend time in a transport box or vehicle (Figure 7.3). However, wild or non-domesticated animals will be much more stressed by human proximity, confinement and transport and so these stressors should be evaluated against other options, such as chemical restraint.

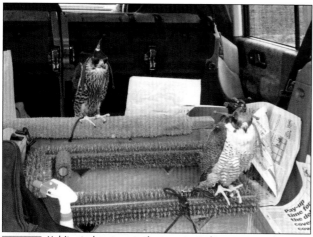

7.3 Habituated raptors can be transported in a car securely.
(Courtesy of John Chitty)

Puppies and kittens

Owners of new puppies and kittens should be advised to expose their young pets to car journeys, carriers and the veterinary clinic to reduce the likelihood of a negative emotional or behavioural reaction in the future. Puppies should be allowed to sit in the car regularly, get used to being safely and comfortably restrained, and then go for short journeys. For carriers, simply leaving it out in the house allows the puppy or kitten to become accustomed to it and not see it as dangerous or something to be feared (Figure 7.4). Young pets should be brought to the veterinary clinic for routine checks, which should be a positive experience.

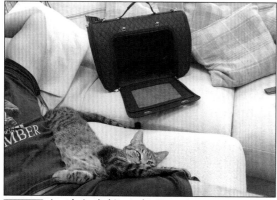

7.4 A cat being habituated to its carrier.
(© Hayley Walters)

Cat carriers and transport boxes

For many animals such as cats, rabbits and exotic pets, the carrier only appears moments before the animal is placed in it for transportation to the clinic. Often the owner is aware of the animal's predicted flight reaction to seeing the box or fight reaction when attempts are made to place the cat inside it. As a result, the cat may arrive at the practice in a stressed state after fighting with the owner to avoid being placed in the carrier, and may even have toileted within it. Exotic pets may be susceptible to escape or draughts in insecure boxes. In all cases, boxes should be large enough to contain the animal and bedding, and should have a lift-off top half to facilitate easy access.

For animals that have a pre-existing negative association with the veterinary clinic, more active training may be required. In these situations, it is essential that the animal remains calm and not stressed. During training, all non-essential veterinary procedures should be delayed until the patient is calm and relaxed within a clinical setting. Animals cannot learn when stressed, as amygdala activation and increases in circulating cortisol prevent learning processes from occurring in the brain.

Desensitization

Desensitization is a treatment or process that diminishes emotional responsiveness to a negative, aversive or positive stimulus after repeated, low intensity, non-arousing exposure to the stimulus.

In animals, desensitization refers to management of a behavioural problem in individuals that already have a negative association with an environmental event or feature. Once an animal is frightened of a particular stimulus, gentle exposure at a level low enough not to cause an emotional reaction is recommended.

Car journeys

For dogs that only travel in a car to attend the clinic, the stress associated with the perceived unpleasantness of visiting the veterinary practice begins long before the animal arrives in the waiting room. Desensitization of dogs to car journeys may be achieved by initially allowing the animal to simply sit in the car. When there is no negative emotional or behavioural response to this event, the intensity of the stimulus can be increased by turning on the engine and, ultimately, driving down the road. The process must be done slowly to avoid evoking a negative response. Success can be determined by the lack of response from the dog during the car journey (e.g. the dog does not tremble, vocalize or salivate). If a negative response is evoked, then the intensity should be decreased to the level that the dog was able to cope with and then slowly increased again over time, staying below the reaction threshold.

Counter-conditioning

Counter-conditioning is a training technique that pairs a positive reward with an aversive experience to change an emotional state.

In animals, counter-conditioning involves the creation of new, more positive emotional associations to a previously fear-inducing event. This can be achieved by presenting the animal with something that it really enjoys, such as treats, stroking or a game, in the presence of the previously feared stimulus. It is very important that the animal remains calm throughout the counter-conditioning process, as once it is stimulated the animal will be unlikely to take or participate in the offered reward. The exposure to the stimulus must always be of low enough intensity to not evoke a negative response and for the animal to enjoy the offered reward.

Rewarding experiences

Car journeys can be paired with, for example, delicious treats initially and then, eventually, arrival at a place the dog enjoys walking. Cat carriers with treats placed in and around them will help the cat to ▶

Rewarding experiences *continued*

associate the carrier with a more positive experience. Once the cat enters the carrier, the door can be closed for a few seconds and then opened again. The time the door is closed for can gradually be increased and, provided there is no negative response from the cat, the carrier can then be picked up and eventually carried around the house (see Figure 7.4).

Therapeutics

For patients with significant pre-existing anxiety around visiting the veterinary practice, and where procedures cannot be delayed to facilitate a counter-conditioning programme, veterinary surgeons should consider prescribing appropriate pre-visit anxiolytic medication. In addition, significant anxiety can prevent an animal from responding appropriately to counter-conditioning and so this may need to be reduced through the use of medication in order for the programme to be successful. Medications such as benzodiazepines, gabapentin or dexmedetomidine may be used in conjunction with low-stress handling techniques (see 'Low-stress handling and restraint', below) to maximize patient welfare and compliance during essential visits. Animals with anxiety should not be sedated without anxiolytics, as this is likely to exacerbate emotional fear and stress responses even if motor responses are inhibited.

Appointment times

Owners of anxious or fearful animals should be offered appointments at quieter times. Owners of dogs that are particularly fearful of being in the clinic can be asked to wait outside and to walk their dog, if this is possible and is something that helps the dog feel more relaxed. Owners of noisy, boisterous or aggressive dogs should also be given appointments, where possible, at a time when there are few or no other animals present so that they do not become more aroused themselves or cause other animals to feel stressed. Species-specific clinics can also help to reduce the distress many patients experience when at the clinic and should be considered where possible, particularly if the clinic sees a range of species. Clinics for prey species such as rabbits, rodents, some reptiles and psittacines could potentially be held together, but ideally predatory species such as dogs, cats, raptors, ferrets, and predatory reptiles should be separate. Where flexibility is limited, waiting areas separated according to predator/prey status rather than according to exotic/non-exotic status and visual barriers should be used, and waiting times should be minimized.

Clinic design and flow

Consideration should be given to the overall design of the clinic, where possible. Many practices occupy older buildings that have been modified to become veterinary clinics; in these cases, structural alterations may be limited but it can be possible to implement small design changes. Consideration should also be given to the 'flow' of patients through the clinic, to minimize the need for backtracking and reduce patient exposure to potentially stressful stimuli.

For example, the reception area and waiting room should lead directly into the examination rooms. Ideally, the examination rooms should have a second door leading to the preparation area. The preparation area should lead to the surgical area and the hospital wards. Quarantine or isolation areas should be easily accessible from the preparation and storage areas, but separate from other areas of the practice to facilitate appropriate biosecurity measures and help prevent disease transmission. Where changes in floor level occur, ramps are usually preferable to steps for older or less mobile patients.

Entrance and outside areas

Entrances and outside areas should be kept clean and obstruction-free. On-site parking facilitates access for patients with limited mobility and allows evaluation of very fearful patients outside of the clinic.

Reception area and waiting room

There should be separate waiting rooms for cats and dogs in the clinic and, ideally, a third area for exotic pets. Where this is not possible, a partition should be considered so that cats and dogs cannot see one another. Olfactory stressors, such as strong disinfectants and the urine of other animals, should be kept to a minimum and calming smells such as lavender or synthetic pheromones used. Noise should also be minimized and background music should be of slow tempo and not loud.

Dogs

Some dogs that present at the clinic will be suffering from osteoarthritis or other painful disorders. A padded, wipe-down mattress should be provided in the waiting area for painful or arthritic canine patients to lie on whilst they wait. Owners may be encouraged to bring their dog's bed for them to sit on in the waiting room or if they suspect that their pet will be admitted as an inpatient, to help increase its comfort with familiar smells from home.

Cats

Cat carriers should never be placed on the floor as this can be traumatic for cats who are already scared and unable to perform their natural behaviour of running and hiding. It can also be extremely distressing if, when on the floor, their carrier is approached by a dog. Providing shelves or units for cat carriers to be placed on can help a cat to feel more comfortable whilst waiting for their appointment. In the absence of shelves or units, owners should be encouraged to place the carrier on a chair or sit with it on their lap (Figure 7.5). Reception staff should ask all owners to do this. Space on the reception desk should also be left free for carriers to be placed whilst the owner is paying or booking their next appointment.

Exotic pets

Rabbits and small mammals: Ideally, rabbit and small mammal clinics should wait until dogs and cats are not present, or a separate exotics waiting area should be provided. Rabbits should be transported in a cat carrier or crate where the lid can be entirely removed, and small mammals may be transported in secure draughtproof carry cases. They should not be transported in cardboard boxes as these are not secure. These species

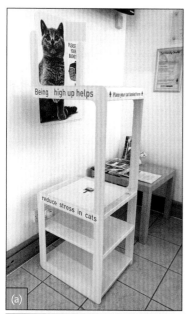

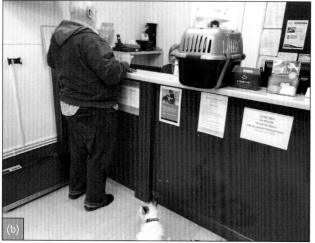

7.5 Cat carriers should never be placed on the floor; if bespoke shelving (a) is not provided, carriers may be placed on the reception desk (b) or held by the owner.
(a, © Heather Bacon; b, © Hayley Walters)

should always be transported with bedding such as hay and food and ideally some leafy vegetables to provide moisture. It is important that these species are kept warm. They will generally feel more secure at floor level as they are often unused to being held at height. Carnivorous small mammals such as ferrets are better placed in the cat waiting area rather than the exotics waiting area and so reception staff should be trained to ensure that all 'exotics' are not lumped together.

Reptiles: As ectotherms, reptiles can quickly chill and so owners should ensure they arrive at the clinic in a secure, draughtproof container on clean newspaper or a similar substrate, ideally with a warm (not hot) water bottle or similar. Waiting times should be minimized.

Fish: Fish should arrive at the clinic in a secure transport tank filled with water from their main tank; acoustic and thermal shock risks should be minimized by careful handling.

Birds: Birds should be transported in a species-appropriate secure cage or box with newspaper or a similar substrate, perching opportunities and easy access for handling. Bird cages should be covered prior to arrival and during waiting to minimize responses to visual stressors. Waiting times should be minimized and birds should wait

away from cats and dogs, with their cage or box placed on a high shelf with a view of the owner (Figure 7.6). Birds of prey should be hooded and jessed and kept away from cats, dogs, rabbits and small mammals.

Wildlife: Where possible, wildlife species should be seen *in situ* at a rescue centre rather than brought to the clinic. Wildlife brought in by the public should be admitted for evaluation as soon as possible rather than kept waiting. In all cases, appropriate advice should be given where zoonotic disease is possible (e.g. in bats). Sensory stimuli, such as noise and light, should be minimized.

Zoological species: Where possible, zoo animals should be examined at the zoo; however, some general practices may work with smaller zoos requiring surgical or diagnostic services only available at the clinic. In these cases, the animal should be assessed to decide whether chemical restraint or habituation programmes are required prior to crating. Crates should be secure and escape proof but appropriately ventilated. Sensory stimuli should be minimized. As much as possible, zoo animals should not wait for veterinary assessment with domestic pets due to the potential stressors involved, including attention from interested domestic animal owners.

Examination rooms

Veterinary examination or consultation rooms have traditionally contained the same equipment, regardless of the species being examined. This includes an examination table, computer station, sink and drug/equipment storage. This type of design facilitates the automatic placement of an animal on an examination table and discourages non-invasive assessment or individual patient handling.

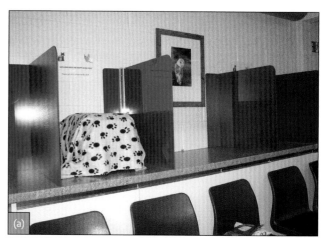

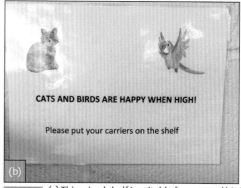

CATS AND BIRDS ARE HAPPY WHEN HIGH!

Please put your carriers on the shelf

7.6 (a) This raised shelf is suitable for cats and birds, with screening between patients. (b) Signage encourages use by owners.
(Courtesy of John Chitty)

With simple changes to the design of the examination room, veterinary clinics can help facilitate client communication and enhance patient welfare.

Dogs, cats and exotic species should be allocated separate examination rooms, and these rooms should be equipped accordingly to facilitate assessment of the specific species. These changes will help improve patient comfort, reduce unfamiliar and frightening experiences (such as being placed on an examination table), allow the veterinary surgeon to observe normal behaviour and movement, and facilitate client engagement and history-taking during the consultation. It is important that all staff are trained to knock and wait for a response prior to entering consulting rooms where animals such as birds or cats may be roaming and could potentially escape.

Dog examination room

The set-up for an examination room for dogs (Figure 7.7) should include the following:

- Removal of the examination table and placement of a comfortable wipe-clean mat
- Hypoallergenic dog treats and toys
- Dog appeasing pheromone plug-in
- Weighing scales (if not in the waiting room)
- Computer and desk with chair for the veterinary professional
- Two chairs for clients
- Sink for handwashing
- Basket muzzles for restraint where indicated.

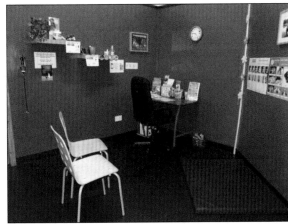

7.7 An example of a dog examination room that supports low-stress handling, with toys, treats and a ground-level mat.
(Courtesy of Claire Corridan)

Cat examination room

The set-up for an examination room for cats (Figure 7.8) should include the following:

- Installation of shelving to allow cats to move around and explore the space
- Hypoallergenic cat treats
- Cat facial pheromone plug-in
- Cat-specific weighing scales
- Computer and desk with chair for the veterinary professional
- Two chairs for clients
- Sink for handwashing. ▶

Cat examination room *continued*

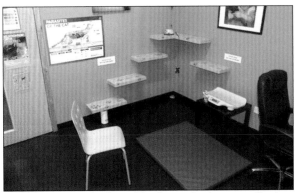

7.8 An example of a cat-friendly examination room, allowing clear communication between the vet and client(s) with a safe and appropriate environment for the cat to explore.
(Courtesy of Claire Corridan)

Exotic pet examination room

The set-up for an examination room for exotic animals should include the following (Figure 7.9):

- Window blinds and locks and secure ventilation outlets
- Light dimmer
- Small weighing scales such as those used for cats
- Small weighing scales with increments of 1 gram
- Computer and desk with chair for the veterinary professional
- Two chairs for clients
- Table to facilitate handling
- Sink for handwashing
- Towels for restraint where indicated
- A calculator
- A net (for catching escapees)
- Exotic-specific equipment including small syringes and narrow gauge hypodermic needles, feeding tubes, small blood collection tubes, and dropper bottles for dispensing medication.

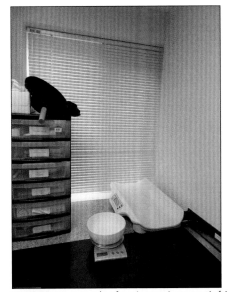

7.9 An example of equipment in an exotic-friendly examination room, including a net and two sizes of scales.
(Courtesy of John Chitty)

Avoid taking animals out of the examination room and into 'prep' for procedures that you may not wish the client to observe (e.g. blood sampling). The patient has already had to acclimatize to the waiting room and then the examination room; taking it into yet another room, where there is often a lot of noise, activity, and potentially other animals being treated, does not help keep the animal calm. It is better to ask the client to leave the examination room, once you have everything you need prepared, and allow the animal to remain in there, on its bed, whilst the procedure is carried out (with assistance as necessary).

Case example 1: Puppy consultations

Staff should be encouraged to discuss behaviour at the time of the first or second vaccination or puppy health check appointment. Behavioural pathology is a significant health and welfare problem for domestic dogs and commonly results in relinquishment or even euthanasia. There is much veterinary staff can do to mitigate the development of behavioural pathologies. It must be remembered that it is much easier to train good habits than un-train bad habits.

Socialization is a complex process but an essential part of puppy development and raising well-behaved dogs. Owners must engage in a varied and ongoing socialization programme including a variety of sounds, smells, environments and social experiences between the ages of 8 and 16 weeks. In particular, it is important for veterinary staff that puppies are habituated to the veterinary clinic and to having all aspects of their body touched – including their ears and feet.

Covering all aspects of socialization in a routine consultation can be challenging. Using the simple acronym CREAD, veterinary staff can easily remember the most important subjects to discuss with an owner when they come in with their puppy (Walters, 2019):

- **Children** – young dogs must be positively exposed to children from as early as possible
- **Recall** – dogs are more likely to suffer from behavioural problems if they do not get off-lead exercise, but must be kept under control and safely recalled
- **Eating** – puppies should learn from an early age that hands are for giving, not taking away food
- **Alone time** – puppies should be exposed to time on their own gradually from an early age
- **Dogs** – being sociable and well behaved around other dogs is vitally important to a dog's welfare.

Children

Guaranteed child-friendly breeds do not exist. Children are unpredictable – they move differently, look different, smell different and sound different to adults. To encourage good relationships between puppies and children, gentle positive exposure is recommended. The puppy can learn from early on that children are not something to be feared, and children must learn that puppies must be treated kindly and calmly.

The following advice should be given to owners to encourage good future relationships between children and dogs:

- **Provide a safe retreat** – a canine sanctuary (e.g. a crate) that is off limits to children
- **Teach children 'gentle hands'** – ask a toddler to practice stroking a teddy before letting them near the puppy for the first time (owners should explain that puppies can be hurt just like children and so are not the same as teddies) and to use the backs of their hands (so they cannot then grab!)
- **Children must be sitting** – make it the rule that children must sit before they can stroke the puppy and that the dog gets to approach them. If the puppy wants to move away they can and must not be chased; do not force the puppy to sit still
- **Offer treats** – special tasty treats that only the child gives. Gently throw them to the puppy and allow them to approach the child. Feed from hands (not fingers) if puppy is gentle
- **Practice quiet puppy talk** – high-pitched screams are a no. Make it fun for the children to see if they can talk in a quiet voice and move in a non-jerky way that entices puppies to come closer for treats or cuddles
- **Active supervision is key** – simply being in the same room is not enough. Owners must learn to understand the dog's body language and pay attention to signs of anxiety or avoidance before escalation to aggression.

Recall

It is estimated that dogs are around 70% more likely to suffer from behavioural problems if they are not given off-lead exercise. Therefore, it is hugely important that puppies learn the recall request from an early age. Advice that veterinary professionals may give to owners on training recall includes:

- Ensure that the puppy knows its name so that they know you want their attention. Simply say their name and reward
- Choose a word or whistle as your recall cue that you use only when you want your dog to return. It should be short
- Start in your garden with some high-value treats. Get your puppy's attention with their name, use your recall cue and take a step away from them. As they return to you, reward with praise and a tasty treat
- Gradually increase the distance between you and your dog in the garden
- Add in some distractions!
- Progress to outside the garden using a harness with a long line
- Let them move away from you before using your recall cue
- If they ignore you gently guide them back to you with the long line and reward them once they are with you
- If they did not need the gentle pull on the long line then make a big fuss of them and reward with high-value treats so they build up a really positive association with coming when called ▶

Case example 1: Puppy consultations *continued*

- You want your dog to learn that coming back to you straight away is really rewarding
- Continue to reward recalls throughout the dog's lifetime – recall can easily be lost if you inadvertently punish the dog (e.g. by always putting the leash back on when the dog returns).

Eating

Food guarding can be a major problem with pet dogs. Unfortunately, it can start before they even arrive at their new owner's home as feeding time with their siblings may be stressful and competitive. Traditionally, owners were taught to show dogs 'who's boss' and to take food away from the puppy whilst eating. However, this can create problems where none may have previously existed or reinforce the notion that food must be guarded. The following advice should be given to owners:

- Calmly drop some treats near your puppy while they are eating from their bowl then walk away
- Repeat this whenever your dog is being fed from their bowl
- Progress to dropping food into an empty bowl
- Never take the bowl away from them whilst they are eating
- Hands are for giving, not taking away.

Alone time

Between 20% and 40% of dogs presented to behavioural referral clinics are diagnosed with separation-related disorder (Bradshaw *et al.*, 2002). Puppies must be taught from an early age that it is okay to be left alone, to prevent the phenomenon of 'Velcro dogs' (dogs that follow owners from room to room in the house, including the bathroom) and dogs that are destructive or house soil or vocalize when the owner goes out. Set puppies up for success – teaching calm behaviour whilst alone is an essential part of socialization.

- Reward the puppy for being calm and relaxed on its bed.
- Give the puppy something delicious and time-consuming to eat (e.g. a puzzle feeder or frozen Kong® toy).
- Move away from the puppy gradually, progressing to just a few metres, to leaving the room, to leaving the house.
- Build up the time left alone in very small stages, a few minutes at a time, so the puppy does not notice.
- Keep departure and arrival behaviours to a minimum so as not to reinforce the notion that life is so much better when the owner is present.
- If the puppy does follow the owner out of the room, do not reinforce this with eye contact or attention. Instead, advise the owner to be as boring as possible so that it is not worth the puppy's while to follow when not asked to.

Dogs

Meeting other dogs must be a positive experience, so carefully introduce puppies to a variety of adult dogs as well as other puppies.

- Ensure these dogs are safe around puppies as a bad experience is often worse than none at all.
- Carefully monitor the puppy playing with other dogs.
- Intervene if the puppy starts to annoy other dogs or other dogs get too rough.

Ensure the puppy is only exposed to healthy, vaccinated dogs until immunizations are complete. However, do not advise that the puppy is isolated; poor socialization is a significant risk factor for further behaviour problems developing.

Hospital wards

Hospitalization can be a stressful experience for patients and providing a suitable environment can help reduce anxiety. The need for a suitable environment is included in the Five Welfare Needs (see Chapter 1) and the needs of an animal do not change when it is admitted to the clinic (Figure 7.10). For specialist species, you should consider whether you have the appropriate expertise and equipment to provide a suitable hospital environment, or whether you may be better off triaging, stabilizing and providing first aid then referring. For extremely stressed and anxious animals, anxiolytics should be considered but there are many other simple and inexpensive steps that can be taken to ensure that patient welfare is safeguarded (see 'Low-stress handling and restraint', below).

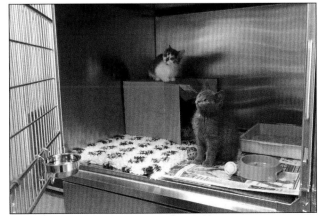

7.10 An appropriate cage set-up for two kittens.
(© The Jeanne Marchig International Centre for Animal Welfare Education)

Short-term inpatients

Dogs and cats: If possible, dogs and cats should be housed in separate wards. If this is not feasible, they should be housed as far apart as possible and be unable to see each other. Patients of any species should not be housed facing one another, as being stared at and unable to escape can be very stressful for an animal. If the ward set-up is such that the cages are situated opposite each other, then try and house the patients so that there is an empty cage opposite each animal.

All cats should be provided with a box/igloo or a stiff blanket to hide in as this may help them to feel safer. They must also have access to a clean litter tray. If a cat chooses to sleep in its litter tray, then a second one should be provided.

The age and temperament of the animal should be taken into account when selecting the appropriate location in the hospital ward to house them. If the animal is old, sleepy, shy or frightened, then they should be housed in the quietest area of the ward to make them more comfortable. If the animal is young, highly sociable or bored, then they should be housed in a high-traffic area so they can watch what is going on and people can say 'hello' regularly.

The hospital ward should be quiet with dimmed lights and the lights should be turned off at night. Where possible, nobody should enter the hospital ward between midnight and 6 am to allow patients the opportunity for uninterrupted sleep. Not getting enough sleep each night can affect an animal's physical health as organ, muscle and immune systems are repaired during sleep.

The animal's cage should be cleaned only when it is dirty (unless the patient has an infectious disease). The cage should not be disinfected, and bedding need not be refreshed every day unless it is soiled (it is unlikely that the owner does this at home). Dogs and cats rely heavily on the smells around them to feel secure and if the cage is constantly cleaned with disinfectants, then these smells are overpowered.

The patient's daily routine should be as predictable as possible (e.g. start each day at the same time, provide meals at the same time daily and provide regular toileting opportunities). Predictability reduces stress, which in turn can decrease patient recovery times.

The animal's name should be used, rather than 'the diarrhoea dog' or 'the nasty fracture cat'. This helps to create a relationship with the patient and can reassure the animal as their name is familiar.

Clean drinking water and food should be provided to all patients unless medically contraindicated. Active steps should be taken if the patient is inappetent. The following questions should be considered:

- Does the animal not like the food being offered?
- Does the food need warming?
- Has the food gone stale?
- Is the patient too sick to eat?
- Is the animal too scared or stressed to eat?

Dogs and cats will often eat after they have been stroked (Figure 7.11). This simple interaction is often enough to change the emotional state of the animal and encourage them to eat. When stroking a cat. they usually prefer to be stroked where their facial glands are located (base of their ears, under their chin, and around their cheeks) as opposed to their back, tail base and stomach. Avoid the top of the head when stroking dogs, as it can feel threatening, and use gentle strokes under the chin or down the chest. Toileting may also stimulate eating and so animals should have regular toileting opportunities.

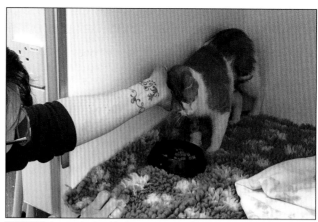

7.11 Inappetent cat being encouraged to eat.
(© Hayley Walters)

Pain scoring should be performed when the temperature, pulse and respiratory rate (TPR) of the patient are checked and then again after any pain relief is administered to check whether it is sufficient. Where possible, TPR checks, pain scoring and drug administration should be undertaken at the same time, as this will minimize the number of times the patient is disturbed and allow plenty of opportunities for rest.

If an animal is chewing at their bandage or constantly licking their wound, then the area should be thoroughly inspected and pain scoring undertaken. Licking and chewing is a recognized sign of pain on the Glasgow Composite Measure Pain Scale for both dogs and cats (see Chapter 2). Avoid the temptation to simply place an Elizabethan collar on the animal.

Recumbent patients should be provided with extra-padded bedding (Figure 7.12) and turned at least every 2 hours to prevent discomfort and pressure sores. This will require two people for animals weighing over 15 kg and must be undertaken with care.

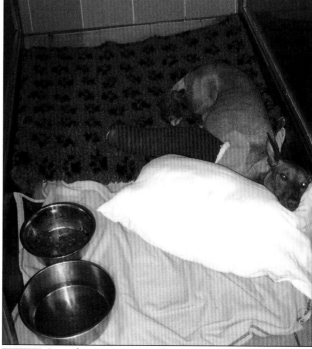

7.12 Recumbent patient in a well-padded kennel.
(© The Jeanne Marchig International Centre for Animal Welfare Education)

The patient should be taken out of their kennel/cage for treatment if they are not scared to leave. The kennel/cage ought to be a safe place where the animal can relax, not where frightening and painful procedures occur.

Tender loving care (TLC) is important (Figure 7.13). Patients require positive human interactions in the form of playing, stroking, grooming or just company. Animals cannot be broken down to simple biological functions: they are sentient beings whose psychological health is just as important as their physical health. TLC is a form of treatment and should not be viewed as work avoidance.

When admitting an animal to the practice, the owner should be asked to provide information about its personality and preferences (see Chapter 2). Relevant questions include:

- Where do they like to toilet? When did they last go to the toilet?
- What litter do you use? What kind of litter tray?
- What and when are they fed at home? Do they have any favourite treats?
- Do they prefer a flat bed or a nest bed or den?
- Are they sociable, friendly, nervous or aggressive, and do they prefer to be left alone?
- What do they like and dislike?

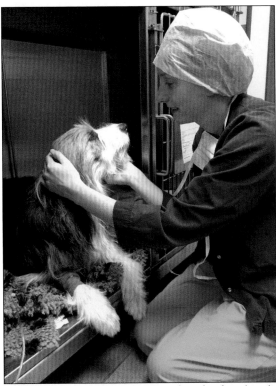

7.13 A nurse providing a moment of comfort for a dog who needs it.
(© The Jeanne Marchig International Centre for Animal Welfare Education)

Barking dogs in kennels

Dogs that constantly bark when in kennels can be testing, but it is not advisable to bang on the door of the cage or to shout at the animal to be quiet, as this will often increase their distress further. Inpatients are totally dependent on the veterinary staff to meet all their needs, so instead the motivation for their behaviour should be determined. The following should be considered: ▶

Barking dogs in kennels *continued*

- How is their day going?
- What can they see, hear and smell?
- Are they comfortable with other dogs?
- Have they been hospitalized before? If so, what type of experience did they have?
- Are they barking because they are excited, frustrated, guarding, bored, scared or because they cannot cope with being on their own?
- Are they in pain, do they need the toilet or are they hungry?
- Do they have what they want?
- If you were the owner of the dog, what would you do? How would you want them to be treated?

Exotic pets: Ideally, clinics should have a separate ward area even for common exotic pets such as rabbits and small mammals – these are prey species and can easily become stressed if housed near carnivores such as cats and dogs. For occasional patients, the far end of the cat ward may be a pragmatic compromise, but clinics that regularly see a wider variety of exotic pets should invest in a designated exotics ward furnished with a range of solid-fronted kennels, vivaria, incubators and other appropriate exotics housing and husbandry equipment (Figure 7.14). Exotic pets often need warmer temperatures, especially if unwell, and so exotics wards should be kept at a higher ambient temperature (usually around 25°C) with specific supplemental heat provided to individual patients as required. Thought should also be given to humidity and ventilation parameters, and the ward design should accommodate the ability to clean using techniques such as fogging. Visual barriers should be placed between patients and enrichment provided, as many exotic species have complex needs (Figure 7.15). Ideally, exotics wards should be fitted with viewing cameras that allow remote assessment of patients. Most exotic pets will change their behaviour in the presence of humans and remotely assessing pain behaviour in birds or small mammals, for example, is more accurate as they will mask these behaviours in the presence of people. Thought should also be given to nursing care provision, to minimize trafficking odours between prey and predator species and *vice versa.*

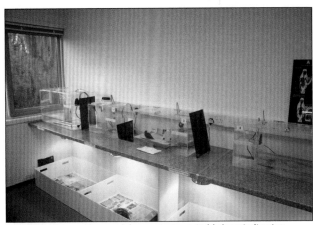

7.14 This exotics ward demonstrates suitable hospitalization facilities. Birds are housed off the ground in enclosures with controlled temperature and humidity parameters. Visual barriers are placed between each enclosure. Tortoises are housed in separate large enclosures on the floor, which are easy to disinfect and provide visual barriers and suitable ambient parameters.
(Courtesy of John Chitty)

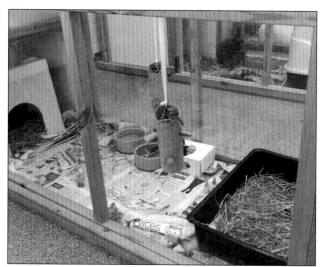

7.15 Hospital inpatients should be provided with species-appropriate enrichment. These hanging cardboard tubes filled with food offer cognitive and physical stimulation.
(Courtesy of Abi Discombe)

Rabbits and other small mammals: Species such as rabbits, rodents and guinea pigs need secure facilities and, as prey species, they require a feeling of safety from potential predators (cats, dogs, raptors, ferrets, reptiles, etc.). These species will feel safer if housed at floor level, but if this is not practical they should be housed in a solid tank or similar enclosure (Figure 7.16). They should be provided with hiding spaces such as tunnels or houses, and house rabbits should have access to litter trays. All housing and furnishings should be chew proof and regularly checked for damage that could injure a patient or

lead to escape. Specific nutritional requirements should be provided for, including vitamin C for guinea pigs and long fibre for rabbits. Liquid fibre diets, such as critical care formula, should be in stock and ideally fresh greens should be provided to stimulate appetites. Consideration should be given to socially housed or bonded animals; for example, rabbits may be kept in pairs even if only one requires hospitalization (Figure 7.17). Ferrets should be housed separately from prey species and should be placed in the cat ward rather than the rabbit ward if other areas are not available (Figure 7.18).

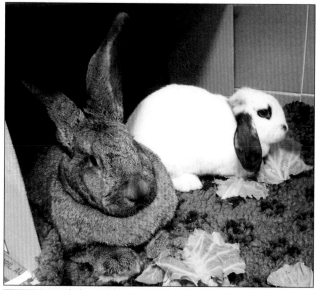

7.17 Bonded companion rabbits can be an important part of the treatment plan for hospitalized rabbits. Interactions and social time should be carefully monitored when the rabbits have experienced any time apart. Note the soft blanket, which is often given to giant breeds experiencing skeletal discomfort and pododermatitis.
(Reproduced from the *BSAVA Manual of Rabbit Medicine*)

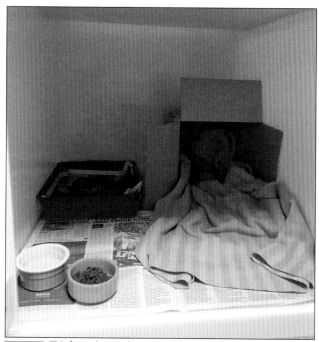

7.18 This ferret hospital cage provides a comfortable bed/hiding area for the ferret to burrow into, a litter tray, and clean fresh water and food.
(Courtesy of Abi Discombe)

7.16 This hospital enclosure has been set up for a rat or similar rodent. It provides a hiding place with bedding, fresh water and food, and a tunnel which can be used for hiding or to facilitate low-stress handling.
(Courtesy of Abi Discombe)

Reptiles: Secure vivaria with appropriate substrate, humidity and temperature gradients should be available for reptile species (Figure 7.19). Supplementary heat provided through the use of safe and secure means to reduce the risk of overheating, thermal burns or under-heating is essential (Figure 7.20ab). In addition, ultraviolet (UV) lighting producing UVB light of an appropriate wave-length should be provided (Figure 7.20c). The use of simple plastic tubs to house reptiles is unacceptable. Ideally all reptiles should be hospitalized in spaces large enough to allow for exercise and movement and to provide a range of environmental options. Most reptiles will benefit from warm water bathing opportunities, which can help with conditions such as dehydration and dys-ecdysis (Figure 7.21). It is essential that good biosecurity is maintained for reptiles, and individual facilities should be available. Reptile housing areas should be suitable for fogging with F10 or similar disinfectant. Appropriate fresh food (including live invertebrates where required) should be available for herbivores, insectivores and carnivores, and should be of good nutritive quality.

Birds: Birds require housing in a warm secure environment. Any windows should be fixed and ceilings low. Any poten-tial perches, such as wall light fittings or mouldings, should be removed to prevent perching of escapees, and windows and ventilation outlets should be secured. Individual cages should allow for nebulization of medicines, changes to temperature and humidity, and increases in oxygen con-centration; most birds admitted to veterinary clinics are severely unwell and should be treated as critical care patients. If permanent housing is not available, birds can be hospitalized in incubators or brooders in a quiet environ-ment (Figure 7.22). Enrichment should be provided for avian patients unless medically contraindicated. Thought must be given to the needs of particular avian species; for example, psittacines will require different housing and perching facilities to raptors, which will have different needs to waterfowl or passerines. Additionally, considera-tion should be given to proximity and predator–prey relationships when housing a variety of avian species, as housing predators near prey species will be stressful. Birds should not be housed in line of sight of other birds as this

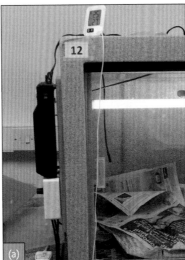
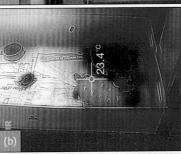
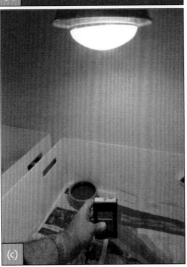

7.20 (a) Temperature monitoring of ectotherms is essential to ensure vivaria stay within the preferred optimum temperature zone – fridge thermometers can be useful for this purpose. (b) An infrared camera can be a useful tool to check that a thermal gradient is available in reptile housing, and to avoid over- or under-heating. (c) Ultraviolet meters are important for ensuring UVB is provided at an appropriate intensity.
(Courtesy of John Chitty)

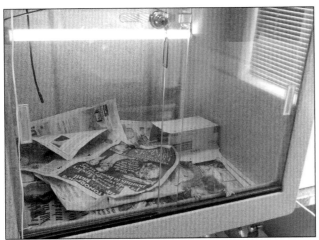

7.19 A simple vivarium can be easily adapted for different reptile species. Newspaper provides an easily cleaned substrate that will not damage skin and disposable cardboard hides provide refuge. As always, fresh water should be provided. Thermal monitoring ensures the preferred optimum temperature zone is maintained and ultraviolet light should also be provided.
(Courtesy of John Chitty)

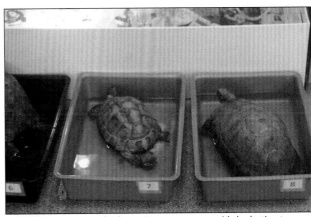

7.21 Warm water baths are important to provide hydration to hospitalized tortoises. Each tortoise should have its own bathing tray that is labelled and cleaned to prevent cross-infection.
(Courtesy of John Chitty)

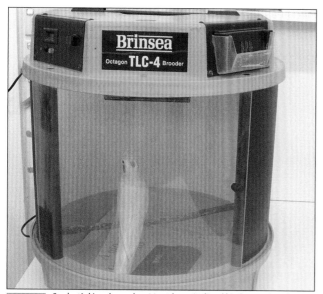

can be stressful and encourage display behaviour. Bird housing areas should be suitable for fogging with F10 or similar disinfectant.

The practice should keep a range of soft crop tubes and species-appropriate foodstuffs, including diets for carnivores, omnivores, frugivores, insectivores and granivores. Diets should include the option of 'unhealthy' food such as sunflower seed diets as these may be needed to encourage feeding.

Wildlife and zoological species: Patients such as foxes, deer, badgers and hares require specialist handling and secure facilities (Figure 7.23). Kennels may sometimes be adapted to house zoo and wildlife species (Figure 7.24) but, where possible, they should be relocated to specialist wildlife rehabilitation facilities. Consideration should be given to specialist diets, experienced handling and appropriate ambient parameters, recognizing that human proximity, noise and bright lighting are likely to result in stress and potentially further injury.

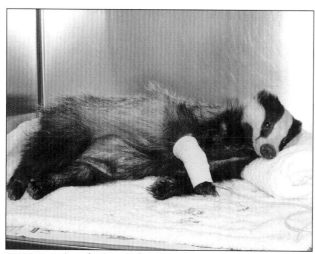

7.23 Badgers (*Meles meles*) can be temporarily housed in large secure dog kennels for initial treatment, but will need to be moved to larger pens for longer-term hospitalization.
(Reproduced from the *BSAVA Manual of Wildlife Casualties*)

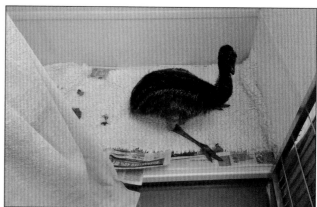

7.24 This young emu is comfortably housed in a walk-in kennel in a quiet area of the clinic, with blankets used to provide visual barriers on the kennel doors.
(Courtesy of John Chitty)

Long-term inpatients

All inpatients should be provided with the facilities described above. Most animals that are housed in the clinic for longer periods of time will need additional consideration given to their welfare needs.

Dogs: In addition to a predictable daily routine, and the requirements described for a short-term inpatient, long-term inpatients will benefit from novel experiences and environmental enrichment. Decreased mental health has been reported in long-term hospitalized human patients and it would be reasonable to assume that the same thing can happen in dogs.

- Owner visits – some animals benefit from regular visits from their owner. If it is safe and the animal is not distressed when they leave, visits from the owner should be encouraged.
- Longer walks – where possible, long-term inpatients should be taken on a longer more interesting walk at least once a day to prevent boredom, maintain muscle tone and improve overall quality of life.
- Scatter feeding – it should be remembered that free-roaming dogs spend a large portion of their day searching and scavenging for food. This is a natural behaviour that is not afforded to most dogs as they are fed from bowls. Scattering dry food around the kennel or run area encourages natural behaviour, makes use of the animal's time and provides mental stimulation. The use of puzzle feeders and Kong® toys may also be beneficial in this regard (Figure 7.25).

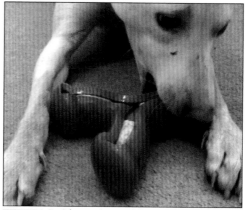

7.25 Enrichment is a useful tool for long-term inpatients.
(© Hayley Walters)

- Medication – for patients that are stressed within the inpatient environment, or are at risk of further injury due to activity, medical management should be considered. Medications such as gabapentin, trazadone and dexmedetomidine may be useful for alleviating acute anxiety and facilitating recovery.

'Special nurse'

- This is a member of staff designated to be a 'substitute owner' for a patient. They may be a veterinary nurse, animal care assistant or another member of the team. This person should only be involved in positive aspects of the patient's care, such as walking, feeding and stroking; they should never be associated with unpleasant or aversive experiences.
- Unpredictable carers who are sometimes associated with pleasant experiences (e.g. stroking) but occasionally also perform aversive procedures create emotional conflict, resulting in stress and reducing the patient's ability to relax. The role of the 'special nurse' is to create a predictable person who the patient can relax around, thus reducing the potential for long-term stress and supporting good patient welfare and a speedy recovery.

Cats: Feline long-term inpatients require everything described for short-term inpatients but, where possible, the following can also be considered:

- The largest cage in the clinic should be made available to allow for more choice and movement
- A scratching post for nail maintenance and the performance of natural behavioural repertoires
- Different height options within the cage in the form of shelving or a cat tree
- Extra hiding places should be included if practical
- Feeding enrichment in the form of scatter feeding, hiding food, treat dispenser balls, or placing food in various locations and heights around the cage should be considered, if the cat's condition allows, to encourage mental and physical stimulation
- Play time with fishing rod toys can increase mental and physical stimulation
- Grooming sessions, with gentle brushes, can improve the bond between patient and staff and help to relax the cat.

Exotic pets: Exotic patient hospitalization is fairly specialized. Whilst temporary accommodation can be provided for occasional short-term exotic patients, long-term patients should be housed in specialist exotic facilities such as referral centres, exotic veterinary practices, or wildlife rescue and rehabilitation facilities. First opinion general practitioners should aim to provide for exotic patients as per the guidance in the previous section, but should always consider referral to a more suitable environment for longer-term patients.

Preparation and treatment areas

The preparation and treatment areas should be quiet, clean, organized and not too brightly lit, and the doors should be kept closed to avoid noise coming through from other areas of the clinic (e.g. the hospital wards). Practices should be mindful of the presence of different species in the preparation area and should aim to keep species separate as much as possible.

Low-stress handling and restraint

Low-stress handling techniques can help reduce the potential of a frightened or 'trigger stacked' (see below) animal reacting aggressively towards veterinary staff when being handled. It must be remembered that much of what an animal undergoes in the clinic is unpleasant and, when combined with being in a strange environment with different smells, sights and sounds, it is unsurprising that they may not cooperate and/or attempt to escape (see Figure 7.32). What some veterinary staff may interpret as naughty behaviour is usually just a very frightened animal doing what it can to escape an aversive situation. Animals that struggle, bite and scratch are much more difficult and dangerous to handle.

The perspective of the animal visiting the veterinary clinic and being examined needs to be taken into consideration and the experience made as positive as possible. The use of minimal restraint and low-stress handling techniques may be a little time-consuming initially but, eventually, will be worthwhile in terms of both time and having a compliant animal that cooperates rather struggles and fights.

Trigger stacking

It may sometimes appear that an animal's aggressive reaction has come out of nowhere and its response is completely disproportionate to the situation. However, it should be remembered that when numerous stressful events occur simultaneously or within a short period of time, they can collectively decrease an animal's coping tolerance – this is known as trigger stacking (Figure 7.26). It is possible, therefore, that during a seemingly benign procedure, an animal has experienced so much prior stress that it simply cannot cope and bites. Many animals can cope with one stressor or trigger, but when several stressors are 'stacked' on top of each other, what are deemed 'out-of-character' reactions may occur.

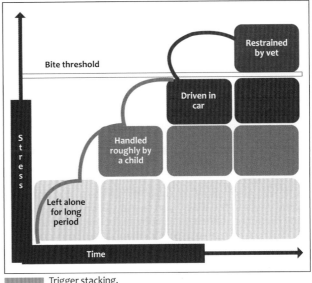

7.26 Trigger stacking.
(© Heather Bacon)

- The physiological response of the animal to stress may mean that sedatives and anaesthetic drugs are less effective, resulting in higher doses having to be administered, which could be harmful to the patient.
- The animal may anticipate that any future interactions with veterinary professionals will be unpleasant and escalate its behaviour, making it even more difficult or dangerous to handle. If this occurs, it may not be possible to even touch the animal, let alone perform a clinical examination.
- Each visit to the veterinary clinic will become more stressful for both the animal and the veterinary staff. This can be upsetting for the owner and may deter them from bringing the animal to the clinic, which could compromise the health and welfare of the animal.

Behavioural responses to stress

In general, animals respond to stressful stimuli in one of two ways: actively or passively (Figure 7.27). However, regardless of the type of response shown by the animal, the underlying cause is often a state of anxiety and so attempts should be made to mitigate potential stressors.

Active responders
• Often at front of kennel/cage
• Stands on hindlegs in an attempt to climb
• Paws people passing the kennel/cage
• Pacing
• Attention-seeking vocalization
• Displays aggressive behaviour
• May be destructive

Passive responders
• Immobility
• Often attempts to hide
• Quiet with no vocalizations, although may hiss or growl if approached
• Shows a lack of interest in the environment
• Shows a lack of maintenance behaviours, such as feeding and grooming

7.27 Active and passive behavioural responses to stress.

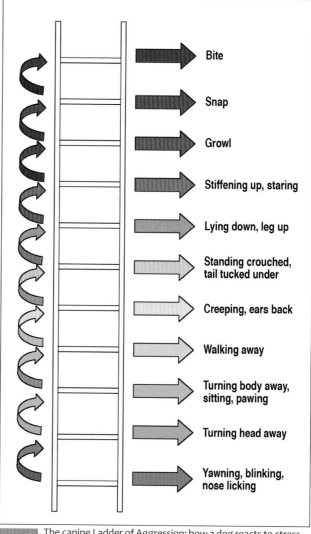

7.28 The canine Ladder of Aggression: how a dog reacts to stress or threat.
(Reproduced from BSAVA Manual of Canine and Feline Behavioural Medicine)

Dogs

Dogs will show specific behaviours that indicate anxiety (e.g. lip licking, yawning out of context) and if these behavioural signs are not heeded, then they will progress to threat-repelling behaviours in an attempt to mitigate potential threats and create a space between themselves and a perceived threat. Threat-repelling behaviours include moving away, growling and an escalation into aggressive behaviours. The behavioural response to stress in dogs is often referred to as the 'ladder of aggression' (Shepherd, 2009; Figure 7.28). By recognizing the early signs of anxiety and stress, veterinary staff can take steps to help reduce stress and anxiety and prevent escalation to more overtly aggressive behaviours.

Cats

Cats will also show specific behaviours that indicate anxiety (ears to the side, head slightly down, pupils dilated, body crouched, tail close to body or flicking). If these signs are ignored or not recognized then, like dogs, cats may have to escalate to the more obvious hissing, scratching, tail thrashing and biting. By learning the early subtle signs of anxiety, handling of a stressed cat can be tailored to that individual and dangerous outcomes prevented.

Exotic pets

Rabbits: Rabbits are prey animals and generally find handling to be stressful, so any handling should be brief and use appropriate techniques. Stressed rabbits may freeze, back into a corner, attempt to hide or lie down, thump with their hindlimbs and they are also prone to sudden jumping, so should be supported at all times during handling. You may also notice an increased respiratory rate, dilated pupils and taut muscles. Stressed rabbits may be at risk of gastrointestinal stasis.

Small mammals: Guinea pigs, chinchillas and other rodents are commonly seen in veterinary practice and require careful handling. When stressed these species may hide, vocalize, become immobile, chew at their own fur, or display aggressive behaviours or altered feeding or activity patterns. All of these species may show 'escape behaviours' such as bar chewing and digging when stressed. Rats may secrete porphyrin from their Harderian glands when stressed, resulting in pinkish staining around the eyes.

Reptiles: Reptiles are a diverse taxonomic group and different species may show different signs of stress. These may include hyperactivity, hypoactivity, escape behaviours (e.g. glass-striking), anorexia, head-hiding, inflation of the body, freezing, hiding, hissing, panting, pigment change, aggression, rigid coiling in snakes and cloacal evacuations (Warwick *et al.*, 2013). Lizard species may show tail autotomy if stressed.

Fish: Stress responses in fish are relatively understudied. However, common signs are exhibited across different species. These may include hiding behaviour, flitting or darting behaviour, stereotypical swimming patterns, surface gasping and reduced food intake.

Birds: Stressed birds will attempt to escape and so require careful handling, as they may easily injure themselves or others. Signs of stress in birds include wing flapping, pecking/biting and lunging (especially in psittacines and passerines), footing (raptors), vocalizations (especially screaming), lack of vocalization and immobility, feather picking and bar biting.

Wildlife

Wildlife comprises a diverse range of species; for many, signs of stress and fear may be extrapolated from other related species (e.g. foxes may show stress signs similar to dogs, wild rabbits and hares may show stress signs similar to domestic rabbits). In all cases, it should be remembered that human presence will be extremely stressful, and that any veterinary intervention will likely require an invasion of the animal's natural 'flight zone'. The flight zone is the distance within which a person can approach an animal before it moves away. Invasion of this zone is extremely stressful and will trigger a flight response, so any interactions should be minimized, and the animal should be secured in a location where injury risks are mitigated. Other stress signs include aggression, hiding and reduced feeding or grooming behaviour.

Zoological species

Zoo animals comprise diverse taxonomic groups and may include many of the species groups discussed above. For safety, many zoo species will require chemical immobilization to facilitate examination, and so handling stress is limited. However, these species may instead face stress in response to darting and chemical immobilization. Stress signs seen across a range of species include escape behaviours, aggression, hiding, stereotypy and tonic immobility. To avoid stress, zoo animals should be habituated to the close presence of keepers and veterinary staff and trained to participate in husbandry procedures using positive reinforcement operant conditioning (see Chapters 3 and 6). This approach can facilitate a wide range of clinical procedures such as physical examination, auscultation, radiography, ultrasonography and sample collection with minimal stress. It can also be used to ensure a calm, smooth induction of anaesthesia where more invasive procedures are needed, by training the animal to participate in injection of anaesthetic drugs.

Handling techniques

Ensure that the environment is as calm and quiet as it can be. Aversive smells, loud noises, slippery surfaces, and the presence of lots of people and other animals should all be avoided. Ensure you have everything that you will need already prepared and available so that you do not need to keep leaving and re-entering the room. You should have a plan formed for what you want to do

and should have explained it to anyone assisting you in the procedure. Talk kindly and reassuringly to the animal, without a high-pitched or excited voice, and use smooth, slow body movements rather than quick, jerky movements. Use the animal's name to reassure it. Allow the animal to sniff your outstretched hand before attempting to touch or stroke it, to give it the chance to smell what you are about. Observe whether the patient is willing to come close to you or is trying to create distance where the 'reward' would be for you to move away. Take your hand away if the animal cowers from you, allowing it to believe it is being listened to and has some control over the situation. Spend some time with the patient before you do anything that may cause them stress.

During examinations, consideration should be given to low-stress handling techniques (see below) and appropriate location for the examination; for example, try and examine cats within their baskets or on their beds (Figure 7.29), and try and keep dogs on the floor (Figure 7.30). Basic changes like this not only reduce patient stress but may also result in more accurate clinical assessments as the impact of stress is reduced and parameters such as blood pressure and body temperature are more likely to be indicative of clinical status. Patients should be desensitized to unfamiliar objects (e.g. allow patients to sniff stethoscopes before auscultation) and the necessity of performing aversive procedures should be considered (e.g. is rectal temperature taking always clinically indicated?). Additionally, veterinary surgeons should use treats and other rewards to build positive welfare experiences with their patients (Figure 7.31).

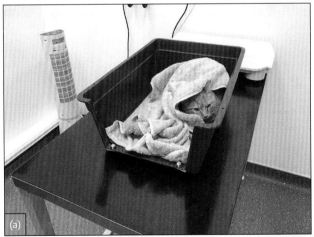

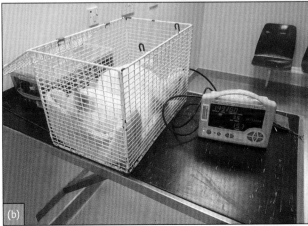

7.29 Cat examinations may be facilitated by (a) low-stress handling techniques and (b) in-basket examination.
(© The Jeanne Marchig International Centre for Animal Welfare Education)

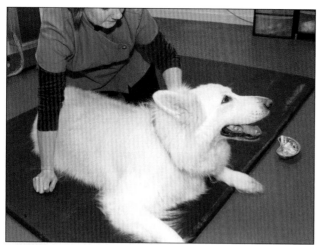

7.30 A relaxed and comfortable dog being examined during a consultation.
(Courtesy of Claire Corridan)

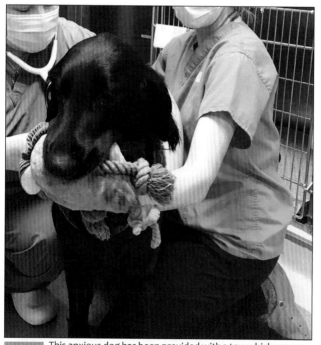

7.31 This anxious dog has been provided with a toy, which serves as a reward and distraction during a clinical examination. Low-stress handling is also being employed.
(Courtesy of Jess Davies)

Many routine procedures, such as blood sampling or blood pressure monitoring, can easily be performed within the consultation room with the owner present, rather than taking the animal into the preparation area – this is often less stressful for both the owner and patient.

Low-stress handling techniques

- Identifying the surfaces, sights, sounds and smells in the veterinary clinic that increase stress in patients and creating a calmer, safer and more secure environment is essential for a successful handling experience.
- Approach and handle the animal in a relaxed, non-threatening manner, recognize when an animal is fearful or anxious and adjust behaviour accordingly. ▶

Low-stress handling techniques *continued*

- Recognize that the way an animal is approached, picked up, restrained and moved from one place to another affects their perception of the veterinary professionals and their willingness to cooperate, so must be done calmly and in a positive manner.

See 'Useful websites' for resources on low-stress handling techniques.

Choice and control

It is well recognized that offering animals control over their daily husbandry and the opportunity to make their own choices can have a positive impact on welfare. These principles can easily be applied within the veterinary clinical environment. Top tips for improving welfare during consultations include:

- Use a quiet room with minimal noise, people and strong smells
- Do not immediately examine the animal – use the history-taking time to allow the pet to acclimatize to the environment: open the cat cage, let the dog sniff, etc. whilst you build rapport with the owner and take the history – patients will relax if they feel that their owners are relaxed
- Increase comfort and minimize slippery or hard surfaces by providing a bed for patients to sit on
- Approach in a non-threatening manner and crouch down to dogs to say 'hello' – ideally let them approach you
- Use the animal's name to reassure it
- Avoid direct eye contact
- Take the top half off cat carriers and leave cats in the base, where possible, rather than drag or tip them out
- Allow cats to explore the consulting room whilst you take the history from the owner
- Build a relationship and seek voluntary participation
- Offer your hand to be sniffed before touching the animal
- Take time to bond with the animal using gentle stroking and talking calmly before you start the examination
- Ensure you have any equipment needed within arm's reach before starting to handle or restrain the animal
- Use long slow strokes, which are more calming than short rapid touches
- Use food rewards and tactile contact to reinforce and reassure
- Use minimal restraint and low-stress handling as much as possible
- Wrap cats in towels if you think they are going to scratch or bite you
- Relax your hold on an animal if it stops struggling – this is its reward for behaving
- Encourage owners to habituate patients to common physical handling (e.g. handle feet and toes, ears and all aspects of the body). This is an important part of puppy and kitten socialization
- Offer owners desensitization and counter-conditioning programmes if their animal is fearful or anxious about being in the clinic
- For exotic pets, keep lighting low and noise to a minimum and ensure all equipment is prepared in advance to facilitate minimal handling
- Birds and rabbits may be wrapped in towels to facilitate handling; hawks may be hooded.

Commonly used non-controlled drugs, including vaccines, should be easily accessible from the consultation room to minimize back and forth movement, which can be potentially stressful for patients and presents an escape risk.

Dogs

Dogs should be approached in a non-direct manner and not backed into a corner, as they may feel like they cannot escape and may exhibit threat-repelling behaviours (e.g. growling; Figure 7.32). Instead, approach in a non-direct manner, use their name, crouch down to their level and do not stare at them too much (Figure 7.33). Immediately stroking the top of their head can feel intimidating or threatening to some dogs, so it is advisable to stroke them under the chin first. Many veterinary professionals like to put dogs on a table to examine them, but this is usually very unnatural for a dog, may alert them that something unpleasant is about to happen and can be slippery and frightening. How often is a dog placed on a table at home? Where possible, leave dogs on the floor, place a blanket down for them to sit on, and kneel down next to them. If

they enjoy sitting on your knee and being cuddled, then you can also allow this. Treat all dogs equally regardless of size – do not immediately pick up or restrain small dogs.

Use the minimal amount of restraint you possibly can. Holding dogs tightly can be frightening and can alert them that something aversive is about to happen; it can also make them struggle in panic, which makes handling more difficult. Instead, restrain them gently and use a calm voice

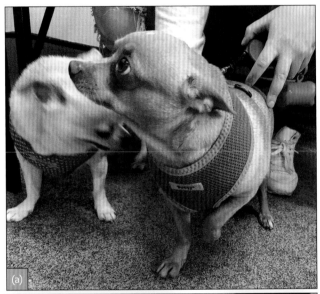

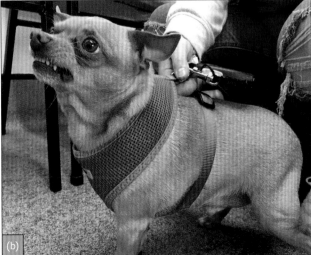

7.32 (a) This Chihuahua is demonstrating calming and threat-averting behaviours. Note the paw lift, 'whale eye' (whites of the eye showing) and ears pulled back. (b) The Chihuahua has now escalated to growling as its previous appeasing behaviours have not resulted in the desired outcomes. See also Figure 7.28.
(© Hayley Walters)

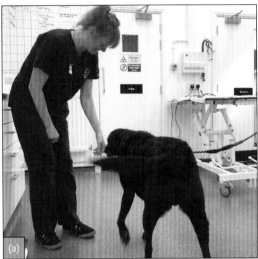

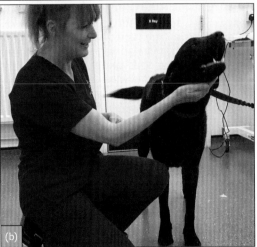

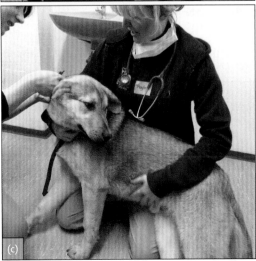

7.33 (a) A dog being allowed to approach and sniff an outstretched hand. (b) A dog being stroked under the chin. (c) A dog being gently restrained on a knee.
(© Hayley Walters)

to reassure them. Using long, slow strokes can also help to relax them. Vigorous stroking and speaking in a loud, high-pitched voice can upset the dog. If it is not contraindicated, then offer tasty treats to help build a relationship and relax the dog. If you do need to do something aversive, such as giving an injection, then hold the dog using a suitable restraining technique, use the minimal amount of restraint possible, then distract the dog by scratching pleasantly (for example, behind the ears) or by offering more treats. If the dog is boisterous, aggressive or struggling against your minimal restraint and you do need to hold the dog more firmly, then ensure you still use a suitable restraining technique and if the dog does stop struggling, relax your hold on them – this is their reward for behaving.

For dogs that are anxious or frightened but still handleable in the clinic, it is advised that a desensitization and counter-conditioning programme be put in place. Invite the owner to bring the dog in regularly to receive fuss and food rewards from staff, if they find this enjoyable, and for nothing negative to happen. When keeping dogs in for procedures, it is often less stressful for owners to leave first rather than the veterinary surgeon attempting to lead a dog away from the owner.

Cats

Many veterinary professionals will take a cat out of its carrier to examine it, but this can cause distress to the cat when they are suddenly exposed, and they may behave aggressively. A frightened cat naturally either wants to hide or run away, but can resort to scratching and biting if unable to do either. If the design of the cat carrier allows, simply take the top off the carrier and leave the cat in the base of it. Most of a cat examination can be done with the cat in the base of the carrier with a towel or blanket on or next to the cat for it to hide if it feels the need. Allowing the cat to hide in a towel, in the base of the carrier, as you examine each body part helps enormously in making the cat feel a bit safer and therefore less likely to scratch or bite (Figure 7.36). If the cat is happy to walk out of its carrier then having a blanket on the table is more pleasant for the cat than sitting on a cold, hard table. It is unadvisable to scruff a cat and pull them out of their carrier. Being pulled out of the carrier they were hiding in by the skin and placed on an examination table, surrounded by strangers in an unfamiliar, brightly lit room is daunting for a cat. Scruffing is only done 'naturally' on three occasions: a

---

Difficult dogs

Some dogs may have had too many negative experiences in the clinic for them to be handled at all. If this is the case, and there is no time for a desensitization and counter-conditioning programme or the procedure cannot be postponed to another day, then chemical restraint should be used. This applies to both small and large dogs. However, due to their size and weight, some veterinary professionals may attempt to overpower small dogs rather than sedate them and this can compromise welfare, as well as endanger the safety of staff. It should be remembered that due to trigger stacking (see above), the more an aggressive dog is handled, the worse its behavioural responses will become during this and future visits to the clinic, and that as a consequence higher doses of sedatives or anaesthetics will be required.

Walking sedation

'Walking sedation' may need to be performed if the animal is too dangerous to restrain for the administration of an intramuscular injection of sedatives. Walking sedation is achieved by asking the owner or a member of staff to walk the dog on a lead, whilst a colleague experienced in administering intramuscular injections waits at a safe distance. The dog should be muzzled (Figure 7.34). The dog will be aroused and distracted by the sights and smells of the clinic, allowing the pre-calculated dose of sedatives to be administered into the lumbar epaxial muscles as they walk past the waiting staff member (Figure 7.35).

Take the dog to a quiet, preferably darkened, area of the clinic and either place in a kennel and observe from a distance (leaving the lead on) or allow the owner to sit with the dog whilst the sedative takes effect.

This technique means the dog has not had to struggle and fight with staff to be examined, has not had a traumatically stressful experience that will make it more difficult to handle next time, and all the staff have stayed safe. If the animal needs to be hospitalized then they should be left with a muzzle on (provided they can still pant, vomit, eat and drink with it on – a Baskerville Ultra Muzzle® allows this), a harness on and lead attached coming out of the cage door, and a sign on the cage advising other members of staff that the dog may bite.

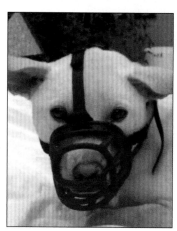

7.34 A dog wearing a Baskerville Ultra Muzzle®.
(© Hayley Walters)

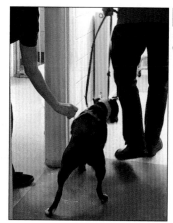

7.35 Walking sedation being administered.
(© Hayley Walters)

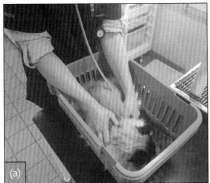

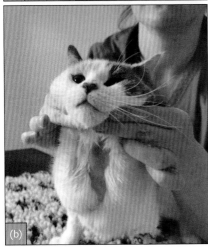

7.36 (a) A cat being allowed to stay securely in the base of its carrier for examination. (b) A cat being gently restrained for blood sampling; note it is placed on a bed and minimal restraint is being used.
(© The Jeanne Marchig International Centre for Animal Welfare Education)

mother carrying her kittens, mating or fighting. Some cats will freeze when they are scruffed, making them easier to handle, but other cats get upset and/or annoyed by it, which may make them more difficult and dangerous to handle. It is an aversive technique and should only be used as a last resort. If you go in rude and grumpy with a cat, you will get rude and grumpy back! All cat handling should be done gently, using minimal restraint, and efficiently to reduce the handling time. Once a cat feels like it has been handled too much, it becomes much more difficult to restrain.

Exotic pets, wildlife and zoological species

Clinics seeing a lot of exotic pets should invest in continuing professional development (CPD) to ensure that staff are confident and comfortable using safe, low-stress handling techniques for a range of clinical and husbandry procedures. Many exotic pets benefit from light sedation or inhalational anaesthesia to facilitate safe and low-stress handling (e.g. during beak or tooth burring, or nail trimming) and this may need to be costed into procedures in order to encourage use of low-stress techniques. Environments should be kept warm and quiet with low light levels as much as practicable.

Many birds will benefit from the use of a towel to facilitate handling and prevent injury in case of an escape attempt. Care should be taken to keep the wings against the body, but restraint should not be so tight as to impede respiration. In psittacine species, care should be taken to ensure that the head and beak are controlled; for birds of prey, handlers should be mindful of the talons and use appropriate gauntlets as required (Figure 7.38).

Rabbits may also be restrained with towels and should not be lifted unless necessary, as lifting induces a panic response (Bradbury and Dickens, 2016). When necessary, rabbits should be carried with the full length of the body supported. Stress can be reduced by allowing them to tuck their head into the crook of your arm. Historically, the 'trancing' of rabbits has been used as a restraint technique. Trancing is the process of inducing a state of tonic immobility in rabbits – usually by turning them on their backs. This technique induces the rabbit's 'play dead' immobility response that would be used to avoid predation; this causes elevated stress hormones and may be

Difficult cats

Much like dogs, some cats have had too many negative experiences to allow themselves to be handled. A towel can be used to wrap the cat in and can make them feel more secure and happier to be handled. Most cats tolerate it well and if the towel is placed quickly and efficiently before the cat has escalated to full-on scratching and biting, then a successful outcome usually ensues. If the cat is still behaving aggressively or appears visibly distressed, then chemical restraint is the best option. With the cat wrapped in a towel (Figure 7.37), or in a squeeze cage, or gently pushed to the back of its cage with a thick towel, give an intramuscular injection of a sedative, place the cat in a quiet, preferably darkened, cage and allow the sedative to take effect. If using a squeeze cage, the cat should be squeezed only for the duration of the injection and then the pressure immediately released. Do not cover the cage with a towel as it is important that the cat is observed in case they become unconscious in a position that obstructs their breathing.

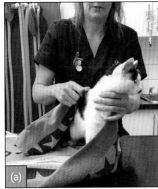
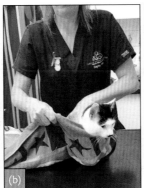
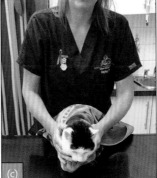
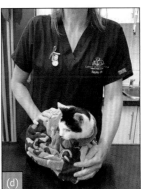

7.37 (a–d) Four-step process to restrain a cat in a towel.
(© Hayley Walters)

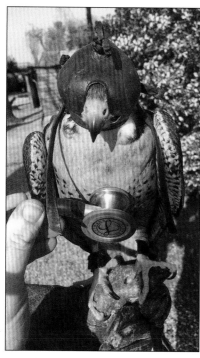

7.38 This kestrel has been trained to sit on the handler's glove and accept auscultation. The use of a hood helps to prevent any environmental stressors occurring and the examination is taking place outdoors in a quiet area away from cats and dogs.
(Courtesy of John Chitty)

detrimental to welfare. Thus, rabbits should not be turned on their backs and the practice of trancing should not be used as a restraint technique (McBride *et al.*, 2006; Rosewell, 2015).

Small mammals should be cupped or may be encouraged into a clear plastic tunnel for handling and examination. The use of tail or ear restraint is not acceptable. Care should be taken to ensure that chinchillas are gently restrained to avoid fur slippage.

Reptiles should be handled carefully to prevent injury (Figure 7.39); particular care should be taken to ensure that sharp claws do not snag on clothing. Larger snakes require two-person handling; a clear plastic tube can facilitate full body examination. Venomous snakes should only

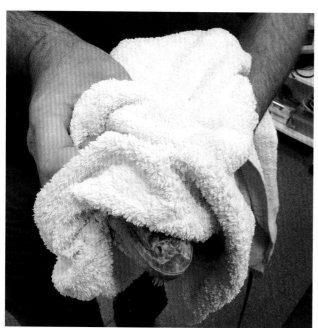

7.39 Towels can facilitate low-stress handling of many different species. This image shows a towel being used to reduce noise and light, whilst also safely securing the limbs of this green iguana.
(Courtesy of John Chitty)

be handled by trained experienced practitioners with the appropriate risk assessments in place. Reptiles should never be chilled to facilitate handling or minor procedures because whilst this may slow their metabolism and result in immobility, the process is stressful and does nothing to mitigate the pain experienced or any fear associated with the procedure.

Wildlife and zoo animal species will require chemical restraint to facilitate safe and low-stress handling. Where possible, the use of operant conditioning in zoo mammals should be encouraged to facilitate low-stress administration of injectable sedatives (see Chapter 6).

Clinical and presurgical procedures

Clinical and presurgical procedures are typically performed in the preparation and/or treatment areas of the practice. These are among the most frightening areas of the clinic for animals because they are no longer with their owner, they cannot hide in a kennel/cage, they are exposed to an alien environment of strange smells, noises and machinery, and they often experience pain and unpleasant procedures in these locations. The following can help maintain welfare standards during clinical and presurgical procedures:

- Beds/bedding should be placed on the examination table or floor for all procedures, if possible, to offer a feeling of comfort and security. The bed/bedding can be provided by the owner or be from the hospital ward if the patient has been admitted
- Low-stress handling techniques appropriate to the species should be used at all times (see 'Low-stress handling and restraint', above)
- For non-emergency patients that are undergoing anaesthesia and that are difficult to restrain, premedication prior to intravenous cannula placement is recommended. This will not only make the patient easier to handle but also reduce their stress levels. Premedicated patients should be kept calm and quiet. Anxious patients may require reassurance and tactile contact to allow the medication to take effect. The use of anxiolytics, with or without premedication, can also be of benefit in these patients
- When preparing the limb for intravenous cannula placement, it should grasped and held throughout the entire procedure (i.e. the limb should not be released between clipping of the fur, swabbing of the insertion site and placement of the cannula; Figure 7.40). Dogs and cats often resent the repeated grasp and release of their limb, so everything should be undertaken in one smooth movement where possible
- Any patient undergoing a surgical or painful procedure (e.g. bandage changes, radiography in animals with pre-existing osteoarthritis) should be given appropriate pain relief prior to the procedure (see 'Pain and pre-emptive analgesia', below)
- All patients should be well hydrated at all times. For patients undergoing sedation or anaesthesia, water can be provided until the animal is premedicated or sedated. There is no need to withhold water prior to this time. Ideally, any animal undergoing sedation or general anaesthesia should receive intravenous fluid therapy to provide normal fluid maintenance

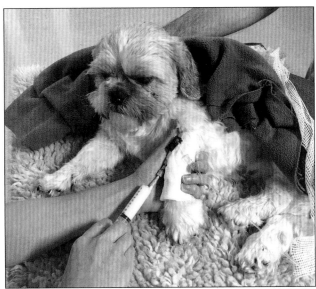

7.40 A dog having an intravenous injection on a comfortable bed whilst the paw is continuously held.
(© The Jeanne Marchig International Centre for Animal Welfare Education)

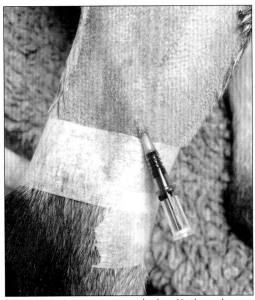

7.41 An intravenous cannula placed in the saphenous vein of a dog.
(© The Jeanne Marchig International Centre for Animal Welfare Education)

requirements, maintain adequate blood pressure and account for any fluid losses that may occur during surgery (e.g. blood loss, evaporation). Dehydration is an extremely unpleasant feeling and can also lead to hypotension, impaired cardiac function, infection and kidney failure

• Animals that are hungry have compromised welfare, so ensuring that food is withheld prior to sedation or anaesthesia for the minimal time possible is important. Gastric transit time for dry or solid food is approximately 6 hours, so this the recommended fasting time for adult dogs and cats. Withholding food for longer than 6 hours is unnecessary and this should be taken into consideration when planning procedures and feeding regimes.

Anaesthesia and analgesia

Anaesthesia is a state of unconsciousness induced in an animal. The three components of anaesthesia are *analgesia* (pain relief), *amnesia* (loss of memory) and *immobilization* (lack of movement). An adequate plane of anaesthesia and comprehensive analgesia, ideally using a multimodal approach, are prerequisites for surgery in any species.

Patients should be well hydrated and normothermic prior to and throughout any procedure. It is important to maintain patent intravenous access when using injectable anaesthetic agents to ensure anaesthetic depth is easily maintained throughout the procedure and to provide vascular access in the case of an emergency. An intravenous catheter should be placed in an appropriate vein for the species (often the cephalic or saphenous vein), following clipping and thorough cleaning of the access site, and stabilized using tape (Figure 7.41). The patient can then be safely induced through this access point and anaesthesia maintained during the procedure.

Care should also be taken to reduce patient anxiety prior to the induction of anaesthesia; low-stress handling techniques should be used and the environment should be calm and quiet. Anaesthetizing highly anxious animals increases the required dose of anaesthetic agents, as well as the safety risks associated with anaesthesia due to the level of circulating catecholamines. Anxiety prior to induction may also increase the risk of dysphoria on recovery (see 'Postsurgical analgesia, rest and recovery' below).

Anaesthesia should be routinely monitored and analgesic efficacy assessed throughout the surgical procedure. Pain responses under anaesthesia are often confused with a light plane of anaesthesia, and patients showing signs of pain may have their anaesthesia increased rather than additional analgesia provided. It is important to remember that inhalational anaesthetics such as isoflurane have no analgesic properties and so simply increasing the flow in a painful but anaesthetized patient will not reduce the risk of wind-up or minimize postoperative pain; additional analgesia must be provided instead. Figure 7.42 shows how to distinguish between inadequate analgesia and inadequate anaesthesia.

Inadequate anaesthesia	Inadequate analgesia
Eye position central	Eye position ventral
Palpebral reflex present	Palpebral reflex absent
Jaw tone present	Jaw tone absent
Swallowing	Not swallowing
Moving	Not moving
Vocalizing	Not vocalizing
Increased heart rate, blood pressure and respiratory rate	Increased heart rate, blood pressure and respiratory rate

7.42 Distinguishing between pain during surgery and inadequate anaesthesia.

Pain and pre-emptive analgesia

Pain is a complex phenomenon and has a huge impact on animal welfare, but is one of the areas of veterinary medicine that the profession is well equipped to deal with. Each individual animal will experience pain differently and recognizing pain in some species, particularly the less familiar exotic species, may be more challenging. Regardless of species, pain is best managed early and aggressively; it is much more difficult to control pain once it is well established than it is to manage pain before it becomes severe. Whilst this may not always be possible in real world situations, it should be remembered that when it is, preventing pain should be the aim of the analgesia plan. Surgical pain is 100% predictable and therefore a good analgesia plan should be in place for every patient, regardless of species, prior to undertaking any procedure.

The term 'pre-emptive analgesia' refers to the treatment of pain using analgesic drugs before the introduction of a noxious stimulus (i.e. surgery). Reducing the nociceptive input to the spinal cord reduces peripheral and central sensitization and therefore also reduces peri- and postoperative pain and hyperalgesia. Drugs commonly used in pre-emptive analgesia include:

- **Local anaesthetics** – block impulse conduction in nerve fibres. Cheap, readily available and extremely effective when used correctly, but often underused
- **Ketamine** – helps to prevent the 'wind-up' phenomenon, helps potentiate postoperative pain analgesics, provides good somatic analgesia but poor visceral analgesia, and is a very useful drug in patients undergoing major surgery where a chronic pain state or neuropathic damage is a risk (e.g. limb or tail amputation)
- **Opioids** – decrease the perception of and the reaction to pain, and also increase pain tolerance. Opioids bind to receptors in the nervous system, inhibiting the release of excitatory neurotransmitters in the brain and spinal cord, thereby reducing the pain associated with a noxious stimulus without interfering with motor function
- **Non-steroidal anti-inflammatory drugs (NSAIDs)** – exert antipyretic, anti-inflammatory and analgesic effects
- **Gabapentin and amitriptyline** – useful drugs to treat the neuropathic components of pain that are not targeted by licensed products. The cascade and rationale for prescribing should be considered.

When prescribing analgesics, the type of pain being experienced is important; pain may be caused by inflammation (inflammatory pain), tissue damage (nociceptive pain) or nerve damage (neuropathic pain). An individual may experience several types of pain concurrently and different medications may be required to adequately manage each. Different classes of drugs act at different sites along the pain pathway and thus can often be safely used in combination to provide optimal analgesia (Figure 7.43): the term multimodal analgesia is given to this approach to treating pain. Combining different classes of analgesic drugs ensures a more effective and enhanced management of pain,

Nociceptive	Inflammatory	Neuropathic
NSAIDs	NSAIDs	Gabapentin
Opioids	Steroids	Amitriptyline
Tramadol*	Opioids	Nortriptyline
Paracetamol	Paracetamol	Local anaesthetics
Local anaesthetics		Ketamine
Ketamine		Amantadine
Gabapentin		

7.43 Categorization of commonly used analgesic drugs according to the type of pain they are effective in treating. Note: not all medications suggested are licensed and veterinary surgeons should use their own clinical judgement and adhere to the prescribing cascade. * = efficacy is questionable in some species. NSAID = non-steroidal anti-inflammatory drug.

and the resulting synergistic effect allows lower doses of each individual drug to be administered, thereby reducing the possibility of side effects.

The *BSAVA Guide to Pain Management in Small Animal Practice* is a useful resource for pain management in cats, dogs and exotic pets.

Exotic pet first aid and analgesia provision

Regardless of the species, all RCVS veterinary surgeons are required to 'take steps to provide 24-hour emergency first aid and pain relief to animals according to their skills and the specific situation.' (RCVS Code of Professional Conduct for Veterinary Surgeons, 1.4). This means that withholding first aid or pain relief is unacceptable in veterinary practice, but it unfortunately remains a recurrent problem observed by experienced exotics veterinary surgeons when receiving referrals from first-opinion practices. Guidance for first aid provision and analgesic drug doses for a range of exotic species are available from a variety of sources including the *BSAVA Manual of Wildlife Casualties*, the *BSAVA Manual of Exotic Pets*, and the *BSAVA Small Animal Formulary Part B: Exotic Pets*. Traumatic injuries or disease process that are painful in mammalian species can be assumed to be painful in other species, and patients of all species should be appropriately stabilized and medicated as required to safeguard their welfare.

First opinion veterinary surgeons should also be able to triage urgent signs in exotic pets, many of which will mask their clinical signs. Exotic pets should be seen immediately if they are exhibiting:

- Injury from a predator, or other significant injury (e.g. from a lawnmower or car)
- Profuse blood loss
- Acute respiratory distress
- Inability to stand or reluctance to move/fly
- Acute enlargement or swelling of any body part
- Absence of feeding or faeces/urine/urate production (non-reptiles).

Surgical procedures

There may be pressure on the surgical team to perform procedures as quickly as possible, especially in a busy clinic. However, although shorter procedures may reduce the chance of infection from air contamination, there are many risks to patient welfare if surgery is rushed. The priority during the procedure is to be thorough, not fast. In order to minimize the risks to patient welfare, veterinary surgeons must remember to follow Halsted's seven principles of surgery.

Halsted's seven principles of surgery

- Gentle handling of tissue.
- Meticulous haemostasis.
- Preservation of blood supply.
- Strict aseptic technique.
- Minimum tension on tissues.
- Accurate tissue apposition.
- Obliteration of dead space.

Gentle handling of tissue

Tissues should be handled as gently as possible, as rough handling increases postoperative pain and the risk of infection. The surgical team should be familiar with all the equipment and instrumentation required for a particular procedure to ensure that they are used for their intended purpose and do not cause unnecessary trauma to delicate tissues. Surgical incisions should be made in a single motion by applying firm pressure with a clean sharp scalpel blade. Multiple cuts should be avoided when making the incision. Ideally, as small an incision as possible should be made, whilst ensuring adequate visibility, with the understanding that the incision may need to be extended if complications arise. All needles to be used during the procedure should be sharp, as blunt needles cause much more damage to the tissues.

Haemostasis

Careful and secure ligation of large vessels controls haemorrhage and prevents blood loss. Haemorrhage from small vessels may be adequately controlled by the application of haemostatic pressure until clot formation occurs.

Preservation of blood supply

It is important to use the right suture pattern and apply the correct tension. Suturing should result in gentle apposition of the tissues but the soft tissues should never be crushed by the sutures. Sutures that are too tight actually impede healing by restricting blood supply to the incision site and increase the risks of catastrophic wound breakdown and significant pain postoperatively. By ensuring that tissues are not crushed, and with the support of intravenous fluid therapy to ensure adequate tissue perfusion, correct suturing will preserve and maintain the blood supply to all the tissues in the body, allowing adequate tissue healing to occur.

Strict aseptic technique

Inadequate aseptic technique during surgery will increase the risk of perioperative infection, a potentially devastating complication.

Minimize tension on tissues

If the soft tissues are under tension when they are brought together to close the incision, then healing is reduced due to the impact of tension on the vascular supply to the tissues. Additionally, tissue tension will be painful for the patient and result in an increased risk of wound breakdown postoperatively.

Accurate tissue apposition

The tissue layers must be adequately apposed or brought together when suturing. The tissue edges should be touching to enable wound healing, but must not be squashed together as this damages the cells and the blood supply to the area, which will delay wound healing and can result in necrosis of the tissue edges.

Obliteration of dead space

If there is dead space, which is a gap created by surgery, a seroma may form. Dead space is commonly created when surgeons undermine the subcutaneous tissues; this may increase the risks of seroma formation, which can result in pain and infection.

Paediatric patients and small exotic species

Due to their size and predisposition to hypoglycaemia and hypothermia, paediatric and small exotic patients will have increased anaesthetic and surgical risks. Many of these risks can be reduced by providing good pre-, peri- and postoperative care, or referring to more experienced clinicians.

Warmth

It is very important to ensure paediatric and small exotic patients are at the correct body temperature prior to surgery. A heat mat, a nest-type bed, thick blankets and a kennel in a warm, draught-free room should all be provided for young patients. Exotic animals should be kept in a warm, draught-free room with access to safe nesting/bedding material. If the animal is still suckling, then it should remain with its mother and siblings until it is premedicated. This ensures warmth from the mother is maintained until the last moment. Thought should be given to shallow water bowls so that the patient cannot submerge itself and become cold.

A heat mat, Bair Hugger™ or 'hot dog' should be used during anaesthesia and, where possible, blankets wrapped around the animal. Bubble wrap can be bandaged on to each paw or baby's socks placed on each paw to help maintain heat. Body temperature should be taken and recorded every 15 minutes throughout surgery and active warming commenced for mammals if their temperature drops below 37°C.

Withholding food

Paediatric patients (16 weeks or under) must not be starved for the same mandatory 6 hours as adults prior to anaesthesia or sedation. Blood glucose levels can quickly drop dangerously low in a young animal that is not eating, so a period of only 2–4 hours is recommended. Blood glucose should be tested prior to premedication or sedation using a glucometer. A healthy cat or dog will have a blood glucose of around 4.4–6.6 mmol/l. Repeated blood samples should be taken and tested every 30 minutes during and after the procedure. Food should be offered as soon as the animal has regained full consciousness and is able to remain in sternal recumbency.

Similarly, most exotic patients are not routinely starved before surgery. For most bird and mammalian species, food consumption should be encouraged upon recovery and prokinetic medication may be helpful, especially in rabbits. It is essential that pain is well controlled to encourage normal feeding activity.

Sleep

Young animals need more sleep than adult animals, up to 20 hours a day. Consideration should be given to this when kennelling and treating paediatric patients.

Postsurgical analgesia, rest and recovery

Dysphoria

Anaesthesia should be maintained until the surgical procedure is complete, and the veterinary team should endeavour to ensure that the patient has a comfortable and smooth recovery from the anaesthetic. 'Dysphoria' or 'emergence' is where animals emerge from anaesthesia in an anxious state. Dysphoria is usually characterized by rigid limbs and ataxic locomotor activity, and patients may also vocalize. Animals that experience dysphoria are often in a state of anxiety and confusion and, because of their lack of motor control, may be at risk of physical injury in addition to their negative emotional experience (Figure 7.44). The risk of dysphoria can be reduced by reducing stress and anxiety prior to anaesthetic induction and ensuring a calm quiet recovery from anaesthesia. Animals that experience dysphoria during anaesthetic recovery may benefit from mild anxiolytic sedation until their anxiety has reduced and muscle rigidity has passed.

Pain

All patients benefit from objective postoperative pain assessment; even with multimodal preoperative analgesia, it is still possible that patients may experience postoperative pain and so their individual responses to analgesia must be assessed. The Glasgow Composite Measure Pain Scale and the Colorado Feline Acute Pain Scale are useful tools

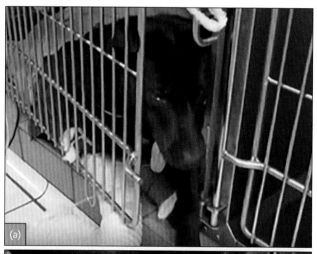
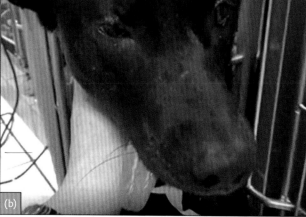

7.44 (a–b) A dysphoric dog attempting to escape from the kennel despite a lack of any limb or even tongue control.
(© The Jeanne Marchig International Centre for Animal Welfare Education)

in evaluating acute postoperative pain in cats and dogs, and grimace scales are available for pain scoring in small mammals such as rabbits, rats and mice (see Chapter 2). Common postoperative signs of acute pain include:

- Noticeable change in behaviour compared with preoperative period
- Reduced activity, reluctance to move or hunched/tense movement
- Increased facial or body tension
- Hiding or reduced interaction
- Licking or paying attention to the incision site
- Vocalization
- Facial grimace.

When behavioural changes indicative of pain are recognized following neutering procedures in dogs, the animal's analgesic support should be re-evaluated, particularly for animals that appear more 'passive' and are hiding away (Bacon *et al.*, 2019).

Whilst tools such as crates and Elizabethan collars are useful to restrict activity and support surgical recovery, they do not offer analgesic action and so should always be used in conjunction with effective analgesics. Elizabethan collars also obstruct normal behaviours such as sleeping, eating and grooming, are stressful for both pet and owner, alter auditory ability, and do not address the cause of wound interference. Considerate clipping and preparation of the surgical site, delicate tissue handling, pre-emptive and multimodal analgesia, and adequate postoperative pain relief will all aid in negating the need for Elizabethan collars. When necessary, Elizabethan collars should be used judiciously – ideally, soft collar options should be offered and the collar should be removed to facilitate eating, drinking and grooming. Elizabethan collars can negatively impact welfare (Shenoda *et al.*, 2020), so the risk of wound interference should be balanced against the welfare impacts of the collar.

The definition of pain used by the International Association for the Study of Pain (IASP) is "An unpleasant sensory and emotional experience associated with, or resembling that associated with, actual or potential tissue damage" (IASP, 2011). Thus, in addition to the medical management of the pain experience, veterinary clinics should also mitigate the emotional and sensory experience of pain. The emotional response to pain may be manipulated by the provision of a comfortable, quiet and calm environment that allows the patient to sleep and rest and which is free of threatening stimuli such as noises, aversive odours and predatory animals. Additionally, human comfort and reassurance, palatable food, toileting and hiding opportunities, and for longer term patients, appropriate enrichment, can all help to support positive emotional wellbeing and mitigate the pain experience.

Outreach and communications

The Federation of the Veterinarians of Europe (FVE), American Veterinary Medical Association (AVMA) and Canadian Veterinary Medical Association state that "Veterinarians are, and must continually strive to be, the leading advocates for the good welfare of animals in a continually evolving society" (FVE, 2018). As part of this role, veterinary surgeons should engage with pet owners, policymakers and the general public to promote good welfare practice and mitigate the potential for welfare harms.

Veterinary professionals may utilize a range of different techniques to engage with and educate clients about animal welfare problems. For example, television screens in veterinary clinic waiting rooms can share educational videos, and noticeboards, posters and leaflets can promote good practices in pet health and welfare. Social media provides a good way for the veterinary team to reach new and existing clients with welfare messages. Specific topics that may be of interest to veterinary clinics engaged in promoting good animal welfare include:

- **Animal welfare basics** – the Five Freedoms (see Chapters 1 and 2) and the duty of care that pet owners have to meet these needs for their pet. Resources such as the People's Dispensary for Sick Animals (PDSA) Animal Wellbeing (PAW) Report highlight key deficiencies in pet animal welfare in the UK
- **Responsible pet purchasing** – advice on sourcing a pet from a reputable rescue centre or breeder, and on researching appropriate species and breeds for the prospective owner's set-up. Common pitfalls such as buying 'designer' breeds or those prone to multiple health problems may be highlighted. Useful resources such as the Animal Welfare Foundation (AWF)/British Veterinary Association (BVA) puppy contract or the PetSavers guides on puppies, kittens, rabbits and guinea pigs could be provided (Figure 7.45; see 'Useful websites')
- **Understanding behaviour** – educating owners in being able to read their pet's body language can be very useful. For example, it may be helpful for dog owners to become familiar with the 'ladder of aggression' (see Figure 7.28) so that they can recognize the sequence of calming and threat-averting gestures that dogs exhibit with the immediate intention of achieving a reduction in the perceived threat and react accordingly. Resources on appropriate child–pet interactions may also be useful.

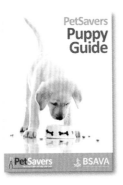 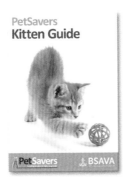 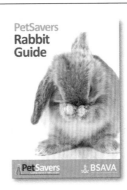 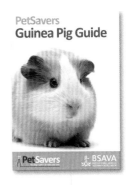

7.45 PetSavers guides to help owners prepare for the arrival of a new puppy, kitten, rabbit or guinea pig are available for members of the public and professionals to download and print out.

Case example 2: Early age neutering

Tristar and Jasmine were 16-week-old intact brother and sister kittens living together in the same house. The owner did not want any more kittens so called the practice to ask if they could be neutered as soon as possible as she could not keep them apart and was worried they would mate. The practice routinely advised that all cats are neutered at 6 months old due to concerns regarding surgical risks in juvenile patients.

The Federation of Veterinarians of Europe (FVE) Position statement on early age neutering collates the most recent research on the pros and cons of neutering in juvenile cats. It recommends that no kitten should be neutered before they are weaned (~8 weeks). This research outlines that common concerns relating to anaesthesia and surgical risks can be mitigated by taking into account the characteristics (size, predisposition to hypothermia and hypoglycaemia) of very young cats and mitigating them as described above. Additional considerations for informed consent include:

- **Growth** – delayed proximal ulnar cartilage closing is seen in females neutered at an early age, but further studies are needed to conclude if slower growth and increased final bone length have a positive or negative impact on a cat's health and welfare
- **Weight** – in terms of weight gain, the harm–benefit analysis seems in favour of early neutering
- **Mammary tumours** – studies indicate that the risk of developing mammary tumours is greatly reduced if cats are neutered before the age of 6 months
- **Urogenital disorders** – the harm–benefit balance between early/late neutering seems equivalent
- **Behaviour** – early neutering in cats reduces several undesirable behaviours, such as inappropriate urination and aggression, but can result in cats being more shy or fearful of humans.

This research alleviated some concerns within the practice about anaesthesia and surgery in juvenile patients and, after discussion with the owner, it was agreed that Jasmine and Tristar would be neutered as soon as possible to eliminate the possibility of unwanted kittens. The practice took into account the extra care needed during anaesthesia and surgery (see 'Paediatric patients and small exotic species', above) and both kittens recovered uneventfully. The practice now routinely performs neutering of cats from 4 months of age, in line with the International Society for Feline Medicine and FVE guidance.

Case example 3: Geriatric patients

Geriatric cats and dogs may well have significant comorbidities – typically senile cognitive dysfunction, dental disease and osteoarthritis. These conditions are often painful, and will become more so if the patient is handled in a way that is not sympathetic to these issues. Additionally, senile cognitive dysfunction can cause confusion and exacerbate feelings of anxiety, leading to behaviours such as aggression. These multiple and sometimes undiagnosed comorbidities, from the patient's perspective, could actually be more of a welfare problem than the problem that is being investigated.

For example, take a 12-year-old cat admitted for blood sampling and abdominal ultrasonography – what other considerations might we want to think about?

- Blood sampling – how will you restrain the cat? Do you need to put pressure on the jaw, elevate the neck or flex or extend the spine? All of these may be painful in an animal with dental disease or osteoarthritis. Could you instead use minimal or towel restraint?
- Restraint for ultrasonography – is the cat relaxed? Would medication facilitate the examination? Do you need to extend the limbs? Will this be painful?
- Hospitalization – is the cat stressed or confused? Can you take some time to reassure them, offer hiding spaces in their kennel and ensure their environmental needs are met?

If the procedures that we are going to perform are painful for the patient then we should be routinely providing analgesia; this applies to many non-invasive procedures, as even radiography, ultrasonography or simply restraint can be very painful or stressful for patients with underlying diseases. Ideally, we want to treat the patient, not the problem. Just because an animal has come in for a particular test or procedure, it does not mean that our veterinary care should be limited to this alone. Consider the welfare issues the animal is facing and prioritize problems according to the animal's welfare, rather than our human perspective.

Prioritizing welfare problems

Jake was a 13-year-old overweight Jack Russell Terrier brought to a busy veterinary clinic for a lump removal. His clinical examination showed severe dental disease with gingivitis, gum recession and calculus. Several incisor teeth were missing, and a carnassial tooth was cracked with pulp exposed. Jake was described as 'snappy' by the referring veterinary surgeon and disliked being restrained for procedures, which generally involved some level of head or muzzle restraint.

Apart from this Jake was in good physical health. As his admission was for a lumpectomy, this was performed. Jake had a lipoma – a non-painful and benign tumour. His dental disease was discussed with his owner but as Jake was uninsured and they had just spent a significant amount on surgery, they were unable or unwilling to treat the dental disease. Jake was seen for a follow-up appointment and whilst he appeared well, his dislike of oral examination was noted. Approximately 18 months after treatment, Jake died from an unrelated illness. His painful dental disease had never been treated.

Ethical dilemmas like this are common in practice: owners may perceive relatively minor pathologies to be problematic – 'lumps' are often a cause for concern because of their potential to have significant health and welfare impacts. However, prevalent and significant chronic pathologies such as dental infections are often overlooked, even when they result in behavioural changes and despite the fact that they may predispose patients to more significant clinical disease and chronic pain. In this case, treatment for Jake was prioritized towards a benign and non-painful condition whilst the dental disease that had caused him significant pain, likely for years, was overlooked or dismissed.

References and further reading

Bacon H (2019) Welfare of geriatric dogs and cats. *BSAVA Congress Proceedings 2019*. Available from: www.bsavalibrary.com/content/congress

Bacon HJ, Walters H, Vancia V and Waran N (2019) The recognition of canine pain behaviours, and potentially hazardous Catch-Neuter-Return practices by animal care professionals. *Animal Welfare* **28**, 299–306

Bradbury AG and Dickens GJE (2016) Appropriate handling of pet rabbits: a literature review. *Journal of Small Animal Practice* **57**, 503–509

Bradshaw JWS, McPherson JA, Casey RA and Larter IS (2002) Aetiology of separation-related behaviour in domestic dogs. *Veterinary Record* **151**, 43–46

Chitty J and Monks D (2018) *BSAVA Manual of Avian Practice*. BSAVA Publications, Gloucester

Fisher S (2015) Bank on it: Building a healthy 'bank' account for our animal friends. *Dogs Trust International Companion Animal Welfare Conference, Porto, Portugal*

FVE (2018) AVMA-CVMA-FVE: vets must be the leading advocates for animals. Available from: fve.org/publications

Hedley J (2020) *BSAVA Small Animal Formulary, 10th edn – Part B: Exotic Pets*. BSAVA Publications, Gloucester

Horwitz D and Mills D (2009) *BSAVA Manual of Canine and Feline Behavioural Medicine, 2nd edn*. BSAVA Publications, Gloucester

IASP (2011) Terminology. Available from: www.iasp-pain.org/resources/terminology

McBride E, Day S, McAdie TM *et al.* (2006) Trancing Rabbits: Relaxed hypnosis or a state of fear? In: *Proceedings of the VDWE International Congress on Companion Animal Behaviour and Welfare*, pp. 135–137. Flemish Veterinary Association, Sint-Niklaas, Belgium

Meredith A and Johnson-Delaney C (2010) *BSAVA Manual of Exotic Pets, 5th edn*. BSAVA Publications, Gloucester

Meredith A and Lord B (2014) *BSAVA Manual of Rabbit Medicine*. BSAVA Publications, Gloucester

Mullineaux E and Keeble E (2016) *BSAVA Manual of Wildlife Casualties, 2nd edn*. BSAVA Publications, Gloucester

People's Dispensary for Sick Animals (2020) *PDSA Animal Wellbeing (PAW) Report 2020*. Available from: www.pdsa.org.uk

Rosewell L (2015) Maintaining standards of welfare in hospitalised rabbits. *Veterinary Nursing Journal* **30**, 290–296

Royal College of Veterinary Surgeons (2020) *Code of Professional Conduct for Veterinary Surgeons*. Available from: www.rcvs.org.uk

Ryan S, Bacon H, Endenburg N *et al.* (2019) WSAVA Animal Welfare Guidelines. *Journal of Small Animal Practice* **60**, E1–E46

Self I (2019) *BSAVA Guide to Pain Management in Small Animal Practice.* BSAVA Publications, Gloucester

Shenoda Y, Ward MP, McKeegan D and Fawcett A (2020) "The Cone of Shame": Welfare Implications of Elizabethan Collar Use on Dogs and Cats as Reported by their Owners. *Animals* **10**, 333

Shepherd K (2009) Behavioural medicine as an integral part of veterinary practice. In: *BSAVA Manual of Canine and Feline Behavioural Medicine*, ed. D Horwitz and D Mills, pp. 10–23. BSAVA Publications, Gloucester

Varga M, Lumbis R and Gott L (2012) *BSAVA Manual of Exotic Pet and Wildlife Nursing.* BSAVA Publications, Gloucester

Walters H (2019) Good intentions and good welfare outcomes. *BSAVA Congress Proceedings 2019.* Available from: www.bsavalibrary.com/content/congress

Walters H (2019) Positive patient welfare: what the RVN can do. *BSAVA Congress Proceedings 2019.* Available from: www.bsavalibrary.com/content/congress

Warwick C, Arena P, Lindley S, Jessop M and Steedman C (2013) Assessing reptile welfare using behavioural criteria. *In Practice* **35**, 123–131

Useful websites

Association of Pet Behaviour Counsellors
www.apbc.org.uk

Dogs Trust Dog School – training classes
www.dogstrust.org.uk/help-advice/dog-school

Fear Free
fearfreepets.com

International Cat Care – advice on caring for cats
icatcare.org

PetSavers – guides for owners of new puppies, kittens, rabbits or guinea pigs
www.petsavers.org.uk/pet-guides

The Truth About Cats and Dogs – free course on behaviour for pet owners
www.coursera.org/learn/cats-and-dogs

World Small Animal Veterinary Association – Animal Welfare Guidelines
wsava.org/global-guidelines/animal-welfare-guidelines

Chapter 8

End-stage care

Lisa Howe and Carrie Kearns

Introduction

Giving clients and their families a positive euthanasia experience is essential for all veterinary practices and veterinary professionals. How the overall process is dealt with will impact how they move through the stages of grief. A traumatic euthanasia experience will result in the client being unable to process events and subsequently impact their long-term mental health. It will also affect client retention and acquisition, with them relaying their bad experiences to family and friends. Handling the euthanasia process compassionately and professionally for all clients should be the primary goal. This can be achieved by making sure that the veterinary team are following a best practice euthanasia protocol, thus ensuring a positive and consistent experience is provided for all.

There are many things we can do to help communicate effectively and compassionately with bereaved pet owners, as well as ways of recognizing the grief process. The way in which we approach euthanasia is of the utmost importance, remembering that it starts from when the client has realized they are facing the potential loss of their beloved pet. If the process is not handled correctly, this can lead to anger and upset; anger will eventually be directed at the practice and subsequently the team that has been directly involved. We must therefore be approachable at all times and especially after the event. This is the time that clients will often need to justify the euthanasia and talk through the events that led to the loss of their pet. Getting the euthanasia process wrong may impact the practice's reputation, but getting it right will lead to the bond between client and practice being stronger than ever.

If we, as a profession, have a better knowledge and understanding of pet bereavement, then we can better support our grieving clients.

The decision to euthanase

Clients may be told that they will know 'when the time comes' for euthanasia. Making sure that clients know when to consent to euthanasia is vital and ensuring that everyone involved is in agreement is just as important. Some family members may discount what the veterinary surgeon (veterinarian) has said and may not be able to come to terms with the fact that their companion is nearing the end of its life. From a professional point of view, we are helping the client to recognize that quality of life (QOL) is more important than quantity of life. Giving a pet more time is worthless if that time is spent enduring procedures or the administration of medications that may cause less than desirable side effects.

Caregiver burden may be a risk not only to the client but also to the veterinary staff who know that the patient is a candidate for euthanasia, but the client is not ready. Caregiver burden in clients may result in a decision being made sooner rather than later, but this can lead to discontent within their household, which may then be redirected at the veterinary team. Some clients may take the view that as their pet was offered certain medications they were obligated to take them. However, it may be that they were prescribed to give the client more time with their pet to make an informed decision. Ultimately, the owner has the final say regarding timing of euthanasia, unless it is a welfare issue, but they have to be in agreement that their pet is suffering and euthanasia is the only humane option.

Quality-of-life scoring systems

There are various QOL scales that can be accessed and used by clients to help them make an informed decision. By asking a client to fill out a QOL scale, they can see by their own admission how their pet is doing. These QOL scales can be adapted to be species specific. A form can be given to all family members, so that the results can be collated and then a decision either way can be made. QOL scales allow the client to log and monitor most aspects of their pet's day-to-day life.

Scoring systems can be adapted to take into account other QOL factors (Figure 8.1) and give the client further indicators to consider, including interactions or attitude and favourite things.

QOL scoring systems can be useful tools in dedicated palliative care/end-of-life clinics. These clinics should be established to help support clients in making a difficult and harrowing decision. Many clients struggle to identify when the right time for euthanasia is, and these clinics can really support them and help them to come to terms with their decision. Many clients will also have further questions they may need to ask, and these clinics can help them to feel they have an important lifeline with the practice and their veterinary surgeon. These clinics can be run by veterinary nurses and any questions can be referred to the veterinary surgeon looking after the pet as needed.

HHHHHMM system

This commonly used scoring system comprises seven indicators:

- Hurt
- Hunger
- Hydration
- Hygiene
- Happiness
- Mobility
- More good days than bad.

Each indicator is scored from 1 to 10, with 1 = poor and 10 = best. The total from each indicator is then added together, giving a sum total. If the total is between 35 and 70, this signifies an acceptable QOL; if the total is below 35, this signifies an unacceptable QOL.

By asking the client to consider each of the indicators in turn and to make an honest assessment regarding each one, they will obtain a better idea of where their pet is in regard to whether they require support or whether euthanasia should be requested. You want your client to appreciate that there will be good days as well as bad, and that there are options available, but they have to realize that if they do not complete the QOL scale honestly then this will have an effect on their pet.

Quality-of-life diary

Below is a weekly diary to keep track of your pet's journey. Please fill in the appropriate number for each category and then add the numbers together. The maximum score is 18. This helps to give a visual understanding of how your pet's illness may be progressing.

Activity of life	Score	Criteria
A: Mobility	2	Good mobility – no difficulty in getting around, enjoys walks or going outside
	1	Poor mobility – difficulty getting up, struggles to get into position to go to the toilet, short walks only
	0	Bare minimum mobility – needs assistance, losing footing, unable to squat/lift leg to toilet, pain medications/anti-inflammatory medications do not help
B: Nutrition	2	Good appetite – still eats food readily
	1	Poor appetite – hand feeding, needs enticing
	0	No appetite – to include vomiting/nausea
C: Hydration	2	Adequate intake – drinking as normal
	1	Poor intake/increased intake – disease dependent
	0	Requires oral hydration or subcutaneous fluids
D: Interaction or attitude	2	Interacts normally without needing prompting
	1	Some interaction or needing to be prompted to interact
	0	Hides away; only gives contact, which may be minimal, when approached
E: Toileting	2	Normal urination and/or defecation
	1	Reduced/irregular urination and/or defecation
	0	None/no or very little output
F: Favourite things	2	Normal favourite activities; no change in demeanour
	1	Decrease in doing their favourite things
	0	No interest in their favourite things
G: Hygiene	2	Enjoying being groomed or grooming self
	1	Not enjoying grooming or not grooming self
	0	Unable to keep clean themselves, complete reliance on you
H: Pain	2	No signs of pain or pain relief/anti-inflammatory medications working
	1	Signs of pain or pain relief/anti-inflammatory medications not working as before
	0	Strong signs of pain – pain relief/anti-inflammatory medications fully explored and no longer working
I: Good days or bad days	2	More good days than bad days
	1	Good and bad days about the same
	0	More bad days than good

Interpretation of the quality-of-life scale is seen from the total scoring:

12–18: Everything is going okay and your pet still enjoys life (and you should too)

6–11: May require intervention, supplementation or adjustment of treatment (contact us to discuss)

0–5: Consider humane, gentle euthanasia (contact us immediately)

8.1 An example of an adapted quality-of-life scoring system.
(Courtesy of Sarah Ramsden)

Understanding the bereavement process

The loss of a pet is a profoundly distressing and emotionally personal time that is felt differently by each individual. Whether it is an adult, an adolescent or a child, the intensity of that grief can be overwhelming. The relationship between humans and animals can be more heartfelt than any other relationship and people are often shocked by the intensity of their grief.

It is important to recognize that your client's pet was a member of their family and had a role in the family dynamic, just as a human member would have. Often the bonds that are formed between animals and humans are as strong, if not stronger in some circumstances, as the bonds formed from human to human. Grief is individual; others in the family may be affected, but this does not mean that every person will be grieving in the same way. Often there are differences of opinion regarding where everyone is at in their grief stages, and this may lead to friction. This is seen especially when family members feel they cannot speak about their own pain for fear of upsetting someone else. The intensity of the grief felt by clients will be determined by:

- The role the pet played in the owner's life
- The length of time the client had the pet
- The age of the pet at the time of death
- The cause of loss – was it due to old age, accident, sickness, euthanasia or disappearance?

Physical symptoms of grief include: headaches, nausea, exhaustion, sleep disturbance, loss of short-term memory, lack of concentration and weight fluctuation. The emotions experienced during bereavement are similar to post-traumatic stress syndrome and this is especially true if the loss is a result of a traumatic event. These overwhelming feelings can last for a while and may be accompanied by a sense of intrusion, helplessness and distress. Reactions to a traumatic or non-traumatic loss will be worse if:

- There is a feeling of wanting to have done more
- The client feels there is little or no support from colleagues, family or friends, or if they are having to cope with several stressful or traumatic events
- The client has an underlying mental health condition.

Psychological response to grief

Knowing the psychological response to grief and the stages your clients will be going through will help you better support them at this difficult time. We have a duty of care to our clients, as well as their pets, and it is very important to know the point at which they should be referred on to a medical professional for further help and support. If you have any concerns about your client's wellbeing, they must be referred accordingly. In addition, putting the client in touch with a local pet bereavement counsellor can help them feel more in control and able to reach out to somebody who is impartial and can allay their fears.

In 1960, Dr Elizabeth Kübler-Ross and a team of psychologists determined that there were five stages of intense mourning (Kübler-Ross, 2014). With regards to pet bereavement, these five stages were adapted slightly in 1990 by Dr Wallace Sife. The stages of grief can be experienced in any order. Individuals must be allowed time to progress through each stage at their own pace, to avoid a detrimental long-term effect on their overall healing. A common emotion clients struggle with is feeling as though their grief is not justified because 'it's only an animal', but it is important for them to understand that their grief is real and justified.

The human–animal bond in zoo, exotic and wildlife species

We are all aware of the strength of bonds between humans and companion animals, but it is also important to acknowledge the strong bonds and relationships formed between humans and exotic, zoo and wild animals.

A loss is a loss no matter the species, and the grief felt may be to a lesser or greater degree depending on the bond. The bond a person had with the animal affects how they react to the loss. It is not just the physical absence that is felt, it is the loss of something from their daily routine.

These relationships, as with companion animals and human-to-human bonds, are based on a series of regular interactions. With zoo and wild animals, it is important that these relationships are managed so they do not have a negative effect on the animal's wellbeing, whilst at all times respecting that they should be treated for the most part as wild. However, repeated interactions with keepers/owners lead to long-term relationships and bonds being formed, and result in a positive sense of wellbeing for both animals and humans. This results in the animal generally being calmer, making it easier to handle and to administer necessary treatments and general animal husbandry to them.

Zookeepers report that the loss is felt just as keenly as with companion animals. Some keepers say that they feel that this is not only because the individual died, but because of the conservational impact of that loss on that species. Keepers also say that they feel a deeper grief, in some cases, when they lose an animal that is not on show or that is not seen as important by the public (e.g. frogs, invertebrates).

The bond between keeper and animal is unique; some animals are safe to be in contact with, whilst others are either not or are only safe to be in contact with if strict safety protocols are observed. When the keeper is unable to touch or enter the enclosure with an animal, the bond that forms is based on respect for the animal and its proximity to a human, through vocal and optical cues and shows of intent. Grief is felt no matter what the species; from invertebrates to megafauna there is a sense of loss when an animal dies. Just as pet owners feel guilt at making the decision for euthanasia, so too do zookeepers, regardless of whether it is their decision or that of others responsible for the collection (e.g. directors). Zookeepers may spend a lot more time with the animals in their care, and unlike domestic pets, many of these animals live for many years.

In contrast, wildlife workers report that, as the animals in their care usually require more care or have a high mortality rate, they felt some loss and grief but not to the same extent as they might with other losses. Although there was a sadness for loss of life, it was not something that affected them long term.

When dealing with the loss of any animal, companion or otherwise, the profound sense of grief can be overwhelming and must be acknowledged so that the person can ultimately, in time, find resolution.

Stage 1 – shock and disbelief

In this stage, the brain's response to intense pain is to generate questions such as 'are they really dead?', 'I don't believe this has happened.' This is usually the first response to death. In some rare cases, the owner may become oblivious to the situation and they can refuse to accept the fact that their pet has died. Clients should be reassured it can take a few days or weeks to come to terms with what has happened.

Stage 2 – anger

Often very soon after the shock of what has happened passes, clients usually find themselves in the anger stage. Anger is a response to the frustration and distress of what has happened. The owner may project that anger at someone or something, needing to find a scapegoat (i.e. the veterinary surgeon, practice or themselves). They are seeking something to hold on to and to fulfil their need to feel in control. It is important to allow a client to express their anger during the grieving process in a constructive way. In some cases, the anger will be justified, such as with foul play or negligence.

Stage 3 – denial

There is a difference between denial and disbelief:

* Disbelief – the inability or refusal to accept something that is true or real
* Denial – the avoidance of something we find too painful. Bereaved people feel numb and will find a way to simply get through each day, avoiding the reality of the loss. Denial helps our brain to cope with the emotional impact of the traumatic event.

There is no set time for your clients to go through the denial stage, but it usually passes quickly as they are forced to accept the reality of their loss.

Stage 4 – guilt

Most clients that require pet bereavement counselling will be stuck in the guilt phase, with anger often feeding into it. This can range from distress to self-blame. Guilt can be one of the longest stages to deal with and can prevent the client's overall healing/resolution. This stage can be identified by the owner expressing the feeling that they could have done something to avoid the loss of their pet: they may be stuck with ruminating thoughts of how the loss could have been prevented (e.g. 'if only I had done something differently', 'if only I had not left him/her', 'if I had picked a different vet'). The client must be helped to realize that hindsight is not to be used as a means of punishment.

If we recognize this stage as veterinary professionals, we can better support our clients, protect ourselves from complaints and avoid possible perceived malpractice. This is why it is important to have a bereavement policy in place for how to deal with such cases. It is very important that the client feels they can approach you after the event, to discuss their feelings and have an open door to communication. Often, they just need reassurance that they did everything possible for their pet and that there was nothing more that could have been done.

Stage 5 – depression

A large number of people who suffer a pet bereavement will understandably suffer with low mood or slight depression. Depression is a normal response to loss, but chronic or severe depression is a medical condition (Figure 8.2). Individuals who have suffered with depressive tendencies in the past or had underlying mental health issues before the loss will be at greater risk. If your client's depression seems to be recurrent or dangerous, then they should be immediately referred to a qualified doctor. If they are having suicidal thoughts or tendencies, they must be referred to A&E straight away or an ambulance called if the client has put the phone down, having told you of their intentions.

* Feeling hopeless or pessimistic
* Insomnia or excessive sleep
* Continuous sad, anxious or negative thoughts
* Loss of interest in hobbies and activities
* Difficulty remembering, concentrating or making decisions
* Loss of appetite or overeating
* Thoughts of suicide or suicide attempts

8.2 Some of the first indicators of depression.

Stage 6 – resolution

Psychologists use the word 'closure' but for the pet bereavement process this is not the correct term. Bereaved people do not want to shut out the loss: they need to find a way of moving on with their lives, being able to look back and draw on the good memories, and embrace feelings of thankfulness for the time that they did have with their beloved pet. How quickly your clients reach the resolution stage is dependent on:

* The personality of the owner
* The pet's role in their life
* How long they had the pet.

A family whose dog lived a long life may reach the resolution stage much quicker than an owner whose pet was their only companion or met a traumatic end.

Client support

Client support begins from the moment that they register their pet. It does not stop when the heart of the patient stops beating. End of life does not mean end of responsibility; end-of-life support is a necessity not a novelty.

Over the years, the approach to end-of-life support has changed for the better, but there is still a long way to go. Unfortunately, there are still some practices that think that as soon as the patient has died and the cremation details have been organized, that that is where their commitment to the client ends. This approach should be discouraged as it can be damaging to the client–practice relationship and, potentially, to the client themselves.

Throughout the lifetime of a pet, no matter the species, veterinary professionals are there to advise the client and assist them with any problems they may have, be it behavioural or regarding preventative protocols. End-of-life support starts from the very first appointment. We are building a relationship of trust and mutual respect. It goes without saying that not every pet will have a dignified death, and that some may die due to accidents or disease.

Clients need support and information from the practice to ensure they make the best decisions for their pet. What may seem obvious to us is only due to the level of knowledge and training we have. Discussing what to do before and after does not have to wait till the patient develops a terminal illness or dies from a traumatic event. Having information on hand at all times for the client to read will help both parties. Clients can be provided with information about the euthanasia process, the cremation options and process, and bereavement support services. By having access to this information before the event, the client may cope better with the loss or impending loss of their pet. Fear is usually the result of the unknown and if we can help to clear up any confusion then this is beneficial to all. Pre-loss handouts are a great way to explain to clients what is expected from the practice and what is expected from them.

Over the years, it has become apparent that a lot of clients were not aware of the process involved with regards to euthanasia prior to the event and, consequently, there were queries as to whether something that happened was normal. This need not be the case – if the client had all the facts to hand to read when they were not in an emotional state, then they would feel better prepared. Euthanasia is not something to be feared, but it is a topic that is often not broached due to the reactions it elicits. Clients are going to experience the loss of a pet at some point, so it makes sense that they are as ready for it as possible.

A handout could contain information regarding the services that the practice or clinic provides. This information could include:

- Cremation options, prices and the details of the crematorium
- Details regarding the euthanasia process itself – do you use sedation? If so, explain why and what may happen when it is used
- Worst case scenarios; for example, vocalizing, vomiting and pacing. By explaining this we are not saying it is the norm but that it is something to be aware of and is normal
- An explanation of how the euthanasia solution of preference works, making sure the client is aware that there is no reversal once it has been administered.

The client needs to be aware of any potential issues that may arise; this need not scare them, but is more of a pre-warning of what may happen. A bereavement pack with the handout in it, containing all the above information and options, is extremely helpful. Suggested reading for adults and children on coping with pet loss should also be included.

There would ideally be a list of sources on pet loss support, such as helplines or numbers and websites for pet bereavement counsellors (Figure 8.3). Recognizing when a client needs extra support is vital. Grief and depression share many common traits and without support a client may go from the sadness of grief to the depths of depression. Be aware of your client and if you feel they need help then offer to let them come in for a chat and refreshments or give them a list of services they can access.

Bereavement packs can also be adapted for children and can provide parents with useful information on how to support their child. When children are bereaved, the most powerful thing we can do for them is to be honest, open and allow them to be able to talk about their feelings in a safe environment. Children find it especially helpful if they can write or draw how they are feeling, and sometimes a simple drawing or a letter to their beloved pet can ease their grief long term.

The most important thing we can give to clients is our time. However, time is precious in a busy veterinary practice and there may not be the opportunity to sit with a bereaved client or to explain the process and options. There is always time to be kind though and to let the client know that you will do your best to make time to talk to them: offer to call them to arrange a time to talk and let them know you are listening to what they are saying. What you say can mean so much in not so many words.

There are phrases that can be used and some that should never be uttered by a veterinary professional (Figures 8.4 and 8.5). Whilst what you say may come with well-meant intentions, we have to remember that we are dealing with grief-stricken clients. Clients who are emotional are probably not thinking straight. It is surprising how the most well-meant words can be taken out of context.

Clients that require additional support

Clients come from all sorts of backgrounds and there will be some with physical disabilities or additional needs who still require support, but the way we provide that support has to be tailored to the individual.

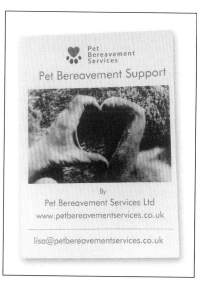

8.3 Veterinary practices should provide clients with information on the pet bereavement support services available to them.

What to say	Why
I am sorry for your loss	You are showing that you see how the loss may affect the client. Showing sympathy to their situation. You appreciate how hard this will be for them
I am/we are thinking of you	This shows the client that you have not forgotten them, that they matter to the practice as much as their pet did
I bet you have some wonderful memories; I would love to hear about them sometime if you want to talk about them	Keeping the memory alive. Clients love to talk about their pets, and knowing someone wants to listen can mean so much to them. They may have no one else that wants to know and this can be upsetting for the client who just wants to talk about them
I am here if you want to talk	The client knows now that you are there if they are struggling; they may not have anyone else to talk to
I'm here to listen if you want to talk about...	You are letting the client know that you do not mind hearing stories about their pet. Some people get irritated and do not want to know, but the client needs to talk about them – it helps their recovery
I want you to know that I loved... And miss... I can't even begin to imagine what it is like for you	The client knows now that the loss of their pet means something to you and the practice. You are also showing the client that you appreciate how hard the loss has hit them but you are not presuming to know how they are feeling and are therefore validating their feelings

8.4   Phrases that may be suitable for use with grieving clients.

What not to say	Reasons to avoid
Time is a great healer	To the client, all the time in the world may never feel long enough to recover
Give it time	This phrase does nothing to validate or sympathize. It just suggests that the client will be okay in time
I remember when my pet was put to sleep	This turns the attention to you. The client may feel uncomfortable opening up about their own loss if they feel it could cause upset. Clients may also feel that they have not been heard. Clients do not need to know your story; they need their own to be acknowledged
I know how you feel	We do not know how they feel. We know how we would feel but that is not the same. It comes from a good place but is not helpful
At least...	This phrase cannot be ended in a way that will help the client, and should be avoided
Don't cry	The client has a right to feel and express their pain. Being told otherwise may lead to the client suppressing their emotions, which can be damaging to their mental health
They aren't in pain now	While true, this phrase is not helpful. It is clear to the owner that the pet is not in pain, but they may question whether they waited too long
It was God's will	Introducing religion can cause more upset than it might alleviate, and is not always welcome
Move on, it is time to let go	There is no time limit to grief. Telling someone to move on when they are not ready is hurtful and invalidates their grief
He/she lived a good long life	Whilst this may be true, the client would like to have spent even longer with their pet. This phrase only serves as a reminder of the good years that are now over
He/she wouldn't want you to be sad	This is just as inappropriate as 'don't cry'; it is not healthy to suppress expression of grief

8.5   Phrases that should be avoided with grieving clients.

Autistic clients

Autistic people may struggle with, for instance, the noise and smells of a veterinary clinic. Whilst there is not a lot we can do about the smells (i.e. animals in general and disinfectant), we can help with the noise to some degree and the waiting time.

Some clinics have undertaken training by the National Autistic Society to enable them to help their clients and their client's children. Some people believe that all autistic people react the same or behave the same. To assume that each person shares the same traits and behaviours is ignorant and does that person a disservice. Most autistic people see the world as very black and white, with no grey area. Therefore, we have to be careful with what we say as well as how we say it, and explain what is about to happen, what may happen and what we will do if something untoward happens.

Do not use euphemisms as this can cause confusion and unnecessary distress. Say what you mean and be clear and concise. Allow the client time to process what you have said and repeat if necessary. Some autistic clients may find it difficult to look at someone speaking to them and also listen and take in what is being said. When someone is listening, they may appear not to be; however, in reality they are only able to take in what is being said if they do not look, as it can be overwhelming.

Having the consultation notes written or typed up for the client may be useful; the client can then go back to this when they get home and can process what was said. Practices that are autism friendly have printed booklets to explain what happens at the veterinary practice – this is ideal for children and adults alike. It may also be useful to have a pre-euthanasia or loss handout for clients to take home, explaining what happens, what may happen and what would be done. Explain in a clear manner without unnecessary jargon or euphemisms. Make it bullet pointed or numbered like a timeline, so that the client knows what will happen and when. It is the unexpected that can cause distress as the client may not know how to respond or what would be expected of them.

Clients with dementia

When you are assisting clients with dementia you must be patient. Be prepared to repeat information even if you have only just given it to the client. There are methods of communicating that will make it easier for you to relay information and for the clients to take in that information. A common misconception is that you have to speak as if talking to a child, using a tone reserved for small children, and that you have to shout to be heard. This could not be further from the truth and to treat someone in this manner is both ignorant and demeaning.

For a client with dementia, they may have difficulty finding words to explain what they mean or they may find it takes longer to process information. This is why it is important to speak clearly, be precise and patient. When addressing the client, try to use their preferred title or their name. Try to avoid using terms such as 'dear, love', etc., as it can come across as patronizing and lead to offence. Using the client's name or preferred title shows that you are respectful of them and is in keeping with a professional consultation.

It may help to be on the same level as the client. If they are seated, you may also want to sit down. It can be quite intimidating to have someone standing over you, talking about things you may be struggling to understand.

Do not assume that your client is unable to hear what is being said. Their brain may be working differently, but they are not necessarily hard of hearing. Shouting or talking very loudly is potentially distressing and is also unnecessary. Speak to them in the tone and level of voice that you would any other client. By all means, if they seem to be unable to hear you then raise your voice slightly. Speak clearly. Say what you mean and try to do so in terms that will be understood.

If you use terms such as 'put to sleep' or 'put down' the true meaning will be lost. You will only cause more questions and upset than you will answer. You may find that your client takes what you have said literally; they may believe that their pet will wake up. It is important that you make sure you explain the permanence of what is to happen, so there is no confusion.

There are some practices that have gone above and beyond to aid clients with dementia. For example, sending the client or their carer a plan of the practice may be beneficial. A floor plan showing the client where they will enter the practice, where the reception desk is, where the consultation rooms are and how to get to and from these areas may be helpful. It can be very confusing to enter a building full of noises and smells, and so if the client knows where to go and how to exit, they may feel more in control. It may also be beneficial to send the client a detailed breakdown of what to expect when they come in. Euthanasia is a daunting and emotionally charged time for anyone, but more so for those with dementia.

Write down the stages, from booking in with reception to what will happen following the appointment, step by step. Maybe mention who the veterinary surgeon will be that they are likely to see. Explain what will happen during the procedure from start to finish: Do you place catheters? Do you do this away from the client? Do you use sedation and, if so, what are the potential side effects? Will a nurse be holding their pet? Can the client be present and can they have some time with their pet afterwards? What is expected of the client and what can they expect from you? How is euthanasia achieved? Is there anything the client needs to be aware of? Potential difficulties should be explained (i.e. no venous access, poor blood pressure, post-mortem reactions such as gasping and stretching or twitching). Anything we take for granted, we need to explain to the owner what may happen, how it happens and what we will do to correct or deal with it. Explain what happens to the pet afterwards and the possible options.

It is crucial that the options are listed, ideally with prices and an explanation. It will make it easier for the client to make a decision based on facts and their financial circumstances rather than emotion. It may be necessary to contact the client or their carer to let them know that their pet's ashes have been returned. You may find that you have to remind the client that their pet has died. This must be done with respect and compassion. To the client this may trigger a memory and they recall the event, or this may sound like the first time they have ever been told.

The reactions may be subtle or intense and the client may need external support from their GP or a pet bereavement counsellor. Having details of external support services available to give to the client will benefit both parties. You are showing you understand the need for such services and the client is now aware that such services exist.

Patience and understanding are vital when speaking to clients with dementia. The world they live in mentally can be frightening, words do not come as easily, names and faces become lost, and sounds and sights can become overwhelming. If you have to repeat information do so as if it is the first time you have relayed that information. You may have said it a few times but to the client it may be like hearing it for the first time.

Clients with physical disabilities

You may have clients that rely on service animals to enable them to navigate their way through their lives, helping them with everyday tasks they cannot manage or keeping them calm and reducing stress. Assistance animals are usually dogs, although a variety of species can be used as emotional support animals.

The type of assistance animal will have an impact on the grief that the client goes through when they lose them. The assistance animal will have been a constant companion. They may have helped the client with tasks most people manage without issue, such as dressing, undressing and picking up the phone. They are social icebreakers and can help people to see the person not their disability. They may serve as an alert to seizures or syncope episodes, or a warning that someone is ringing the doorbell or that anxiety levels are rising and the client needs to get to a safe place.

Imagine having an assistance dog that does everything to make your life a little easier and to help you retain some independence. Imagine being blind and having a dog that guides you and keeps you safe and able to lead your life. Now imagine they retire or die. You would be left alone while waiting for another companion to be assigned to you and then, whilst grieving, you would have to build another bond and relationship with a new assistant. If you can imagine this, then you can understand why the loss of a service animal is so devastating.

The loss is felt in all areas of the client's life: from their day-to-day routine to social interactions, they receive constant reminders that their companion is no longer by their side.

We cannot truly understand what a client is going through, but that does not mean we cannot be sympathetic. The level of support given to grieving clients should be exceptional – they deserve nothing less.

Children

We must not forget that we have clients of all ages and although we speak to adults about family pets, the children are also involved. They are emotionally invested in their pet and may be the reason the family took on the pet in the first place. We must be aware that what we say is being taken in by young ears and minds.

When a pet requires euthanasia, the whole family will be affected and children may have to live with the decisions of adults. They may feel ignored or helpless as their parents or guardians have the final say over the fate of their pet.

Whether children should be present for euthanasia is a decision for their parents. However, if you feel it would be too distressing, you can suggest to parents that it might be best for children to say goodbye beforehand.

It may help to have some information for children to read (with parental consent). There are many good books available: *Megan's Journey* by Janet Peel and *The Invisible Leash* by Patrice Karst are two such books. Children want to know what happens and are naturally curious, but should be protected from the negative side of euthanasia. It can be traumatic for an adult to witness and potentially more so for a child. Children may benefit from a leaflet that explains the euthanasia process and helps to answer any questions. The parents should decide whether this is provided.

With the parents' consent, you may wish to offer the child something they can keep to remember their pet by, such as a lock of fur or the pet's collar.

Elderly clients

Elderly clients' pets may also be old and suffer from age-related illness. They may have had difficulty coming to the practice or may have required home visits. The circumstances surrounding how a pet was acquired will have an impact on the owner's reaction to the loss; the pet may have been the last living link to a deceased spouse or relative. Some pets are bought or adopted to fill an, empty nest, once children leave home. It may be that the pet was taken on as a companion for someone who would otherwise have no one in their life. Pets can become a reason to live; they give people purpose. They are a reason to get up in the morning, a social icebreaker and a companion. When such a pet dies, the owner is going back to an empty house, alone and grief stricken.

When we speak to elderly clients, we should be respectful, and speak to them as we would anyone else. You may find that their hearing is not what it was so, if your normal tone and level is not initiating a response, then raise your voice accordingly. Do not treat your client like a child; they may be older, but they should not be infantilized. They may have brought in a companion that has been by their side for years and it is likely they have been through a lot together.

Losing a pet when elderly may make an owner consider their own mortality; they have seen friends and family pass and seen their pet grow old with them. Some elderly clients may be set in their ways, with old-fashioned beliefs about what is best for their pet. Some clients may have left their pet for too long before seeking veterinary help, but this may be due to lack of knowledge of QOL or because they have had no external support to bring in the pet sooner.

Some elderly clients may be struggling financially and this will have an impact on their grief as they may wish to choose a cremation option that is financially unavailable to them. Therefore, it is important to ensure that all cremation options are listed with current prices attached and that staff try to recommend a suitable option.

How to provide a positive euthanasia experience

We are not taught how to be empathetic and caring during euthanasia appointments or what to do to try and comfort distraught clients: we all learn over time. We should take pride in the service we provide to clients when many are at their most vulnerable.

Euthanasia must be offered with care. It is a decision to be made between the veterinary surgeon and client and is not simply based on science. We must provide supportive care to clients, showing sympathy and empathy for the difficult decision they are facing. Treat each owner and their pet as individuals; respect their intense bond and try to make their experience unique.

The veterinary team should be sympathetic and convey empathy to the client. Do not be openly judgmental or uncomfortable with the decision, unless you are certain you will not euthanase the animal. Discomfort from the veterinary team can lead to profound guilt and prolong the grieving process.

It is the veterinary surgeon's role to explain and discuss euthanasia with the client but, in reality, some clients find it difficult to raise the subject with the veterinary surgeon or ask questions. The rest of the team should always be approachable and on hand to answer any questions clients may have. Palliative care/bereavement clinics can be a great way for clients to feel they have made an informed decision, and the aim of these is to prepare the client for the impending loss by providing support, trust and reassurance that they are doing the right thing. Some clients need to repeatedly clarify QOL indicators, which can be addressed in these dedicated clinics rather than in a short consultation. Qality-of-life scoring systems (see above) can be very helpful for these clients.

Prior to the euthanasia appointment

Euthanasia appointments should be booked during quiet periods where possible. An appointment at the end or beginning of the surgery allows the owner and their pet the ambiance they deserve. Sick animals are vulnerable and easily stressed by busy/noisy situations. It also helps to ensure that the veterinary surgeon is not rushed and can dedicate some time to the client and their animal, and the owner has the time they need to say goodbye. Home visits should be accommodated wherever possible.

Make sure that euthanasia appointments are clearly identified in the diary, as the owner will have been building up to this and will not appreciate a cheery "hello"! A kind and empathetic greeting is far more respectful. Remember to be courteous in reception – no laughing or unprofessional conversation should be heard (this goes for reception in general, not just when dealing with euthanasia).

It is important to suggest that the client makes arrangements to have someone accompany them and drive, if possible. They may not expect to need it, but owners are often overwhelmed by the strength of their emotions. This can be dangerous and may cause an avoidable accident, so they should be asked to give this option consideration. Owners should be invited to bring a favourite toy or blanket to go with their pet at the time of the cremation. Try to give the client the name of a member of staff who is familiar with their history, who they trust and can contact with any questions during the lead-up to a planned euthanasia. Just knowing there is someone there to put their mind at ease can be of great comfort.

Make sure all notes are up to date with any relevant information and any decisions/preferences the client may have with regards to euthanasia. A video on the euthanasia process and what to expect, can really help clients prepare mentally; it is a good idea to make one and put it on your practice website to direct people to. Some great examples of practice videos can be found on YouTube.

Arriving for the euthanasia appointment

If it is possible, greet the client as they arrive in the car park and then help them through to the consulting room. If the animal is large, has poor mobility or the client is taking the body for cremation following euthanasia, offer to euthanase the animal in the car.

If you have an available consulting room free when the client arrives, take the client and their animal through rather than sitting them down in a busy waiting room; it can be very distressing for the owner to be surrounded by others. Try to make the client's last memories of their pet and the situation surrounding them as comforting as possible.

Make sure there is a comfortable bed for the animal to sit on and that there are tissues available, and ask whether the client would like a glass of water if they are very distressed. Clients will remember this personal touch and will pass it on to others when reliving their ordeal. Ask the client if they would like to be present during the euthanasia or if they would prefer to wait somewhere quiet. If space is available, a dedicated bereavement room can be a beneficial addition to the practice (Figure 8.6).

At the euthanasia appointment

Walk in with a gentle smile and greet the pet with a positive statement such as 'Hello handsome boy/girl'. It is possible people have been telling the owner for a while how unwell their pet looks, so it is good for them to hear something positive. Try and say positive things, rather than negative phrases like 'it doesn't hurt' or 'he won't be in pain', which can lead the client to overthink the process.

Some clients can get quite offended when a nurse accompanies the veterinary surgeon into the consulting room to hold their animal, as they can feel that this is a violation of their last few moments with their pet. A clear explanation of the process can mitigate this. Where possible, allow the client to hold their animal with the nurse on hand to steady the back end of the pet and raise the vein.

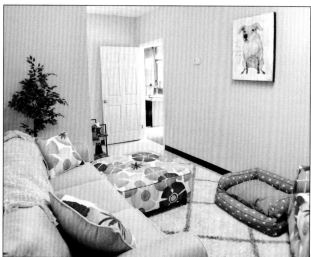

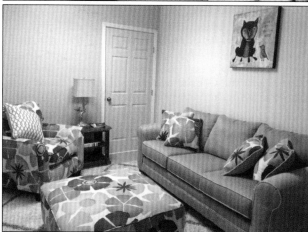

An example of a bereavement room.

The last 15 to 30 minutes the owner has with their animal while it is alive are often the most remembered and precious. If you decide to place an intravenous catheter, consider doing so in the room with the owner, rather than moving the pet to another room.

Discussing the procedure and reassuring the owner are very important. Every client will cope differently: some will want a detailed explanation, whilst others will want it over quickly, but knowing what to expect can prevent a nasty lasting memory and thus allow them to pass through the stages of grief more smoothly and prevent them getting stuck in the guilt stage. Do not be frightened – owners would rather be warned than be unaware. Euthanasia can be extremely distressing and upsetting to see if they are not fully briefed and, in all cases, this prolongs and worsens the grieving process. Explain that euthanasia means 'good death' and that the medication is an overdose of anaesthesia, from which the pet goes to sleep and dies.

Make sure the client is aware of the following:

- That the animal will not close its eyes fully
- That they may gasp as the diaphragm contracts
- That they may twitch or stretch out as the body shuts down
- That they may urinate or defecate as the muscles of the body relax
- That, depending on the reason for euthanasia, on some occasions, the animal may leak a little fluid from its nose.

Explain that if the animal is very stressed or aggressive, we may need to use sedation and that this lowers the blood pressure, so finding a vein can sometimes be a little trickier. There have been some awfully upsetting situations where the veterinary surgeon cannot find a vein and has had to use intracardiac injection.

If you are shaving the animal's foreleg for venous access, ask the client if they would like a little of the hair in a bag for them to keep. Ask the owner to 'keep talking to her/him'. This takes attention away from what you are doing and keeps their focus on their pet. Ask the client if they are happy for you to proceed. There is nothing worse than an owner who was not ready being distressed that their pet has gone before they were expecting it. Once the animal has died and the veterinary surgeon has checked that the heart has stopped, it is important to know when to respect the silence.

When the client is ready, comfort them with a gentle touch on the hand or shoulder; this displays more empathy than words will. Do not conceal any emotion you feel; when clients see that we grieve with them, their emotions become less overwhelming. Ask them if they would like some time on their own with their pet and try to make sure that the area is kept as quiet as possible. If the animal is staying on the premises, tell the client that you will take good care of their pet. This will help reassure them and make them feel more comfortable in leaving.

Once the client is ready to leave, escort them out, using an alternative exit if available; this shows empathy towards their feelings.

A bereavement pack with signposting for counselling services may be a useful resource (Figure 8.7).

After the euthanasia appointment

Follow up the next day with a courtesy call to see if they would like to discuss anything and ak how they are coping. During the grieving process, clients will often need

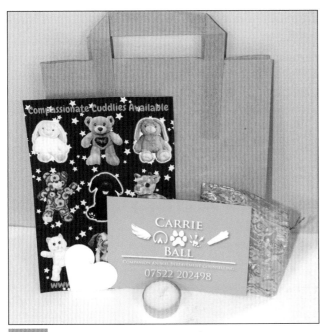

8.7 An example of a bereavement pack.

to repeatedly talk about their pet's death and the circumstances surrounding it. They are far more likely to move though the grief cycle without getting stuck in the guilt and anger phases if they are able to talk about their feelings and concerns. They may just need a reassuring friendly ear to share some memories of their beloved animal.

Condolence cards should be sent in all cases. Make sure that each condolence card is personally written and unique to the animal. Some clients have had multiple pets euthanased over time and have received multiple generic cards. When they receiveed the first card the sentiment and empathy was welcomed, but upon receiving the same card on subsequent occasions, they felt hurt and angry.

Post-mortem examinations

Talking to a grieving client about performing a post-mortem examination/necropsy is difficult but important. It must be handled sensitively, by explaining to the client that a post-mortem examination could be advantageous to look for a cause of death/disease.

A post-mortem examination does not always have to be an invasive procedure. The phrase 'post-mortem' alone can conjure up negative images for clients and worries that their beloved pet will be opened and pulled about and have pieces removed without care. As veterinary professionals, we know that this is far from the truth, that the patient will be treated with respect and the only parts excised will be areas of interest that give cause for concern. Many clients are very scared and upset by the idea when, in reality, it could be as simple as just taking a small sample of liver to send for rabbit haemorrhagic disease testing. Of course, it will not change the outcome for the patient but it may save a bonded partner or larger collection, if a contagious disease is suspected.

When undertaking a post-mortem examination, it is very important to gain informed consent from the client. The RCVS has produced detailed guidance on this subject. This includes guidance on written/oral consent, contractual relationships, confirming the client has understood what

has been said, mental incapacity, dealing with young people and children, and consent forms.

The client's expectations must also be managed, and it may be that a post-mortem examination is undertaken but the results are inconclusive; this must be clearly explained to the client so that it does not come as a shock.

How to approach a client about a post-mortem examination

As when euthanasia is broached, clients may react badly because they do not know exactly what to expect, or do not understand the purpose of the post-mortem examination or what will happen to their pet afterwards. Common questions include:

- Will I get my pet's body back?
- Will I be able to have them cremated or buried?
- What happens during the examination?
- Will they be treated with care?

It is difficult to ease the fears of a client who may be imagining their pet in pieces on a cold steel table. However, we can help to ease their minds by explaining the process, what to expect from us, and why the examination is so important.

In some cases, returning the body following post-mortem examination is not advised. For example, if the pet has to be tested for rabies the patient will be decapitated and the head and brain sent to a laboratory. The practice may offer cremation of the patient and return of the ashes to the client. In this circumstance, it may be best to inform the client of the fact that the brain has to be tested. Some clients may understand what that entails without further explanation, but some may want or need a clearer description and you may have to break the news that the head must be separated from the body. It is best to omit this information if possible as there is no nice way to explain that you must cut off the head of a pet.

There may be a legal obligation to perform a post-mortem examination, in which case the client has no say or chance to consent to the procedure. This may be the case with aggression towards humans (possible rabies) or after other extreme behaviours.

Explaining your reasoning may help a client to come to terms with and readily consent to the procedure. If a condition that may affect other pets in the household is suspected, then the client must be informed.

Let the client know that whilst this death was unfortunate and distressing, there may be a chance that they could prevent further losses if the post-mortem examination goes ahead. It would be best not to allow the client to pin their hopes on this; it may be that no satisfying answer is produced, but if we do not investigate, we will never know.

Clients themselves may request a post-mortem examination to settle their own minds as to what the cause of their pet's death was. You may agree and have your own curiosity about what happened. You may feel this procedure is unnecessary, and then must either dissuade the client from going ahead or perform a procedure that would not answer any query you had not already answered. Veterinary staff must always be mindful that they are communicating with the client in a manner that is professional but compassionate. This is a family pet, someone's companion, and not just an interesting case to research.

How to assist grieving clients

The most important thing we can do is reassure the owner that the emotions they are feeling are a completely normal, natural response to grief. Take the time to understand what role their pet played in their life. Open the door to communication; good communication can improve client retention and prevent complaints/possible perceived malpractice.

Take the time to listen to the griever's deepest concerns and be patient with their story. Allow the griever to share memories of the deceased pet. Share resources that can be a useful form of support such as books, support websites and helpline numbers. Seek medical help if you are concerned for your client's safety or that of others.

Have a bereavement policy in place that staff can refer to. Know where your role ends; refer your clients on to a bereavement counsellor if they seem to be stuck in the grief cycle.

Dos and don'ts

Below are some **dos** and **don'ts** to advise clients following an animal bereavement.

Do:

- Express your emotions to someone
- Accept opportunities to share your experiences with others; they may have something to offer.

Don't:

- Bottle up your feelings
- Avoid talking about what happened
- Be too hard on yourself; you may need time to adjust to what has happened.

Positive coping actions

- **Increasing contact with family and friends.**
- **Starting an exercise programme** – exercise, even in moderation, has a number of positive benefits. Walking, jogging and swimming all reduce physical tension and distract the individual from painful memories or worries.

Negative coping actions

- **Use of alcohol or drugs** – this may wash away memories, increase confidence and induce sleep, but it can cause more problems than it cures by creating a dependence.
- **Social isolation** – by reducing contact with other people may avoid situations that make them feel afraid or force them to acknowledge loss. Isolation will cause major problems, resulting in a loss of social support and friendship.
- **Continuous avoidance** – avoidance of thinking about unpleasant events or about the fact that additional help may be needed keeps away distress but prevents progress in coping with the trauma.

Make a thought diary

Clients may find it useful to write down their thoughts, emotions and reactions regarding the traumatic event so in time they can look back on them and reflect on their feelings. This can also be particularly helpful if they seek some form of further help such as counselling.

Appropriate ways to handle someone who is grieving

Figure 8.4 lists some of the phrases it is appropriate to use during the grieving process.

- 'I wish I had the right words, just know I care' – this shows the person you care and is better than saying the wrong thing.
- Give a hug instead of saying something – a comforting gesture conveys more empathy than words ever will.
- Always listen first (ALF) – 80% listening; 20% talking.

Inappropriate things to say to someone who is grieving

Avoid clichés – pet owners realize that the animal is no longer in pain and that they had a happy life. These examples do not offer any comfort; a simple 'I'm sorry for your loss' is more than enough. Often all a bereaved owner needs or wants is someone unbiased to listen to them. Figure 8.5 details some of the phrases that should be avoided.

- Do not tell someone how they feel – despite your knowledge and experience, you will never really know how someone is feeling regarding their grief unless they tell you.
- 'There is a reason for everything' – we have to be careful not to make assumptions and when you lose something you love it is difficult to hear this. Instead give the bereaved some space to find their own answers.
- 'Aren't you over him/her yet' – people never get over losing a loved one, even an animal, but they learn with time to live with the loss.
- 'You can get another one' – a lot of owners do not want to think of immediately getting another animal; this can be very upsetting.

Supporting bonded animals

It has been widely documented that non-human animals show what we believe to be signs of grief. Whilst they may not react in the same way humans do, they do seem to show some awareness that their companion has died. Some animals will mourn, pine, go off their food and/or show no interest in activities that normally bring pleasure. We may say that they appear to be depressed and even though it is easy to anthropomorphize their experiences the evidence seems to support the idea that they feel a sense of loss. As veterinary professionals, we can help and support our clients to recognize and understand the signs a bonded animal may be grieving following the loss of their companion.

Common signs to look for:

- Sleep pattern disturbance
- Changes in toileting habits
- Changes in appetite/weight loss
- Searching for the companion
- Whining or crying
- Attention-seeking behaviour
- Separation anxiety
- Lost or sad demeanour
- Changes in temperament.

Measures that can help a grieving animal:

- Keeping their routine the same
- Avoiding stress
- Avoiding changes to their environment
- Leaving the other animal's bedding and toys in place for a while following the death
- Using a species-specific pheromone diffuser in the house
- Encouraging positive calm behaviour.

It is widely accepted that animals can benefit from seeing their deceased animal companion following their death. There are obvious exceptions to this, for example, if the animal has died of a contagious disease or if they pose a risk to the living animal or owner.

If an animal is to be buried in the owner's garden, it is important to ensure that the living pet does not see the burial place, as they may try to dig their companion up.

Dogs

Clients may report that after the loss of a companion, the dog that is left behind exhibits signs of mourning. They may vocalize (perhaps calling for their companion), become inappetent or be unwilling to engage in activities they would normally enjoy, akin to grief in humans.

Medical causes should always be ruled out initially, especially if the companion that died from something potentially contagious or congenital, or as a result of something environmental that others may have been in contact with. If there is no medical cause it is reasonable to assume that the dog is indeed grieving the loss of their companion and they need support.

It may be necessary to develop new routines to adjust to the loss, for example different walking routes, changing the times of exercising or changing meal times. This is done to try to take the remaining dog's mind off the fact their companion is missing. However, some dogs may need the stability of the routine they have always had and so it would be best to support them in some other way. Pheromone and essential oil diffusers can have a positive effect in helping dogs to cope with upheaval in the home.

There are differing opinions as to whether more attention should be offered to a dog that appears to be grieving. Some suggest that it encourages unwanted behaviour and increases the likelihood of separation anxiety. However, grief is recognized as an emotional response rather than simply a behavioural change; therefore, what would probably be more helpful is to give attention, comfort, rewards and reassurance. Separation anxiety is an understandable response in a dog that has seen a companion leave and not return.

If possible, it may be helpful to let an animal see the body of their companion. This seems to provide a form of what humans would call closure. They can investigate the corpse to satisfy themselves that their companion cannot be roused and that they smell and look different, and this helps them to carry on with their lives. They may be withdrawn for a while, but at least we have removed the uncertainty from their loss.

Cats

Cats can and do live quite happily in multi-cat households, but they have subtle interactions that we as humans may not fully appreciate. For example, when a cat from a multi-cat household dies, surviving cats that were seemingly reserved may become more playful, outgoing and affectionate. This is not to say that they were necessarily unhappy when their housemate was alive, and it may help to tell owners this.

For those cats who seem to withdraw when they lose a companion, it may be that the deceased cat was the more confident animal and it may help to tell owners this.

Social small mammals

Small social animals such as guinea pigs and rabbits benefit from observing and investigating the body of a deceased companion. It may be less stressful for them to realize for themselves what happened and that their mate has not suddenly disappeared; these animals are naturally prey species and so a sudden disappearance of a companion may cause unnecessary instinctive stress. There is evidence that rabbits should be given 3–6 hours alone with the body of their bonded companion. As the hours pass, the owner may observe a change in the rabbit's behaviour, as they realize their companion has died. Similar behaviour can be observed in guinea pigs.

The introduction of another companion may help, especially if the loss has left them on their own. Careful introductions must be made as bonding can take time.

Horses

Horses and other equids have been known to investigate the bodies of stablemates or other known individuals when they die by nudging with a hoof, biting, pushing and pulling. Vocalizing is also common – it seems they try every way possible to make their companion get up. When this does not work, they realize that their companion has died and react accordingly.

Some horses can become quite withdrawn and 'depressed'. As herd animals they may be concerned that there is danger about, or it may be that they just miss their companion. Owners often place the rug of a deceased stablemate over the door of the surviving animal's stable so that they can smell it and stay with it until they have 'accepted' the death.

Non-domesticated species

Non-domesticated species of animals have shown that they are aware of death and that they can respond to the loss of a companion. For most wild animals, reactions seem to be based more on the survival of the group rather than grief. This is not to say that they do not appreciate that they have lost a member, but that there is no time to mourn, and group survival depends on moving forwards. Examples of potential grieving behaviours by non-domesticated animals include:

- Elephants have been known to stroke the bones of other elephants and they have been recorded acting in a manner which, if human, would be sad and mournful (e.g. heads hung low, slow movements)
- Primates have been shown to react badly to the loss of a family member. Jane Goodall documented the case of Flynn, a wild chimpanzee who lost his mother Flo. He went off his food, searched all the places his mother was normally found and eventually succumbed to illness due to malnutrition and neglect
- Corvids have been observed to hold almost funeral-like rituals when they come across a dead individual, and other birds such as ducks and swans have been known to die shortly after the loss of a mate or family member (Cudmore, 2015).

Evidence that non-human animals, and especially fellow mammals, show signs of grief or at least acknowledgement of death, highlights that we should do more for bereaved animals in our care and support them through their losses.

Reptiles and invertebrates

The brain formations of reptiles and invertebrates are very different to the mammalian brain and they lack structures linked to emotional grieving responses in the latter. Their focus seems to be on their basic needs of survival.

Supporting veterinary professionals

There is a tendency to focus solely on client support when discussing pet bereavement, but we must not forget to identify when we as professionals also need help. We frequently act as a listening ear/shoulder to cry on for our clients and their emotions, and in time the toll of this burden may become unbearable. Sadly, there is a high incidence of suicide within the veterinary profession. It is important that staff feel supported at all times. Staff should be able to voice their feelings and concerns to their colleagues without feeling intimidated or judged. We are regularly exposed to traumatic situations and events and expected to cope and carry on. At times, we have to follow up a euthanasia by putting a smile on to see the next appointment. Sometimes, we push our emotions down so that we can move through the day. But identifying the need and asking for help must be embraced across the veterinary profession, and we should lean on each other for emotional support. At the end of the day, we are all human and can only take so much before we reach breaking point, and there is no shame in asking for help. See Chapter 10 for more information on support for the veterinary team and the 'Useful websites' section at the end of this chapter for contact details of support groups mentioned in this chapter.

There are several good support groups on social media: The Unity Community on Facebook is one and there is also a support group for veterinary and zoo workers who see loss on a regular basis and need somewhere to talk to others in the profession. The Pet Bereavement Support for Vet Staff Facebook group is another safe place to talk to other professionals about the losses faced and to help others by listening and understanding.

Vetlife provides an independent, confidential and professional free helpline for the whole veterinary community, with 24/7 phone and email help. They can help with a wide range of issues, such as employment worries, compassion fatigue, stress and depression, performance anxiety, financial issues, and complaints. They provide financial help to veterinary surgeons, veterinary nurses and their dependants. The British Veterinary Nursing Association (BVNA) also has a helpline that deals with legal and employment advice and can signpost for other queries. The BVNA's Daphne Shipman fund can provide financial assistance to their members (including for students, registered veterinary nurses and associates. This information should be displayed in a prominent place in every practice, making sure all staff are aware of the service. If you or a colleague feel as though you require help, don't delay – there is no shame in asking for or seeking support.

Regular debriefings may be beneficial, especially if there have been a lot of losses in a short space of time. It is important to ensure that you know your team, that you know who may need support, and that your team know who or where to go to when needed.

Training

There is no excuse for poor or lack of end-of-life support for clients. There are numerous resources and courses that are readily available to help staff to help their clients. One such provider is Innovet CPD Training. Innovet CPD Training is a company that offers a wide range of continuing professional development courses for all members of the veterinary team, including the The Pet Loss and Bereavement Support Advisor course, which states: "Grief affects people's mental health and general wellbeing and it is our responsibility to be able to recognise when a client requires our validation of loss and further support" (Innovet CPD Training, 2022). This course helps teams to provide more proactive compassionate care, to have a deeper understanding of the bereavement stages, to spot the early signs of compassion fatigue and ease the emotional trauma and the resulting client loss. Veterinary staff that have attended or undertaken this course have described how it helped them both personally and professionally. No one inately knows exactly how to support people in varying emotional states. It is something that you learn to do, growing and adjusting the support with experience.

If you are unsure how to support a client then there are resources available that will help you to help them, giving you the tools you need to support your client from first phone call to their pet's last breath and beyond. The loss of a patient affects everyone in some way and, from a business point of view, poor handling of patient loss can lead to client attrition.

Covid-19

For many clients that lost their animals during 2020 and 2021, the Covid-19 pandemic had a profound impact on their grief. Losing a beloved animal at any time can be traumatic and distressing, but these feelings can be heightened by the helplessness and isolation associated with social restrictions enforced during a pandemic. This means that for many clients their grief became more intense. The social isolation that we all experienced may have served as a reminder of their loss. In addition, the loss of routine associated with a beloved animal can fuel grief, as can the loss of general routine caused by a lockdown.

During the Covid-19 pandemic, the risk of suffering complicated bereavement or post-traumatic stress disorder was much higher as a result of the social isolation and the fact that clients may not have been able to access their usual veterinary services or to say goodbye to their pet in the way they would have liked.

Complicated grief
- Persistent focus on the loss
- Intense, daily longing
- Feeling that life is meaningless
- Replaying aspects of death in mind
- Intense attachment or rejection of reminders
- Bitterness and anger at the world ▶

Post-traumatic stress disorder

- Intense flashbacks
- Recurring nightmares
- Sensory experiences that trigger trauma
- Unwelcome thoughts
- Paranoia and fear
- Anxiety
- Jumpiness

References and further reading

Ball C (2017) *The Last Visit.: A Guide for Veterinary Staff.* CreateSpace Independent Publishing Platform, Amazon

Cudmore B (2015) *Do birds grieve?* Available from: www.audubon.org/news/do-birds-grieve

Innovet CPD Training (2022) *Pet Loss and Bereavement Support Advisor CPD Course.* Available from: www.innovet-cpd.co.uk

Kübler-Ross E (2014) *On Death & Dying: What the Dying Have to Teach Doctors, Nurses, Clergy & Their Own Families.* Scribner Book Company, New York

Sife W (2014) *The Loss of a Pet: A Guide to Coping with the Grieving Process When a Pet Dies, 4th edn.* Howell Book House, New York

Useful websites

Alzheimer's Society
www.alzheimers.org.uk
0333 150 3456

Animal Bereavement Counselling
animalbereavementcounselling.com
07522 202498

Association of Private Pet Cemeteries and Crematoria
appcc.org.uk
01252 844478

Blue Cross Pet Bereavement and Pet Loss
www.bluecross.org.uk/pet-bereavement-and-pet-loss
0800 096 6606

British Veterinary Nursing Association
bvna.org.uk
(Helpline available to members)

Emily Holmes – The Empowering RVN
theempoweringrvn.co.uk
support@theempoweringrvn.co.uk

Guide Dogs – Coping with the loss of your dog
www.guidedogs.org.uk/getting-support/information-and-advice/family-support/coping-with-the-loss-of-your-dog

National Autistic Society – Bereavement
www.autism.org.uk/advice-and-guidance/topics/mental-health/bereavement
0808 800 4104

Pet Bereavement Services
www.petbereavementservices.co.uk
01252 411775

Pet Bereavement Support for vet staff
www.facebook.com/groups/cballpetlosssupport

Samaritans
www.samaritans.org
116 123

Vetlife
www.vetlife.org.uk
0303 040 2551

Following the loss of a pet, some clients may have associated safety measures and lockdown restrictions with their suffering, as they were unable to access their normal veterinary service for their pet at the end. The policies and processes made necessary due to Covid-19 were understandably distressing, but there are things we can still do as veterinary professionals to help give our clients a positive euthanasia experience while abiding by such restrictions, whether imposed by Covid-19 or a future incident.

Sadly, there were instances during the pandemic where clients were asked to stay outside while their pet was euthanased. If you ever have a strict 'no owners inside the practice' policy, then consider whether it would be possible to offer euthanasia outside or in the owner's car. This is obviously not ideal, but it can be an option if all the appropriate personal protective equipment (PPE) is being used. A home visit and using the owner's back garden, if they have one, is an alternative option. It may also be possible to adhere to social distancing rules by allowing one owner into the practice to accompany their pet during euthanasia. Of course, they must be wearing the appropriate PPE.

The most important thing is to be compassionate and understanding to clients' feelings at all times. It should still be possible to give your clients time with their pets following euthanasia and this should always be encouraged.

Impact statement

Louise Etheridge

Losing my dear cat Lilly has been one of the most painful experiences I've been through in life. Like everyone, I've had my fair share of struggles and heartbreak, but in terms of loss and grief, it has certainly been the most painful to date.

Having made it to her 22nd birthday and some, and with a number of worsening health problems, I knew deep down that our time together was coming to an end, but somehow I was not remotely prepared for her death or the tidal wave of all-consuming grief that would engulf me, sucking me under into its vortex. Indeed, the physical manifestations of grief felt like a spinning sensation, much like being pulled into a whirlpool. The force of the bereavement did not reveal itself straight away; in the immediate aftermath of loss and in a state of shock, I was simply going through the motions, trying my best to deal with the practical side of arrangements and keep prior work and social commitments. Death doesn't wait for the right moment; it is unabashed in its thoughtlessness, impertinence and inconvenience.

It wasn't until around a week or two following Lilly's passing, after I'd had a chance to be still for a moment and after her ashes were returned to me, that the immensity of her loss really hit. I was completely wracked by self-doubt and became stuck in a seemingly endless cycle of punitive thinking; questioning and obsessing over what I could have done better, imagining different possible outcomes. I became trapped in this cycle of self-blame and self-loathing, constantly ruminating over all the things I believed I had done 'wrong' in managing Lilly's care and quality of life. In the grip of bereavement, grief had managed to convince me I was the worst owner ever, despite the fact I had been told by the two vets I consulted that I was a very diligent owner, that 'letting go' of Lilly had been the right thing for her, and even though everyone around me was telling me that I had done the best I could. But grief does not listen to reason and told me otherwise: I was a terrible caretaker and I should have fought harder for Lilly.

My state of mind was so poor that a friend and her mother decided to carry out an 'intervention' on me and encouraged me to get some help. They were so concerned they even offered a financial contribution to help me

continues ▶

Impact statement *continued*

on this path. I was very lucky to have people like this around me. Unfortunately, the backdrop to my bereavement was, and still is, a very stressful period of my life and the loss only served to push me over the edge of reason.

The intrusive thoughts persisted. Rather than subside, they fed one another, clamouring to be heard. No sooner had I come to a resolution on one of them, than another would immediately arrive to replace it, castigating me for imagined wrongs. Mornings were the worst; it got to the point that I was waking up every day wishing I wasn't alive and longing to be reunited with Lilly, even though I'm not sure that I believe in an afterlife. After a couple of weeks of this mental torture, I finally decided I could not live this way, I had to seek help.

I found Lisa's details through the Ralph site, which had been recommended by one of the vets I had consulted. I was immediately drawn to her profile because of her experience as a veterinary nurse. On a rational level (it still existed somewhere), I knew much of my grief was tied up in what I could have done differently to prolong Lilly's life, rather than simply acknowledging that she was a very elderly cat with multiple health problems. I knew I needed someone who would not only be able to assist me in opening up about my grief, but who would also have a good understanding about the veterinary perspective on the events that culminated in Lilly's death. I felt if I could demystify some of my irrational beliefs around her passing (again, on some level I knew they were irrational), I might be able to make peace with the situation.

Having to make the decision to euthanase a creature you love, your companion and ward, is one of the most difficult and painful decisions to make in life. It is counterintuitive to everything else you have done to protect them, make them comfortable and give them the best quality of life you can. It feels like a terrible betrayal and is accompanied by immense guilt. I immediately regretted it the day after. Of course, in hindsight, there was no other choice. Prolonging her life at that stage would have only been to prolong her suffering, but the grief would not allow me to see that at the time. Only acceptance and healing has allowed me that clarity.

Attending the pet bereavement counselling with Lisa offered me a safe space to air all of these unwanted and intrusive thoughts and finally start to challenge the irrational beliefs that I was holding on to. I had been trying to conceal the depth of my grief from those around me. I felt they might judge me because I was grieving for an animal. Although we are a nation of animal lovers, our society still tells us that it is somehow less acceptable to deeply grieve the loss of a pet, that it is perhaps slightly self-indulgent. I believed they wouldn't understand, and indeed, although most people were very sympathetic, a minority of those around me did not really understand. The words and actions, or inactions, of those few cut very deep at the time.

With Lisa's support I was able to express and explore all of my self-doubts around Lilly's death, as well as my decisions and the care I had provided for her. She assured me that my feelings were completely normal and that many people experiencing the loss of a pet go through a very similar cycle of grief. By having a dedicated space where I didn't feel judged, over time I was able to start to challenge these unhelpful thoughts and to free myself of them. Over a period of around 2 and a half months, these loud and powerful thoughts gradually loosened their hold on me and I began to come to a place of acceptance. I knew I was better when I finally managed to reach the conclusion that I was in fact glad that Lilly no longer had to suffer in her tiny, frail and broken body. She was finally released from all of the pain that she had surely been quietly bearing.

Lisa also introduced me to the idea that I could hold a memorial service for Lilly. I didn't receive the best after-life care from my vet surgery. Although I believe they tried the best they could, being a small practice, they offered a very limited service. Not having the opportunity to access some of the services I now know are on offer also fed into my grief. Realising that I still had the opportunity, even after several months, to mark Lilly's life, made me feel much better about the situation. I'm currently planning a memorial service for her so I can say my goodbyes in a way that's more serene, less rushed.

Writing this, I don't know what my mental state would currently be if I hadn't had the good fortune to find Lisa and embark on a course of pet bereavement counselling. I went from feeling that life wasn't worth living to slowly piecing my life back together. I still experience moments of grief and guilt, it doesn't really leave you, but I now know that they are just thoughts and are generally fleeting.

Grief is a ruthless and relentless beast; it plays tricks on your mind, it desperately wants the outcome to be different and tries in vain to rewrite the course of history. But we cannot change what has gone before and we cannot prolong life beyond what is possible or out of our control. However, understanding our grief and making peace with it is part of the journey to acceptance, and ultimately, recovery.

Chapter 9

One Health

Matthew Rendle and Becky Jones

Introduction

The basic concept of One Health is that the health of people, animals and the environment are intrinsically linked at a local, national and global level (Figure 9.1). Adopting a collaborative, multidisciplinary approach can achieve optimal health for all. It is a concept that has gained momentum in recent years, but this way of thinking is not novel; there are references dating back to ancient times, such as the Greek physician Hippocrates, who acknowledged that human health depended on the environment. The German pathologist Dr Rudolph Virchow first used the term 'zoonosis' in the 19th century in reference to an infectious disease that could be passed between humans and animals. Other notable figures that have contributed to this movement include William Osler, Robert Koch and James Steele. It is, however, Dr Calvin Schwabe who is credited with coining the term 'One Medicine', stating a need for medical and veterinary collaboration when dealing with zoonotic diseases. The evolution of this term to 'One Health' was a response to the impact of a rapidly growing human population and accelerating changes to the ecosystem. Notably, it was the link between these and the growing number of emerging and re-emerging infectious diseases that established the One Health concept as the advocated approach to addressing these threats.

The human–animal–ecosystem interface

The world's population is growing by 1.1% annually – approximately 83 million people – and is expected to reach 11.2 billion in 2100. Within this growing population is an increase in the ageing and vulnerable, who are more susceptible to disease and ill health. The ageing population currently accounts for 12.3% of the global population and this is expected to rise to 22% by 2050. The exponential growth of the human population has also led to an increase in food animal and companion animal populations. Food animal population growth is impacting livestock management and leading to more intensive farming and increased deforestation. It is also causing a lack of genetic diversity, increasing potential for disease outbreaks.

Expanding urbanization and the global movement of both humans and animals is increasing contact between humans, domestic animals and wildlife with a growing impingement on natural areas, in turn increasing the spread of infectious diseases and disrupting the ecosystem (Figure 9.2). Biodiversity underpins all life on earth and the loss of plant and animal species is having significant consequences for the health of all; the protective effect of biodiversity is being lost. Pollution, climate change and natural disasters are also having a significant impact; increasing temperatures and fluctuating rainfall are affecting food supplies, leading to increased vulnerability to disease.

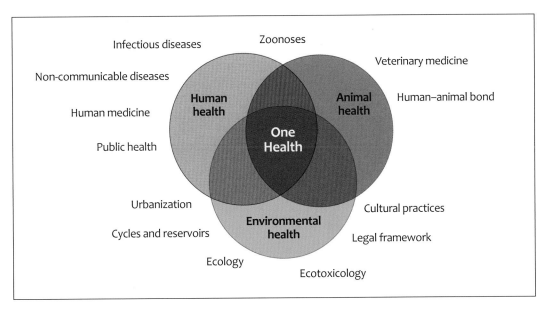

9.1 The One Health concept.
(Redrawn after Destoumieux-Garzón et al., 2018)

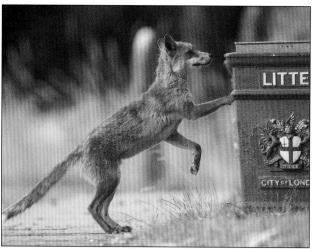

9.2 Red foxes are frequently studied as they are a wildlife reservoir for several important diseases of humans and domestic animals, including the rabies virus and the fox tapeworm (*Echinococcus multilocularis*) in continental Europe.
(Jamie Hall/Shutterstock.com)

These factors are also affecting the population and distribution of many species and have created a perfect opportunity for microorganisms to adapt and cross species lines. This potentially means that microorganisms could infect humans directly, negating the need for another species to act as a host. Added to this is the increasing threat of antimicrobial resistance in these pathogens.

The situation is evolving so rapidly that the infrastructures needed to manage the increasing threat are not up to date, contributing to this complex challenge and highlighting further the need for the collaborative and multidisciplinary approach of One Health.

Infectious disease is still very much the driver for the One Health agenda but there is also a focus on other global issues: food safety and food security, climate change, antimicrobial resistance, and ecosystem health. The lack of a formal definition for One Health means that there are different interpretations of the concept. As awareness and adoption of the concept grows, so too does the scope of issues considered to be relevant (Figure 9.3). The definition of health has expanded to encompass mental health and welfare as well as disease. All groups of

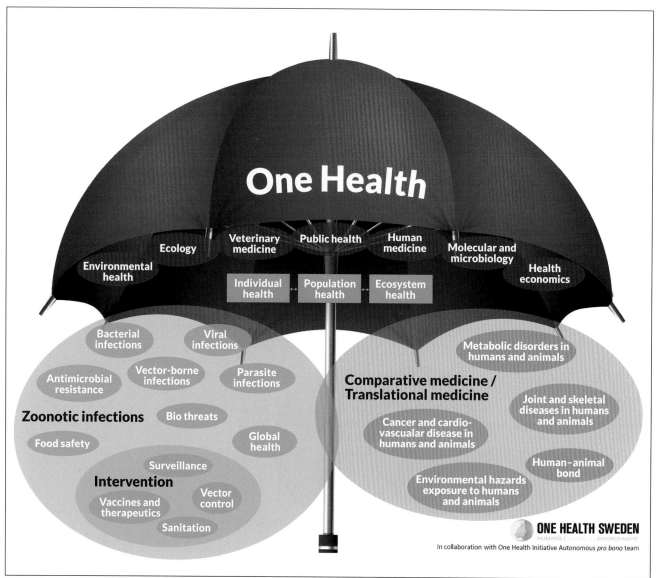

9.3 The One Health Umbrella highlights the breadth of factors to be considered when taking a holistic approach to human, animal and environmental health.
(© One Health Sweden in collaboration with the One Health Initiative)

animals – livestock, wildlife and companion animals – are now included within this triad, with the environment encompassing anywhere that these animals and people meet across the world. We are all existing in a complex and interdependent relationship.

The opportunities presented through collaborations under this umbrella are vast but often there is a bias towards the benefits for the 'human' component of this triad. For One Health to be truly beneficial for all, it is critical that the needs of the animals and the environment are also fully considered. It is important that this collaboration promotes the ability to better understand issues from all perspectives; to be able to act and implement change, fully acknowledging the benefits and implications for all involved.

Global One Health issues

Zoonoses and emerging/re-emerging infectious diseases

Many factors (see Figure 9.1) contribute to the increasing threat of infectious disease. New diseases continue to emerge and old ones re-emerge due to problems such as antimicrobial resistance (Figure 9.4). Zoonotic diseases (Figure 9.5) are estimated to account for 75% of all emerging infectious diseases. The impact of zoonoses presents a global challenge for both public health and the social economy. Successful management depends on multidisciplinary collaboration, education at all levels, continued research, and robust surveillance programmes and healthcare infrastructures.

Infectious disease is a potential concern for anyone in contact with animals and animal products. However, the risk is not unidirectional. Reverse zoonosis is possible, in cases such as meticillin-resistant *Staphylococcus aureus* (MRSA). Anthropogenic changes are also causing devastating infectious disease outbreaks in animals; for example, toxoplasmosis in marine animals and white-nose syndrome in bats. The prevalence of several diseases, including zoonoses, has been shown to be greater in wild animal populations living in urban areas compared with those living in more rural or natural environments (Figure 9.6). The interaction of environmental factors with an infectious agent and its host is known as the epidemiological triad. Knowing how these components interact enables identification of disease causality; each disease demands a unique interaction between the three components (Figure 9.7).

The bushmeat trade is a very active worldwide problem and is often run by organized crime gangs rather than desperate, financially destitute people. The variety of species traded is unknown. The carcasses are dried or smoked to preserve them and are often dismembered and tightly packed together; visual identification of species is impossible in most cases, and species identification using DNA is expensive and time consuming. Prosecutions are rare, as identifying the primary source of the exports is not possible. The handling and consumption of bushmeat represents a significant zoonotic risk, as the disease prevalence in these animals is generally unknown.

Live and wet markets exist in many parts of the world, and are prominent in parts of Asia, Africa and Latin America; they provide animals for direct consumption or for use in traditional medicine. A huge variety of species is held live, often without food and water, in cramped, dirty conditions. Animals are often handled extremely roughly and are only killed by the vendor at the point of sale, often with no consideration for animal welfare (Figure 9.8). These markets must be considered a significant risk to human health. Very little control on what can be traded is in place and some high-profile or endangered species, such as pangolins, are only traded, under the counter, to known local buyers and often command a very high price. In some cases, these markets have existed for hundreds of years and are of cultural significance, but as our understanding of animal welfare, disease transmission and viral magnification has evolved these wet markets have mostly remained unchanged and are extremely concerning in the context of One Health.

Historically, responses to these diseases have been as a result of their detection within the human population, and this is generally an emergency response and investigation before the source of infection is understood. Often, this involves control of the animal reservoir with techniques such as culling, quarantine, vaccination and vector control. However, this approach does not identify the root cause of the disease; for example, increasing impingement of natural areas is leading to a 'spill over' of disease from wildlife to domestic animals and then on to humans.

Routes of transmission

The importance of assessing potential vectors (living sources of disease transmission) and fomites (inanimate items that act as sources of disease transmission) in any environment or situation should not be underestimated. If there is little or no evidence, one should always extrapolate from the published data.

Possible routes of transmission can be exacerbated by many factors (Figure 9.9). Legitimate travel is common worldwide and often well-meaning people act as vectors; even conservation biologists have played a part in these routes of transmission, for example, the spread of chytridiomycosis around the world on clothing. One must always assume the worst and apply the precautions associated with known pathogens and parasites.

Food safety and food security

Food safety and food security are complicated subjects, as a balance needs to be maintained to provide enough food for the population without compromising the nutritional content and safety for the end consumer. Freezing is one proven way of reducing the risk of ingestion of pathogens, but often reduces the quality of the product. The temperature and duration of freezing are important; some pathogens, such as *Escherichia coli* require a minimum of 2 weeks at –18°C to be eradicated consistently. Recently, hypochlorite (NaOCl; bleach) has been added to poultry products in some countries to reduce the pathogens present in that product; the long-term impact of this attempt to mitigate risk to the end consumer is as yet unknown. The use of genetically modified crops is becoming a reality due to the increasing population's demand for food; again the long-term problems this might cause are not fully understood, but it is recognized that the use of pesticides and fertilizers in an agricultural environment can have a negative impact on flora and fauna, which creates an ethical One Health conundrum.

Antimicrobial resistance

Antimicrobials are essential for human and animal health; therefore, antimicrobial resistance poses an increasing and urgent threat. Antimicrobial resistant infections are

Global map of significant and new emerging infections in humans: spread to new areas since 1998

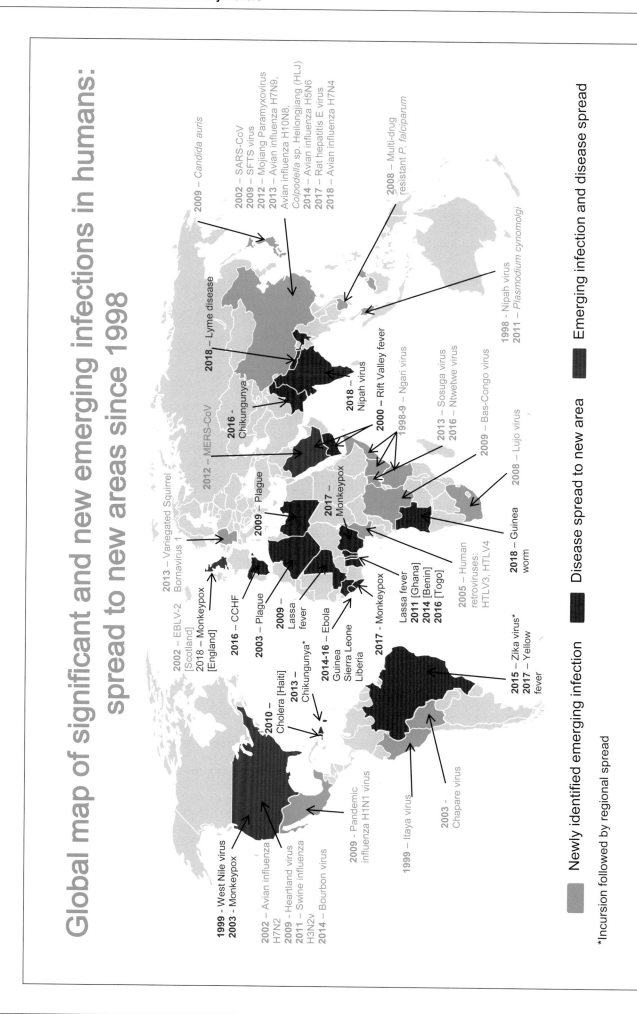

Newly identified emerging infection

Disease spread to new area

Incursion followed by regional spread

Emerging infection and disease spread

*Incursion followed by regional spread

9.4 Map of emerging and re-emerging infectious diseases detected in humans since 1998.
(Contains public sector information licensed under the Open Government Licence v3.0)

2009 – *Candida auris*

2002 – SARS-CoV
2009 – SFTS virus
2012 – Mojiang Paramyxovirus
2013 – Avian influenza H7N9,
Avian influenza H10N8,
Colpodella sp. Heilongjiang (HLJ)
2014 – Avian influenza H5N6
2017 – Rat hepatitis E virus
2018 – Avian influenza H7N4

2008 – Multi-drug
resistant *P. falciparum*

1998 – Nipah virus
2011 – *Plasmodium cynomolgi*

2018 – Lyme disease

2016 –
Chikungunya

2012 – MERS-CoV

2018 –
Nipah virus

2000 – Rift Valley fever

1998-9 – Ngari virus

2013 – Sosuga virus
2016 – Ntwetwe virus

2009 – Bas-Congo virus

2017 –
Monkeypox

2009 – Plague

2008 – Lujo virus

2005 – Human
retroviruses:
HTLV3, HTLV4

2018 – Guinea
worm

2013 – Variegated Squirrel
Bornavirus 1

2002 – EBLV-2
[Scotland]
2018 – Monkeypox
[England]

2016 – CCHF

2003 – Plague

2009 –
Lassa
fever

2014-16 – Ebola
Guinea
Sierra Leone
Liberia

2017 – Monkeypox

Lassa fever
2011 [Ghana]
2014 [Benin]
2016 [Togo]

1999 - West Nile virus
2003 - Monkeypox

2002 – Avian influenza
H7N2
2009 – Heartland virus
2011 – Swine influenza
H3N2v
2014 – Bourbon virus

2010 –
Cholera [Haiti]

2013 –
Chikungunya*

2009 – Pandemic
influenza H1N1 virus

1999 – Itaya virus

2003 –
Chapare virus

2015 – Zika virus*
2017 – Yellow
fever

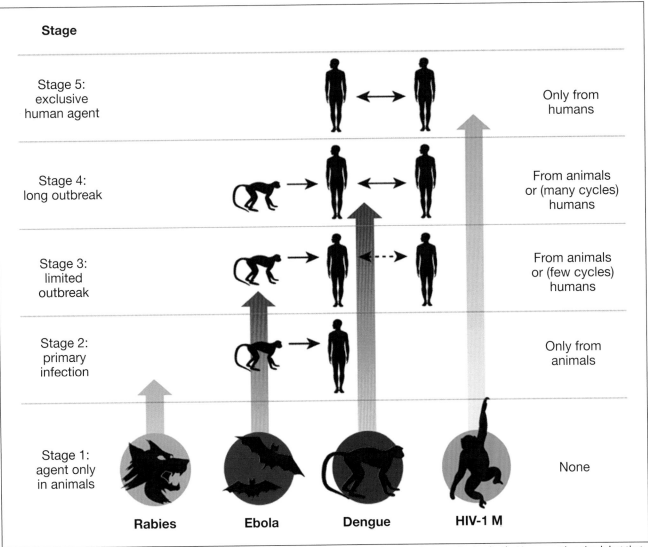

9.5 The five stages through which pathogens of animals evolve to cause disease in humans. Stage 1 = A microbe that is present in animals but that has not been detected in humans under natural conditions. Stage 2 = A pathogen of animals that, under natural conditions, has been transmitted from animals to humans but has not been transmitted between humans. Stage 3 = Animal pathogens that can undergo only a few cycles of secondary transmission between humans, so that occasional human outbreaks triggered by a primary infection soon die out. Stage 4 = A disease that exists in animals, and that has a natural cycle of infecting humans by primary transmission from the animal host, but that also undergoes long sequences of secondary transmission between humans without the involvement of animal hosts. Stage 5 = A pathogen exclusive to humans.

(Reproduced from Wolfe *et al.* (2007) with permission from the publisher)

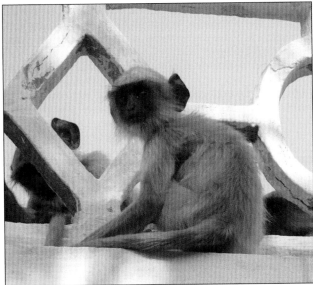

9.6 Primates venturing into houses for food in India are at greater risk of communicable disease than their rural counterparts.

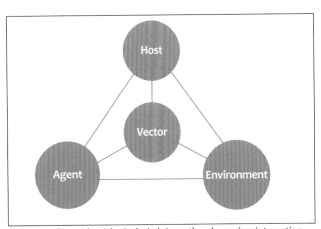

9.7 The epidemiological triad. An outbreak requires interaction between an agent, a host and the environment. The agent may be any potential pathogen (e.g. a virus or bacterium). The host is any organism that carries the disease, with or without clinical signs. The environment refers to any factor influencing the spread of the disease that is not part of the agent or host (e.g. temperature, population density). In vector-borne diseases, the vector is often related to all three components of the triad.

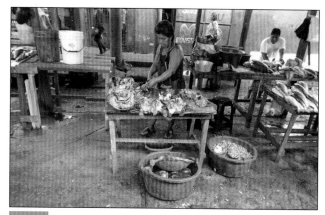

Wet market in Peru selling live and dead turtles.

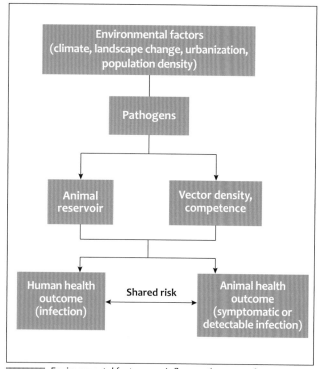

9.9 Environmental factors can influence the route of transmission of pathogens via animal reservoirs and vectors.
(Data from Rabinowitz *et al.*, 2008)

and tuberculosis are global issues, and drug resistance is starting to affect treatment for other high-profile diseases, such as human immunodeficiency virus (HIV) and malaria. Bacterial resistance to last resort antibiotics is also on the increase; for example, resistance to a last-resort treatment for *Klebsiella pneumoniae* has spread across the world.

Antimicrobial resistance affects all species and, as such, there are many organizations collaborating to jointly tackle this threat at a global and national level. Co-ordinated action is needed at a local level too; education of both healthcare professionals and users of antimicrobials is essential. Studies show that understanding the implications of inappropriate antimicrobial use is key to increasing compliance in both human patients and pet owners. In 2012, the BSAVA and the Small Animal Medicine Society (SAMSoc) developed the PROTECT ME guidelines on responsible antibacterial use (updated in 2018), which are intended to support veterinary practices with their decision-making (Figure 9.10). More recently, the British Veterinary Association partnered with other veterinary and medical healthcare professionals to design the poster *Are you antibiotic aware?*, which is designed to be displayed in both veterinary practice and doctors' surgery waiting rooms (Figure 9.11; see 'Useful websites'). The key messages regarding responsible antibiotic use are the same for both humans and animals:

- Not every illness requires antibiotics
- The right antibiotic needs to be used for the right illness
- Always finish the prescribed course.

Vaccine hesitancy

Vaccination currently prevents 2–3 million deaths per year in humans, and it is estimated that a further 1.5 million deaths could be avoided with an increased uptake. Vaccine hesitancy is defined as the reluctance or refusal to vaccinate despite vaccine availability. The World Health Organization considers vaccine hesitancy to be one of the top 10 global health threats; outbreaks of vaccine-preventable diseases, such as measles and diphtheria, are increasing. This is not just a concern for human populations; there has been a significant decline in pet vaccination too, potentially predisposing pets to the same risk of declining protection from life-threatening diseases, such as distemper and parvovirus. Vaccine hesitancy also increases the risk of outbreaks of zoonotic vaccine-preventable diseases, such as leptospirosis and rabies.

Vaccine hesitancy has many influences, including an individual's own views and past experiences, as well as wider political and sociocultural factors. Anti-vaccination campaigns, via the internet and social media, have contributed to misinformation and negative messages. For example, anti-vaccination campaigners have previously voiced concerns regarding links between vaccination and autistic behaviour in dogs. However, there is no scientific evidence to suggest that autism occurs in dogs, or that there is a link between autism and vaccination (BVA, 2018). Anti-vaccination is not the only reason for vaccine hesitancy; other factors include complacency, lack of knowledge, inconvenience and cost. Ironically, the success of vaccination programmes in eliminating or reducing diseases is another contributing factor for vaccine hesitancy; people question whether vaccinations are still required when the diseases no longer appear prevalent.

estimated to cause an annual 700,000 deaths globally, with this figure expected to rise to 10 million by 2050. The term 'antimicrobial' includes antibiotic antiviral, antifungal and antiprotozoal drugs. Antibiotic resistance is the biggest threat currently, but resistance has also been reported in other drug categories, such as antivirals used for influenza strains. Antimicrobial resistance is a naturally occurring process, a result of mutation of microorganisms in response to exposure to a drug. It is being accelerated by factors such as inappropriate use of antimicrobials, poor infection control, inadequate hygiene and sanitation, and international travel.

Without effective antibiotics, even minor surgical procedures could become high risk. Resistance to first-line drugs used to treat *Staphylococcus* infections is already widespread; the cost of healthcare for patients with resistant infections is high, due to the increased duration of illness and the need for additional treatment and use of more expensive drugs. Drug-resistant *Escherichia coli*

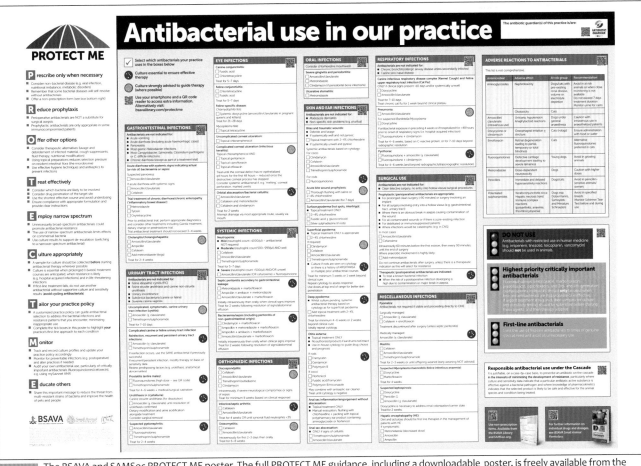

9.10 The BSAVA and SAMSoc PROTECT ME poster. The full PROTECT ME guidance, including a downloadable poster, is freely available from the BSAVA Library (see 'Useful Websites').

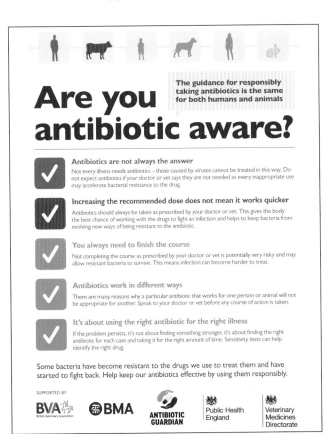

9.11 The BVA *Are you antibiotic aware?* poster for veterinary practices.
(Reproduced with permission from BVA)

Successful and continued reduction in the prevalence and incidence of vaccine-preventable diseases is dependent on a high enough uptake level to protect communities through herd immunity. Some countries have introduced laws making vaccination mandatory, but this is controversial and potentially counterproductive. Individual decision-making regarding vaccination is complex; increasing confidence and awareness of the importance of vaccination is dependent on building trust and providing credible information. Education has again been shown to increase compliance; veterinary and medical healthcare professionals need to enhance opportunities to promote and raise awareness of the importance of vaccination to ensure the continued protection of the health of both humans and animals.

Titre testing can be offered as an option for owners that are apprehensive about vaccination. It involves taking a small blood sample to identify levels of antibodies. If sufficient levels of antibodies are present, this indicates adequate protection against the disease. This needs to be repeated at several intervals throughout the animal's life and costs are considerably higher than standard vaccination courses.

The Small Animal Veterinary Surveillance Network (SAVSNET) collects data on the prevalence of canine parvovirus and other vaccine-preventable diseases in dogs and cats; veterinary professionals are encouraged to contribute to this data collection (see 'Useful websites').

Air pollution and climate change

There is a close relationship between air pollution and climate change, and both present a global challenge. The extraction and burning of fossil fuels is driving climate change and is also a key source of air pollution. Carbon dioxide (CO_2) is considered a major contributor, its levels acting as a barometer for climate change and effects of air pollution. Commonly referred to as a 'greenhouse gas', rising CO_2 levels trap sunlight within the atmosphere, leading to climate instability and changes such as rising temperatures and increased rainfall. Rapid reduction of CO_2 emissions is vital but not sufficient on its own; there are other air pollutants that also have a significant impact. Black carbon (or 'soot', produced when fossil fuels are burnt) is the second greatest contributor to global warming, closely followed by methane, which reacts with other pollutants to form ozone. Unlike CO_2, which has an atmospheric lifespan of more than a hundred years, these remain in the atmosphere for much briefer periods. Reductions would therefore have a significant and immediate effect on both climate change and the associated risks to health due to exposure.

Exposure to air pollution is having a direct impact on the prevalence of non-communicable disease (see 'Non-communicable diseases'). Black carbon is particularly dangerous as the particulate matter it is composed of can penetrate the lungs and bloodstream. Low–middle income countries are more at risk of 'household pollution' because of exposure to damaging pollutants from cooking and heating with polluting fuels such as coal, wood, dung and kerosene. Children are also especially vulnerable; exposure to these pollutants early in life can have long-lasting effects on their lungs.

Air pollution and climate change also impacts the ecosystem, affecting biodiversity and damaging habitats, which leads to a further worsening of the effects of these changes. All species have the capacity to adapt to environmental change but it is the pace at which these changes occur that has such a negative impact on their viability. Environmental stressors not only cause degradation of habitats, but also compromise the reproductive parameters and immunocompetence of species, ultimately threatening their health and survival. The decline of one species can also impact another, for example those that rely on other species for food. Extreme weather as a result of climate change significantly alters the number and distribution of many species, pathogens and vectors.

Other anthropogenic changes have also led to an accumulation of pollutants, such as organochlorines and heavy metals, in both land and water environments, presenting yet another threat to species health and survival. Among those most susceptible are marine mammals, amphibians and birds.

Non-communicable diseases

A non-communicable disease (NCD) is one that is not transmissible from one person/animal to another. These diseases tend to be chronic; a result of genetic, physiological, environmental and behavioural factors. It is estimated that NCDs are responsible for 71% of all global deaths, with cardiovascular disease being the leading cause, and they are more prevalent in lower income countries. There is a huge socioeconomic impact associated with NCDs; early detection can result in better outcomes for patients as well as significantly reducing healthcare costs. Companion animals are predisposed to the same NCDs as humans, related to similar contributing factors, due to shared lifestyles and environments. Environmental changes and exposure to toxic substances are important factors in the occurrence of NCDs; air pollution is the second largest global cause (see 'Air pollution and climate change').

Non-communicable diseases include:

- Cardiovascular disease
- Cancer
- Chronic respiratory disease
- Arthritis
- Diabetes
- Alzheimer's disease
- Mental illness.

Risk factors can be divided into two categories – modifiable behavioural risks and metabolic risks:

- Modifiable behavioural risks:
  - Alcohol
  - Smoking
  - Poor diet
  - Lack of physical exercise
- Metabolic risks:
  - High blood pressure
  - Obesity
  - Hyperglycaemia
  - Hyperlipidaemia.

The One Health links for NCDs are multifactorial.

- Environmental factors affect the health of both humans and animals in similar ways.
- Poor health in humans can impact on the health of their pets by reducing the capacity to provide adequate care.
- Lifestyle habits of people can also impact on the health of animals; for example, overfeeding leading to obesity, and passive smoking.
- Animals can have a positive effect on the physical and mental health of people through the human–animal bond.

The human–animal bond and pet ownership

Relationships between humans and animals have existed since the beginning of civilization. The dog is believed to be the first domesticated animal, with earliest fossil records from the Middle East dated circa 12,000 years ago. Since then, there has been evidence of the relationship between humans and dogs depicted in paintings, mosaics and sculptures. Aside from the dog, the cat was the only other known domesticated animal kept for companionship, and it was considered sacred by the Egyptians. The first evidence of the domestication of food-producing animals is around 9000–7000 BC as communities of people became more settled and looked for other ways to obtain their food. As civilization continued to evolve, so too did the relationship between humans and animals, with people utilizing animals for many purposes, including work, service, sport and companionship.

It is estimated that 50% of UK adults own a pet (People's Dispensary for Sick Animals (PDSA), 2020); many households own more than one pet, with dogs, cats and rabbits being the most popular, but there is an increasing diversity of species. People tend to anthropomorphize their pets, developing strong relationships that are akin to those with other humans. Companionship is often stated as the main reason why people purchase a pet but there is a growing body of scientific literature to suggest additional physical and psychological benefits of pet ownership and other interactions with animals. This relationship is commonly referred to as the 'human–animal bond (HAB)' or the 'pet effect'.

Benefits of the human–animal bond include:

* Stress buffering effect
* Reduced blood pressure
* Alleviated social isolation and loneliness
* Increased physical activity (dogs)
* Increased wellbeing – benefits for both physical and mental health
* Improved child health and development
* Healthier ageing.

The variations in how studies relating to the HAB are conducted (e.g. populations, interventions, methods) mean that proving a causal link between the HAB and effects on health is difficult. A review of the effects of pet ownership on human health by McNicholas *et al.* (2005) proposes that there are three potential mechanisms to explain the association (Figure 9.12):

* **Non-causal association** – other cofactors, such as personality, economic and health status influence decisions to own a pet, thus appearing as an apparent link between pet ownership and health benefits
* **Indirect effect** – pets enhance social interactions, which reduces feelings of loneliness and social isolation, therefore providing an indirect effect on health and wellbeing
* **Direct effect** – ways in which pet ownership may exert a direct effect on health, for example, reducing anxiety-related illness and enhancing recovery from serious illness.

The effects of pet ownership on cardiovascular health (CVH) and obesity are among the most researched topics. This is perhaps unsurprising given that cardiovascular disease (CVD) is reported to cause an estimated 17 million global deaths annually, with worldwide obesity tripling since 1975 – an issue once considered more prevalent in higher income countries, but now also affecting low–middle income countries.

Cardiovascular disease

Such is the growing body of literature relating to CVH and pets that, in 2013, the American Heart Association published a scientific statement in which they stated that there was a substantial body of data to suggest that pet ownership, particularly dog ownership, is associated with a reduction in cardiovascular disease factors and increased survival in individuals with established CVD (Levine *et al.*, 2013). Commonly reported findings in many studies assessing effects of pet ownership on CVH include increased activity levels, reduced basal heart rate and systemic blood pressure, and lower reactivity to stress. Psychosocial factors such as social isolation, loneliness and depression were also reported to be reduced, the impact of which should not be underestimated as social relationships are shown to be a significant contributing factor to good health and wellbeing.

Obesity

Obesity is a societal concern and a health issue for both human and companion animal populations. For both, obesity predisposes to a range of diseases including CVD, diabetes, cancer and orthopaedic conditions such as arthritis, as well as potentially decreasing lifespan. There have been numerous studies looking at the impact of pet ownership on reducing incidence of obesity in people: notably, the benefits of a collaborative approach between both veterinary and medical healthcare professionals. See 'Shared health issues' for further discussion of obesity.

Cancer

Cancer is another example of a disease where the HAB is reported to be of benefit, notably with psychosocial factors such as alleviating stress, anxiety and depression. There is also a reported increase in overall emotional wellbeing and a reduced perception of pain associated with animal-assisted interventions (AAI) and cancer patients. For example, one study of two groups of oncology patients – one group that participated in an animal-assisted activity (AAA) session and a control group which did not – showed a decrease in blood pressure and signs of depression in the group participating in AAA when compared with the group that did not (Knisely *et al.*, 2012).

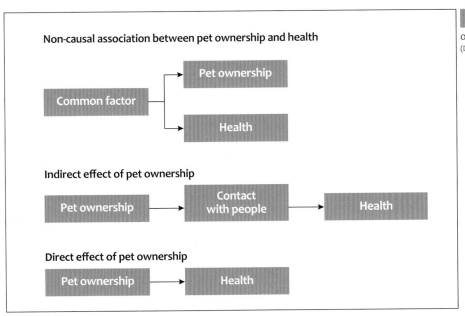

9.12 Proposed mechanisms for association between pet ownership and health benefits for humans. (Data from McNicholas *et al.*, 2005)

In addition to these benefits, there is also research into the use of dogs to detect cancer; the first published study using dogs for detection of bladder cancer was by Willis *et al.* in 2004. It is well recognized that early detection of cancer is key to survival rates. Cancerous growths produce volatile organic compounds, which are believed to have distinctive odours detectable by dogs. A dog's sense of smell is 10,000 times more sensitive than a human's: sensitive enough to detect cancer markers in a person's breath, blood or urine with remarkable accuracy. The use of 'detection dogs' has exciting potential as a low risk, non-invasive method for cancer diagnosis. However, further research is required regarding the effectiveness and reliability of this technique.

Mental health

Mental health refers to our cognitive, behavioural and emotional wellbeing; taking care of our mental wellbeing is important at all stages of our lives. Research suggests that the HAB can be very beneficial in supporting mental health and, as a result, there are an increasing number of animals used for therapy and emotional support to help with mental wellbeing (see 'Animal-assisted interventions').

The positive effects of the HAB on mental health include:

* Alleviation of stress and anxiety
* Reduced symptoms of depression
* Social and emotional development
* Alleviation of loneliness and social isolation
* Alleviation of stress and anxiety in the hospital setting
* Enhanced quality of life
* Calming effect
* Providing a sense of purpose.

Social relationships have a profound effect on mental and physical health; loneliness is a major risk factor for depression and the effects of social isolation on physical health are akin to other risk factors such as smoking. Although often linked, social isolation and loneliness do not always occur together; the absence of social relationships does not necessarily cause loneliness, whilst another person may have many social connections but still feel incredibly lonely. Social isolation and loneliness are considered significant social problems. There is a general perception that these are problems that affect the older generation, but they can affect all age groups and are particularly prevalent in young adults. People can experience social isolation or loneliness for many reasons; these can be long-term factors or sudden changes in circumstances. Examples of factors include:

* Living alone
* Physical or mental disability/illness
* Bereavement
* Societal adversity
* Domestic violence
* Unemployment
* Homelessness
* Significant life events or health crises.

The human–animal bond can provide a way to connect with others, breaking down communication barriers, acting as a social lubricant, and providing companionship in the absence of others. The HAB can provide a buffering effect on stress and anxiety, which has both physical and mental health benefits; blood pressure and heart rate are

reduced and recipients report feeling safer, calmer and happier. The HAB also provides comfort and a sense of purpose and focus that distracts from the recipient's own issues or illness. These effects can be beneficial for both chronic conditions, such as depression and anxiety, or acute, such as recovery or rehabilitation from illness or surgery in the hospital setting. The HAB can also be particularly effective for those that have experienced trauma (e.g. for those suffering post-traumatic stress disorder).

Elderly population

According to Age UK, there are over 11 million people in the UK over the age of 65; half of this population report that their pet or the television is their main source of companionship (Davidson and Rossall, 2015). In addition to the benefits of the HAB associated with minimizing the effects of social isolation or loneliness, pet ownership is also reported to be beneficial in minimizing cognitive decline and motivating physical activity.

Dementia

Dementia is not a specific disease, but a descriptive term for a collection of symptoms, such as memory decline and alterations in thinking and reasoning. Several diseases can cause symptoms of dementia, including Alzheimer's disease, which is a degenerative brain disease causing complex brain changes due to cellular damage. Research indicates that the HAB can improve quality of life for both those living with symptoms of dementia and their carers. Benefits include increased social interaction, improved mood, and reduced aggression and agitation.

Childhood health and development

Introducing children to animals from a young age can have a positive influence on their social and emotional development, even through just the presence of a pet in the household. However, where pet ownership is not suitable, research also suggests that interactions with animals in other ways, through therapy or school visits for example, can have a positive influence on a child's development. Communicating with animals can be a much simpler experience than with another person; animals are less complex, non-judgemental and respond well to non-verbal forms of communication. Children can also develop self-esteem and empathy for others through their interactions with animals (Endenburg and van Lith, 2011). Learning about how to care for an animal from a young age is not only beneficial for building a child's sense of self-worth and confidence, it also helps to develop their awareness of an animal's sentience, which can help promote a respect for the wellbeing of animals throughout their lives.

Education on basic pet needs does form part of primary school education, but some argue that this should be expanded to cover animal health and welfare in more depth. Many charities offer free resources for schools, including school visits/talks and online resources such as structured lesson plans and awards that link in with the school curriculum. Some schools may consider having a classroom pet as an opportunity to teach children about responsibility and empathy towards animals. Research also demonstrates that children feel more comfortable reading to an animal than another person. However, the disadvantages of having a classroom pet far outweigh the advantages. There are health and safety considerations for both children and animals –

for example, injuries and zoonotic diseases. The nature of the school routine will likely also mean that the animals are confined to small enclosures for much of their life and, when they are removed from these, it is likely that they will experience a great deal of stress through multiple handlers and a lot of noise and excitement. The conditions in which they will likely be kept will also prohibit some species from being able to exhibit their normal behaviour, for example if they are usually more active at night. There is also the added consideration of what happens to these animals outside of school hours – overnight, at weekends and during school holidays. It can be exciting for the children to have the opportunity and responsibility of taking the school pet home but, for the animal, this can mean being exposed to another unfamiliar and unpredictable environment. At best, this will cause additional stress for the animal, and at worst it can also put them at risk of poor welfare or abuse. Schools should be encouraged and supported to enhance their children's exposure and awareness of animal welfare by using alternatives, such as charity resources, visits to local farms/zoos and virtual experiences. These activities are far more likely to promote a caring and respectful attitude towards pets than having an animal confined in a cage in the classroom.

Asthma and other allergies: Research suggests that exposure to pets reduces the risk of development of asthma and other allergies, the hypothesis being that a lack of exposure to infectious agents, symbiotic micro-organisms and parasites during early childhood leads to suppression of the developing immune system, predisposing the child to allergic disease.

Autism spectrum disorder: Autism spectrum disorder (ASD) is a complex neurological and developmental disorder; 'spectrum' meaning that different people present with a range of signs. It begins early in life, with most children exhibiting signs within the first 12 months of life, and affects how a person acts, learns and interacts with others. The potential benefits of pet ownership can extend wider than the individual; positive associations have been made regarding relationships between parents/carers of autistic individuals, along with overall benefits to the functioning of the family unit. Other benefits include a decrease in problem behaviours and stress levels, increased independence and improvements in communication ability. As with all HAB relationships, the benefits need to be assessed against the family's individual circumstances and ability to provide adequate care for a pet. Animal-assisted therapy and equine-assisted therapy can also be very beneficial in increasing social functioning (see 'Animal-assisted interventions', below). There are also organizations that provide and train assistance dogs for children with ASD; their role being to help keep the child safe and to have a calming influence, reducing stress levels in social environments.

Homeless people

The homeless population is extremely vulnerable and no different to any other population in benefiting from the strong attachment of the human–animal bond. Homelessness can be an extremely isolating and unsafe experience; the presence of a companion animal can provide a sense of protection against this. Again, this relationship can provide a sense of purpose and responsibility as well as companionship. Pet ownership in this group has also been linked to an increased contact with the wider community; homeless people have reported being treated more kindly and that people talk to them more. Conversely, some have reported being criticized or experiencing negative encounters due to their pet ownership.

Shared health issues

Zoonosis and anthroponosis

The World Health Organization defines a zoonosis as an infectious disease that has jumped from a non-human animal to humans. Zoonotic pathogens may be bacterial, viral, parasitic, or may involve unconventional agents, and spread to humans through direct contact, food, water or the environment. With an increasing number of immuno-compromised humans in the population, instances of zoonosis have also increased. Balancing the mental health benefits of pet ownership for a debilitated person against the zoonotic risk can be incredibly hard, as neither risk can be assessed in a quantifiable and repeatable manner. It is important to make rules in this area as each case is different and needs assessing on its own merits.

Anthroponosis describes a disease that can jump from humans to non-human animals; ethically, this needs considering in the context of pet ownership and One Health. The herpes simplex virus that causes cold sores in humans can be extremely pathogenic and debilitating in some species of New World primates in the family Callitrichidae. Any disease risk analysis around an individual owning a pet should take anthroponosis into consideration.

Obesity

In the past 30 years, there has been an increased prevalence of obesity in both people and animals, despite substantial efforts to address this problem, indicating that effective strategies for weight loss remain elusive (Bartges et al., 2017). Obesity is the most common nutritional disorder in both companion animal and human populations. It is a complex disease involving multiple factors, including diet, physical activity, behaviours, environmental factors, and genetic disposition. Studies suggest that certain dog and cat breeds are more predisposed to obesity, which mirrors human risk factors, where genetics are also believed to play a role. Low socioeconomic status is also associated with a higher prevalence of obesity in people and this can have an impact on pets (Day, 2017). A collaborative approach between human and veterinary healthcare professionals has been identified as a key strategy for tackling obesity (Figure 9.13).

The human–animal bond can be viewed as both a positive and negative influence on obesity. Studies have shown that social relationships and social support are strong motivators for adhering to lifestyle changes, such as diet modification and increased physical exercise. Pets are considered as family members by most owners and, as such, can provide this motivation. Studies show owning a dog is a motivator for increased physical activity and this is of particular value if both owner and dog are overweight or obese (Day, 2017). Conversely, the HAB can also be a contributing factor to obesity in pets – notably due to the anthropomorphizing of pets by their owners. Given this, it is unsurprising that there is a link between pet obesity and child obesity. A similar 'co-dependant' relationship can exist between pets and their owners, and

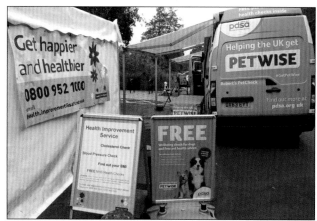

9.13 A key strategy in tackling obesity in both humans and companion animals involves collaboration between healthcare and veterinary professionals.
(Courtesy of Sue Bartlett, PDSA)

children and their parents; pets can be treated as children and as such, can be overindulged, with food used as a form of comfort or reward.

Despite the increasing prevalence of obesity, there is still a reluctance from both human and veterinary healthcare professionals to discuss it, due to the sensitivity of the subject. There are a number of ways in which this may be overcome (see 'Supporting the human–animal bond', below), one of which is focusing on the overall health of the patient, rather than a specific aspect (i.e. their weight). Physical activity, for example, is a vital component of good health with benefits that are much broader than weight loss. Weight management should also form part of a regular preventive health check, which then provides an opportunity for discussion. Discussions should be non-judgmental and sensitive, with an understanding of the factors that have driven the behaviours resulting in obesity. Weight management plans need to be individualized to encourage compliance and account for any specific barriers to success. Diet and physical activity are both important; plans should be goal driven and specific (i.e. type of physical activity and duration). Continuous support from healthcare professionals is required for a weight loss plan to be successful and it should also be recognized that the ongoing maintenance of weight loss is a greater challenge for both humans and companion animals.

Passive smoking

Despite a continuing decline in smoking rates, nearly 1 in 5 adults still smoke with smoking being more prevalent in deprived areas, amongst certain demographic groups and in those people with longstanding mental health problems (Public Health England, 2018). Smokers are at an increased risk of cardiovascular disease, respiratory disease and cancer. However, they are not the only ones at risk. According to the World Health Organization (WHO), smoking is linked to 8 million deaths per year, with 1.2 million related to passive smoking. Passive smoking does not just affect people; exposure has a direct impact on pets too. Pets can breathe in second-hand smoke, but it can also settle on their fur, posing an additional risk when grooming; cats are particularly susceptible. Eating cigarette butts or nicotine products is also a concern, due to the toxins that they contain. Passive smoking predisposes those affected to similar health risks associated with smokers. Vaping is also believed to carry similar risks and there are specific concerns relating to the glass cartridge;

this must be kept out of reach of pets. Ultimately, smoking cessation would be of most benefit in reducing health risks. However, the risks can be lowered by:

- Not smoking in enclosed areas such as the house or the car
- Keeping tobacco products and vaping products out of reach
- Washing hands after smoking.

Pets can act as a sentinel (see 'Animals as sentinels', below) for passive smoking, often showing clinical signs related to the effects far earlier than people. Discussing the effects of passive smoking as part of a preventive health check could be very beneficial. Veterinary practices should also consider participation in 'non-smoking' campaigns, such as Stoptober and World No Tobacco Day.

The Association of Respiratory Nurse Specialists (ARNS), Royal College of Nursing (RCN), Royal College of Veterinary Surgeons (RCVS) and British Veterinary Nursing Association (BVNA) launched a joint One Health initiative on this topic, which involved a press release targeted at the general public and both veterinary and human nursing professionals (ARNS, 2017). The aim was to raise awareness of the impact of passive smoking on pets as an additional motivation for smokers to consider quitting. This generated a lot of media attention and is a good example of how joint collaborations can be of huge value in tackling these types of problems.

Injuries
Dog bites

There are no global estimates of the number of dog bite injuries but studies suggest that they account for tens of millions of injuries annually; children account for the largest percentage of those injured (WHO, 2020). Dog bite injuries can cause physical and psychological trauma. In the UK, the main complication is infection but rabies is obviously a concern in other parts of the world. Experts estimate that dog bites account for over 99% of all instances of rabies in humans (WHO, 2020). Media outlets often sensationalize incidents of 'dog attacks', which can cause hysteria, but dog bites can be the result of far more benign interactions. There can be many complex factors such as misinterpretation of behaviour, fear-based aggression, exposure to unfamiliar surroundings/people and pain. Education on how to interpret behaviour and awareness of situations that predispose to the risk of bites can be useful; for example, The Blue Dog Project aims to provide education to children to increase their knowledge and awareness regarding safer interactions with dogs (see 'Useful websites').

Non-accidental trauma

There is increasing evidence to suggest links between the abuse of people, particularly children and vulnerable adults, and animals. It is also recognized that an animal can be a sentinel for violence within a household (see 'Animals as sentinels'). Veterinary professionals may be presented with a patient with injuries that they suspect could be non-accidental. Under the Animal Welfare Act, there is a duty of care to ensure that the animal's welfare is protected. However, these situations are complex, daunting and challenging. Understandably, individuals may have concerns regarding how to handle the situation. Practices should encourage team discussion on this topic and have a detailed practice policy to ensure that their staff have clear direction on what to do, should they be presented with such a situation. The Links Group (see 'Useful websites') is an organization that raises awareness of the links between the abuse of people and animals. Their resources include a free downloadable veterinary practice guidance document and various training initiatives. They also recommend establishing links with relevant local agencies, such as the police, child protection agencies and animal welfare organizations, for support and advice. Collaboration with relevant organizations can help to identify those potentially at risk and enable action to be taken.

Animals as sentinels

A sentinel event can be defined as "a preventable disease or disability, or an untimely death whose occurrence serves as a warning signal that the quality of preventive and/or therapeutic care may need to be improved" (Rutstein et al., 1983). The classic example of an animal being used as a sentinel is the canary bird, caged in mines, to give an early alert of the presence of toxic gases. Since then, tracking of health events in both animals and humans has been used to detect and manage disease risks. As with humans, exposure to environmental hazards has an impact on the health of animals. In addition, due to their behavioural habits and closer proximity to the environment, animals can acquire the disease and therefore exhibit clinical signs more rapidly, meaning that they can be potential sentinels for threats to human health. However, the challenges in identifying the clinical signs in animals means that the disease is often first detected in humans, with them therefore becoming the sentinel.

Barriers to the successful implementation of using animals as sentinels include professional segregation, data separation and evidence gaps in these links. A potential health threat can only be acted upon if the appropriate link is made. Global organizations are overcoming this with taskforces such as the Global Early Warning System (GLEWS), a collaborative effort to rapidly share disease information about animal and human cases of avian influenza and other zoonotic disease and strategies for global surveillance of avian influenza in wild birds. Monitoring these sentinel events is a critical component of the One Health approach; greater awareness of these links and closer disease surveillance in animals as well as humans is vital. Consideration needs to be given to the common environments and food sources shared by humans and animals as well as the potential for consumption of contaminated animal products.

Supporting the human–animal bond

The human–animal bond is described as a mutually beneficial and dynamic relationship that positively influences the health of both humans and animals. While the benefits for the human are well-documented, there is very little evidence that these benefits are reciprocated. At a societal level, the HAB can promote positive attitudes towards animals which can be beneficial to their welfare. Conversely, this relationship can also lead to conflict between the benefits for the human and the welfare of the animal. For example, with pet ownership, the anthropocentric nature of these relationships can contribute to problem behaviours or obesity issues. Behavioural problems are the leading cause of euthanasia in Western countries and obesity is the most common nutritional disorder (Wensley, 2008). End-of-life decision-making is another example of when the strong bond can impact on the welfare of the pet. Owners can be extremely reluctant to euthanase their pet, especially if they represent an emotional link to their past. Although companionship is often stated as the primary reason for acquiring a pet, there are other reasons; many of which are not conducive to the welfare of the animal:

- **Impulse buying** – according to the PDSA, one in four people do no pre-purchase research and impulse buying of pets is still a significant concern
- **Status or trend** – certain breeds of dog – so-called 'dangerous dogs' – and a growing number of wild or exotic species, for example, are purchased as status symbols. Celebrity pet ownership and the appearance of different species in popular films can also influence decisions
- **Pressure from children** – parents may concede to their dependant's requests without thorough consideration of the longer-term care of the animal, and often with very little or no research into the animal's suitability as a pet
- **Preparing for parenthood or in place of children** – thought to be the primary reason for the high prevalence of pet ownership in millennials; decisions to delay other life choices, such as getting married or having children, are driving decisions to instead get a pet
- **Hoarding** – the pathological and compulsive keeping of large numbers of animals by people that are usually either overwhelmed caregivers or 'mission-driven' rescuers. Some may have exploitative reasons for hoarding, such as financial gains. Hoarders have an inability to recognize the extremely poor welfare conditions of the animals, instead often believing that they have a strong connection and an ability to communicate with these animals. They do not believe in euthanasia on any grounds. If an intervention results in the removal of the animals, hoarders will often resume their collecting very quickly.

Although many people have well-meaning intentions, the lack of research undertaken prior to acquiring a pet can lead to significant issues for the animal's physical and mental wellbeing and can lead to rehoming, abandonment or neglect, which is not quite in the spirit of a dynamic and mutually beneficial human–animal bond.

Research shows that owners educated on the welfare needs of their pets are more likely to ensure that they are met. Veterinary and other healthcare professionals have an opportunity to promote the positive benefits of the HAB whilst providing guidance to counteract the potential negative implications. Under the One Health umbrella, this education can be broadened to help owners understand how their pet's health is intrinsically linked to their own. However, it is imperative that healthcare professionals recognize that how this education is provided is key to success. Often, an owner's actions are led by misguided good intentions; they need guidance that is delivered in a non-judgemental and sensitive manner. Recognizing the strength of the human–animal bond and incorporating this in discussions regarding the pet's welfare can also help to establish trust between the healthcare professional and the client.

Stages of Change model

A patient/client-centred approach is one that focuses on the needs of the patient/client and incorporates their own views. Healthcare professionals need to use appropriate communication methods that encourage the patient/client to consider their role in their own health and wellbeing and that of their pets. This approach builds trust between the patient/client and healthcare professional and increases the potential of successful and sustained behavioural change. Another key element is recognizing when a patient/client is ready to make these changes. The 'Stages of Change Model', also known as the 'Transtheoretical Model', was introduced in the late 1970s/early 1980s by researchers Prochaska and DiClemente (1983). It describes the cycle of stages that a person will go through when modifying behaviour:

1. **Precontemplation** – not ready or willing to change. Interventions usually ineffective but can 'sow the seed' in a compassionate and non-judgemental manner.
2. **Contemplation** – awareness of the problem and intention to consider change. More information and resources can be provided at this stage but, again, a non-confrontational manner should be maintained.
3. **Preparation** – acknowledgement of the problem and seeking professional guidance. The person should be asked how they can best be supported with this. Motivational interviewing is a good technique to use for these conversations.
4. **Action** – significant action taken to address the problem. Regular check-ins, support and encouragement will be needed.
5. **Maintenance** – maintaining success but with the potential for relapse. Need to identify potential threats and how to overcome these.

Vulnerable groups

As discussed, many people have very strong attachments to their pets; they will often prioritize their pet above themselves, sometimes to the detriment of their own health, and the loss of their pet can be emotionally very difficult. There are also specific groups of people with increased vulnerability for whom there are specific challenges and considerations for both the welfare of the person and the animal in their care. For these groups, the level of attachment and dependency on their pets can be even greater:

- Elderly people
- Those with dementia or Alzheimer's disease
- Those with a physical or mental disability
- Those with a sudden health or life crisis
- Homeless people
- Immunosuppressed people.

Having discussions regarding the practicalities of pet ownership for these groups can be very difficult, especially if the owner feels that they are in jeopardy of losing their pet. The thought of needing to go into hospital for treatment or into a care/residential home, for example, can cause a considerable amount of distress. Equally, the owner may have already acknowledged the potential difficulties or decisions that they may have to face with regards to their pet's care and be feeling very overwhelmed and unsure as to what they can do. The following points can be used as guidance for these discussions:

- **Have a sensitive and positive approach** – using the Stages of Change model as a framework to gauge where the client is sitting in terms of openness to have these conversations, the discussion should be framed within the context of wanting to help them to keep their pet as long as possible
- **Seek to understand their situation** – there are many organizations that can provide insight, through resources or training, into understanding the issues faced by people with specific health concerns or disabilities (see 'Useful websites'). At the very least, healthcare professionals should ensure that they take the time to explore and listen to the individual or their family members/carers to fully understand their situation and identify any potential concerns
- **Help them to plan** – consider the practicalities and what can be done to overcome these – what pet/s do they have? Do they present any hazards for their owner? What are the pet's needs? Can they be met by the owner or do they require assistance? Are there any welfare issues of concern? Do they have any family or carers that would be prepared to help? Are there pet aids that would be useful, for example, 'no-bend' pet bowls/car ramps/specific harnesses? Owners with dementia, for example, may benefit from regular routines for walking and feeding, or notes/alerts on mobile phones that can act as prompts. There is a growing number of organizations (see 'Useful websites') that can either provide advice or a voluntary service to help with dog walking/temporary fostering, etc.
- **Be prepared to have those difficult conversations** – the rehoming of their pet may ultimately still be the best solution, if the relationship is having a detrimental effect on the welfare of the animal that cannot be resolved. It may be a decision that needs to be planned for the future, for example, if the owner needs to go into a care or residential home
- **Reach out to other local organizations** – collaboration with other organizations is key to the One Health approach and can help facilitate joint initiatives to support and raise awareness of issues faced.

Homeless people

Living on the streets can present a very different set of challenges. Pet ownership can be a potential barrier for accessing temporary and permanent accommodation, to obtaining employment and accessing healthcare services for both the individual and their pet. Organizations such as Street Vet work in collaboration with other outreach groups to overcome these issues and provide access to free veterinary care, helping to ensure that this human–animal bond can be maintained.

Emotional support and end-of-life decisions

A break in the human–animal bond for whatever reason can be emotionally distressing for both humans and animals but the end-of-life situation is the most traumatic, whether this is the owner or the pet. Considering what will happen to their pet should the owner no longer be around to care for them can cause a lot of anxiety, some of which may be alleviated to a degree by having a plan. Equally, making decisions regarding their pet's end-of-life care can be distressing and one that many owners will avoid for as long as possible. Having support and guidance to plan for this event can help alleviate some of the emotional turmoil. Understanding what will happen at the end and the process for euthanasia may also help.

The range of emotions experienced during bereavement will be similar for many owners but there is no set pattern or timeframe. There are a growing number of organizations that offer bereavement counselling. Healthcare professionals can also undertake their own training and it can be useful for veterinary practices to have at least one member of staff who has undertaken specific training in this area. See Chapter 8 for more information on this topic.

The human–animal bond *versus* other interactions

While every effort may be made to ensure that the bond between owner and pet can be maintained, there will inevitably be situations when pet ownership is not appropriate. Certainly, acquiring a pet solely for the purposes of improving a person's physical and/or mental health should not be advocated, without thorough consideration for the welfare needs of the animal. It should also be noted that the human–animal bond will not be suited to all; some people do not have an affinity with and/or are fearful of animals or certain species.

Immunosuppression

Common immunosuppressing conditions include cancer, autoimmune disorders, metabolic disease and acquired immunodeficiency syndrome (AIDS). Pregnant women are also at risk. Immunosuppression increases the risk of acquiring infectious diseases, which complicates pet ownership. As already discussed, there are significant physical and psychosocial benefits to pet ownership that should not be overlooked in these circumstances. Suggesting the rehoming of a pet can cause significant emotional upset for the owners and is not the recommended approach. A healthy pet is of minimal danger, providing appropriate precautions are taken. Ensuring that the human–animal bond can be maintained is dependent on providing accurate information on the risks and benefits for the owner and establishing a good relationship between the owner, veterinary team and other healthcare professionals involved in the owner's care.

Although there is general guidance that can be applied in these situations, each case should also be individually assessed for specific issues of concern. For example, maintaining the health of the animal is imperative to ensure that the owner's health is not compromised. However, it is also important to ensure that the owner's health status does not compromise their ability to meet the welfare needs of their pet; for example, do they live alone or with others who can assist with pet care? The age of the immunosuppressed person is also of relevance; for example, younger children may not comprehend the importance of adhering to guidelines. Certain species, such as reptiles, birds and other exotic species, also present a higher risk due to an increased susceptibility to diseases such as salmonellosis, so additional consideration needs to be given to the risks and benefits of ownership.

General guidelines for pet ownership when immunosuppressed include:

- Good hand hygiene and avoidance of intimate contact, such as kissing the pet or allowing the pet to lick faces or share the bed/sofa
- Preventive healthcare is essential and should include vaccinations and vector/parasite control
- If a pet shows signs of ill health, these should be addressed promptly
- Care should be taken when dealing with faeces or equipment used for toileting, such as litter trays; these jobs should be delegated to other members of the household if possible. Where not possible, the owner should wear gloves and wash their hands thoroughly
- Food safety is important; ideally pets should not be fed raw diets
- Bites and scratches should be avoided; rough play and any other behaviour that may lead to these types of injuries should be discouraged
- In the event of a bite or scratch, these should be treated as soon as possible
- Existing cuts or open wounds should be covered and, again, good hand hygiene is essential.

It should be noted that some advice may include keeping pets indoors to minimize contact with other animals, which carries the risk of bringing disease into the household. Given that there are other ways that disease/vectors/parasites could be introduced into the household, the authors do not believe this to be necessary. In addition, a restriction such as this could be detrimental for the welfare of the animal.

As well as pet ownership, the use of animals as therapy dogs within other environments, such as a hospital, is increasing as research regarding the benefits continues to grow. The Royal College of Nursing published guidelines *Working with Dogs in Health Care Settings* currently state that "Patients who are immunocompromised or nursed under protective isolation are not to be visited by the animal-assisted intervention team" (RCN, 2019; Figure 9.14).

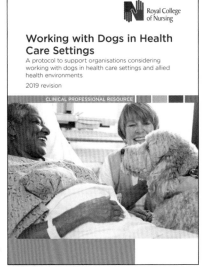

9.14 The Royal College of Nursing publishes clinical professional resources, including *Working with Dogs in Health Care Settings*.
(© Royal College of Nursing)

Some studies have been conducted looking at the duration and type of animal contact required to elicit some of the same positive benefits associated with pet ownership and animal-assisted interventions. Several studies have indicated that merely observing animals can have a positive effect on stress-moderation; some studies have even shown that these effects are evident in people watching videos of animals. There have also been a handful of studies considering the role of soft toys for both those with dissociative disorders and those with dementia. While these alternatives are clearly not a complete substitute for the unconditional love, affection and companionship that a person may receive from an animal, they may be worthy of consideration as an alternative and pose less of a risk than introducing an animal into a situation that may be detrimental to their welfare.

Exotic pet trade

Discussions around the exotic pet trade often involve the use of very emotive language and opinions are frequently based on a small number of isolated cases of exotic pet ownership gone wrong. Undesirable isolated cases occur in dog and cat ownership too, and highlight the importance of education. In a small number of cases, the desire for an exotic pet is based on misinformation, sometimes driven by animals appearing in films, adverts and social media posts. The often unrealistic portrayal of exotic pet ownership needs to be discouraged and more focus needs to be placed on the long-term challenges of keeping these species. One example is the macaw: they are very beautiful birds, but the ones used for filming are highly trained to a level that may not be achievable in a pet's home. Veterinary professionals must encourage exotic pet owners to discuss potential purchases with them, without judging or disrespecting the wants and needs of the owner. Owners need to be able to seek out supportive and proactive veterinary care without issue; if owners are made to feel uneducated or disrespected, they will stop seeking veterinary care, which can only worsen animal welfare. Trying to ban exotic pet ownership is not the answer, this would drive the hobby underground and remove any opportunities for education.

When the importation of wild-caught exotic pets (Figure 9.15) is discussed, passions run high and people

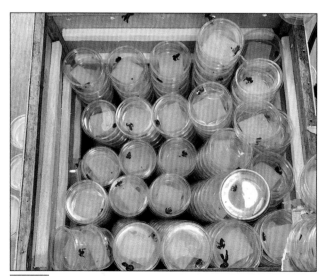

9.15 A shipment of wild-caught frogs.

are quick to judge this trade as inhumane and request that it be banned. However, some consideration needs to be given to the positive socioeconomic impact this trade can have. The focus again needs to be on educating trappers, traders and importers. on how to carry out imports properly and with a high standard of animal care and welfare. If these animals are handled respectfully, they will often do well in captivity. Not allowing this trade would devalue the animals *in situ* and could lead to their welfare being compromised in the wild.

Animal-assisted interventions

Unsurprisingly, given the close historical relationship of humans and dogs, it is believed that the dog was the first species to be used to aid those with disabilities. There are various depictions throughout history of dogs being used to assist the blind, including a fresco that dates to ancient Roman times. Johann Wilhelm Klein was a pioneer for the teaching of the blind and, in 1819, published one of the first textbooks to reference the use and training of dogs to support the blind. After the First World War, with many soldiers returning having been blinded, German doctor Gerhard Stalling explored methods of training dogs to assist them. He opened the world's first dog training school and it is this work that is credited as the beginning of the modern-day guide dogs for the blind and the subsequent growth and development of the assistant dog role.

The use of animals for therapy also has a long history, with official records dating back to the 18th century; animals were used in facilities for the mentally ill and general hospitals to provide social interaction and promote wellbeing. The military have, for a long time, used dogs for therapeutic purposes. It was psychiatrist Dr Boris Levinson who became a pioneer for animal-assisted therapy (AAT) after discovering that his child therapy sessions were more productive when his dog was present. His work led to the establishment of other organizations such as Therapy Dogs International and the Delta Foundation, now known as Pet Partners, who have continued the research and promotion of the benefits of animal-assisted interventions. Since then, there has been significant growth and evolution in both the number and types of assistance animals. Alongside the benefits to the physical and mental wellbeing of the individuals in need, their extended family, friends and carers can also benefit from these interactions. The dog remains the most commonly used assistance animal, but the diversity of species has expanded to include miniature horses, cats, small mammals, birds and exotic species.

Categories of assistance

Clarifying the categories of assistance and therapy animals is not an easy task, especially with the growing expansion of roles, but is important as they perform very different functions and are afforded different legal protections.

Assistance dogs

These dogs are specially trained to provide specific support to an individual. They are working dogs and not classed as pets. However, the strong bond and the companionship provided should not be underestimated; studies show that assistance dogs have a positive influence on self-esteem and anxiety levels and alleviate social isolation. Assistance dogs include:

- **Guide dogs** – supporting those with loss of sight or impairment
- **Hearing dogs** – supporting those with hearing loss or impairment
- **Mobility dogs** – supporting those with a physical disability by aiding mobility and assisting with tasks such as pushing/pulling wheelchairs, opening doors, shopping and laundry
- **Medical alert dogs** – supporting those with medical conditions such as epilepsy or diabetes, alerting them when they are at imminent risk of seizure/hypoglycaemic episode
- **Autism dogs** – supporting those with autism by providing routine, breaking repetitive behaviour and providing comfort in unfamiliar surroundings
- **Mental health dogs** – providing support to those with mental health issues, such as post-traumatic stress disorder (PTSD) or depression.

In the USA, assistance dogs are usually referred to as service dogs. In addition to service dogs, there are now also a small number of miniature horses providing a service as a guide animal for someone with sight loss or visual impairment.

Animal-assisted therapy

The animal and the handler are specially trained to assist healthcare practitioners with delivering specific, goal-driven interventions to aid a person's recovery by promoting improvement in physical, emotional and cognitive function. It is believed that one of the ways that AAT assists with recovery is by providing a strong motivational factor for individuals. For example, one study showed that individuals that participated in AAT had an increased voluntary ambulation treatment participation rate and walked twice as much as those that did not participate in AAT (Knisely *et al.*, 2012). Having an animal present in therapy situations can also enhance emotional safety and reduce anxiety and barriers to the situation.

After dogs, horses are the second most used animal for AAT. Horse-assisted therapy takes several forms:

- **Equine-facilitated psychotherapy** – promotes and practices interactions with horses to assist those with mental health conditions, such as PTSD, anxiety and depression
- **Equine-facilitated learning** – provides emotional and social support through horse-based activities and is particularly effective for young adults
- **Hippotherapy** – uses the movements of the horse to assist with improvements in motor and sensory skills of the patient. The movement of the horse is an essential part of the therapy. Hippotherapy is performed using a specially trained horse and handler alongside a physiotherapist or occupational therapist
- **Therapeutic riding** – performed by a riding instructor under the direction of a hippotherapist with the patient learning specific riding skills. Horseback riding mimics human gait and aids improvements in physical strength, balance and flexibility of the patient, as well as providing social and emotional benefits. It is particularly effective for children with cerebral palsy, Down's syndrome and autism.

Dolphin therapy refers to the therapeutic practice of swimming with dolphins. The patient, usually a child with disabilities, has a one-to-one session with a therapist in a marine facility. The evidence to support this type of therapy is controversial, as is the ethical issue of using captive dolphins.

Animal-assisted activity

This is the most common form of intervention and is usually provided by pet owner volunteers via a charity organization. These animals need to meet certain criteria but do not require specific training. They simply enable a general interaction for the recipient which provides a beneficial, therapeutic effect. Due to this, the diversity of species used is much broader than that used for the other categories of assistance animals. Animal-assisted activity takes place in many different settings, for example, hospitals, care homes, schools and hospices.

- **Dogs** – most widely used.
- **Cats** – can be suitable for individuals who might be fearful of dogs or just prefer cats. They can be more difficult to control and train so are often used in establishments, such as care homes, where they can roam freely.
- **Small mammals** – rabbits, hamsters and guinea pigs are widely used as they offer the same benefits in terms of companionship and improving motor skills but being smaller, they are easier to transport and contain.
- **Reptiles** – require specific care, and this, along with their uniqueness, is a reason for their growing popularity as therapy animals. Caring for reptiles can act as a distraction and build self-esteem, providing a coping mechanism for those with mental health issues, such as PTSD, eating disorders and depression.
- **Birds** – birds, in particular parrots, are also increasingly used, for similar reasons to reptiles. Parrots can also show high levels of empathy and can be trained to talk or perform tricks which further adds to their appeal. Some veterans suffering with PTSD work in sanctuaries caring for abused birds.

Emotional support animals

These are dogs and other animals that provide emotional support and comfort to owners. They must be legally prescribed by a licensed mental health professional (e.g. psychiatrist or therapist). They do not have special training like assistance animals.

Assistance animals and the law

Most countries provide legal protection for assistance dogs and their owners under their respective disability acts; service providers cannot discriminate against people with a disability or because they have an assistance dog. Service providers are required to make reasonable adjustments to accommodate assistance dogs and cannot refuse access except under very exceptional circumstances. Despite this, variation in laws between countries, and even within different areas of the same country, regarding accreditation and regulation of assistance animals still presents a range of issues, including continued discrimination and refusal of access. It is important to note that currently the law only extends to assistance dogs and does not include therapy dogs or other species. The exception to this is in the USA, as the Americans with Disabilities Act (ADA) now includes a separate provision regarding miniature horses, which states that entities covered by the ADA must modify their policies to permit miniature horses where reasonable.

Another exception in the USA is regarding emotional support animals (ESA); these animals do not have the same legal protection as service animals, but there are two federal laws which grant them special rights:

- **The Fair Housing Amendments Act 1988** – enables living and staying at any home/lodging with an ESA, even those that prohibit animals
- **The Air Carrier Access Act** – allows an ESA to accompany their owner into the aircraft cabin.

A growing number of organizations across the world aim to promote and provide access to assistance and therapy animals. In the UK, although many of these are accredited to Assistance Dogs International (ADI) or the International Guide Dog Federation (IGDF), this is not currently a legal requirement. The accreditation process for these organizations is rigorous, ensuring that all aspects, including dog training and welfare, client support and supporting infrastructure, meet a specific standard. The lack of clarity relating to the accreditation and regulatory process poses a risk if less reputable organizations do not adhere to the same standards, potentially compromising welfare and safety of both the person and the animal. There is a current initiative by the Disability Unit (part of the Department for Work and Pensions) that aims to bring stakeholders together to create a Public Access Test (PAT) that would be available for owner–trainer–assistance dog partnerships trained by non-ADI/IGDF organizations, the hope being that this will then lead to a national register of assistance dogs that have either been trained by the ADI/IGDF or have successfully completed the PAT test.

Accrediting organizations for assistance dogs
Assistance Dogs International

Assistance Dogs International is a worldwide coalition of not-for-profit organizations that train and place assistance dogs. Founded in 1986, it is the leading authority in this field and has several regional chapters across the world, each comprising at least five member organizations:

- Assistance Dogs UK (ADUK)
- Assistance Dogs Europe (ADEu)
- Assistance Dogs North America (ADINA)
- Oceania – Australia/New Zealand.

International Guide Dog Federation

The IGDF was formed in 1989 and currently comprises 95 member organizations. In response to the growing recognition of the benefits of animal-assisted interventions, the Royal College of Nursing introduced the first protocol to address concerns regarding bringing animals into healthcare settings – *Working with Dogs in Health Care Settings* (RCN, 2019; see Figure 9.14). These best practice guidelines highlight the precautions that should be taken regarding infection control and health and safety.

Welfare considerations for animal-assisted interventions

As with pet ownership, most literature regarding animal-assisted interventions is focused on the benefits to humans; research regarding the impact on animals is somewhat lacking. Although in some roles, these animals are not classed as pets, they are 'owned' by someone and therefore their health and wellbeing are still dictated by this relationship in the same way as a pet's; for example, the lifestyles and behaviours that they are exposed to can still put them at risk of obesity. In addition, there is a unique array of welfare issues to consider; these vary depending on the type of assistance that the animal is providing. For example, assistance dogs are with their owners all of the time and are expected to perform specific tasks, whereas animals used for AAI will assist with multiple different people and in a variety of different environments; both present different challenges.

At the very least, basic welfare needs (see Chapter 1) and preventive healthcare requirements need to be met. The physical needs of animals, (i.e. the need for food, water and shelter) are often better understood by people; there is less recognition of their social and behavioural needs. Both physical and mental needs require attention to ensure optimal welfare of these animals.

Welfare considerations for assistance dogs

Assistance animals are exposed to many processes and a frequently changing environment to prepare them for their role which presents a unique set of challenges.

Selection and breeding

The need for specific physical and behavioural characteristics means that breeding programmes are still prominent within assistance dog organizations, particularly for the breeding of guide dogs. Labrador Retrievers, Golden Retrievers and German Shepherd Dogs are the most frequently used breeds. Assistance dog organizations will also accept donations or purchase puppies from other breeders. While breeding programmes can provide more assurance in terms of uniformity of physical and behavioural characteristics, there are a number of ethical considerations including the risk of inherited disorders, the welfare of the dogs used for breeding and the welfare of those puppies/adolescent dogs that do not make the grade. The Guide Dogs National Breeding Centre adheres to their own Breeding Code of Ethics, working closely and in consultation with The Kennel Club; other accredited organizations adhere to The Kennel Club Code of Ethics.

Although there has been some success with the training and use of dogs rescued from animal shelters as assistance animals, the lack of a complete history means that there is some hesitancy in deeming them suitable for all assistance animal roles. They tend to be considered more suitable for roles that are less physically demanding and do not require specific physical characteristics, such as hearing dogs or therapy dogs. There is a potential ethical argument for using dogs rescued from animal shelters, providing a new life for them and reducing the need for breeding programmes. However, given the potential negative implications for the welfare of animals used for AAI, it would be wise to adopt a cautious approach to the selection and use of these animals, given that they may have been exposed to certain emotional and physical stressors in the past.

Training and development

Many working dogs have an instinctive motivation to perform tasks; for certain breeds, herding, searching for game or running with a pack of dogs requires little or no reward. In comparison, despite breed selection for specific characteristics, many of the tasks required of assistance dogs are not in line with their innate behaviours; in these cases they can have difficulty understanding the objective of the task. Training, therefore, requires operant conditioning – a learning process in which behaviour is modified by the reinforcing or inhibiting effect of its consequences. Many organizations are now adopting more positive reinforcement training techniques, such as clicker training. However, given the aversive nature of some tasks, there is still the potential for conflict, with the dog receiving a reward for performing a task that it initially neither understands nor enjoys. The training process is also very dependent on the handler's ability and technique; poor handling, rewarding at the wrong time or using punishment can cause confusion and apathy in the dog. There is also the potential for an inexperienced handler to wrongly interpret responses as the dog misbehaving.

Assistance Dogs International publishes standards and ethical guidelines on training that cover the responsibility of trainers, programmes and clients. Accredited organizations are expected to adhere to all minimum standards and to keep up to date on information regarding dog training, behaviour and care.

The training process itself can be a source of stress as it involves many different environments. The puppies spend their first 12–14 months with a foster family and then another 4 months receiving intensive training with the organization. This means that they go from a very social environment to a more isolated one, with periods of kennelling. A good organization will make efforts to address this by providing enrichment and play/rest opportunities. Some will also foster the dogs during the advanced training period to minimize the time spent in kennels.

A gradual introduction into the unpredictability of the role is important to enable the best opportunity for success and to minimize any negative effects. Adequate and appropriate enrichment and rest opportunities are also important components of maintaining the dog's welfare during the training process.

Sources of stress

Assistance animals are exposed to many potential sources of stress, including noise, crowds, unfamiliar people and other animals, unpredictable routines, and insufficient time to rest. It is, therefore, important that trainers, handlers, clients and healthcare professionals are appropriately trained to recognize signs of stress. Motivation of the dog to perform their role can be a good indicator; strong motivation indicates that there is no detrimental impact and, conversely, lack of motivation indicates cause for concern. Assistance animals are trained to remain calm and not react to certain situations so they may not exhibit stress-associated behaviours in the normal way. It is more difficult for them to get away from or avoid situations that they are not enjoying; they are very reliant on the ability of the people around them to effectively interpret this and intervene as appropriate.

Assistance animals also need the opportunity for rest, play and toileting. These factors should be considered if a dog starts to show signs that may be perceived as 'poor behaviour'. For example, toileting in the house may actually be a sign that the dog is not getting enough opportunity outside of the house when they are considered to be working. Apathy may be a sign that the dog is overworked and overtired. It can also be a sign that their physical health is affected, particularly in older dogs.

Specific roles can have different sources of stress; for example, assistance dogs working with children or adults with behavioural or psychiatric health conditions may experience rough handling or even abuse.

Physical stress

Some of the tasks required of assistance dogs can test the limits of their physical capabilities and, in some instances, result in injury or physical strain. One example is the pulling of a wheelchair which is designed to be pushed and is not aligned with the dog's natural movement; this can have an impact on the comfort of the harness, putting pressure on different parts of the dog's body. The force required to move the wheelchair is dependent on many factors, such as duration, distance, floor surface and gradient. Another example is the opening of doors; the dog is trained to take hold of a rope (or similar) that is attached to the door. The dog needs enough leverage and traction on the rope to open the door, which can put pressure on the mouth and teeth and potentially on the joints as they pull and crouch backwards.

In addition, there can be more basic sources of physical stress for the dog. For example, harnesses are routinely used to enable effective handling of the dog by the client. If these are not fitted correctly or the dog gains weight, they can be uncomfortable and cause rubbing. Selecting an appropriate harness requires consideration of the types of tasks that the dog will be performing, to ensure that the harness protects them appropriately. Other factors that can cause physical stress include working conditions (such as duration of working hours, temperatures that they are exposed to, opportunities for rest and toileting).

Ageing and retirement

The cognitive and physical impairment that comes with the ageing process is particularly problematic for assistance dogs, more so than those used for AAT or AAA. Assistance dogs have specific, often physical, roles to fulfil; a reduced ability to perform these has consequences for both the welfare of the animal and the safety of the owner. These animals are heavily relied upon by the owners and so planning for the inevitable ageing and eventual retirement of the animal needs careful consideration. Retirement provides the opportunity for freedom and rest from the stressors and tasks to which the dog was exposed. Conversely, the sudden change from working to not working can actually be quite stressful and confusing for the dog. A slow transition with a gradual reduction of duties would help alleviate this anxiety but this is often not possible due to the level of dependency that the client has on the dog.

Consideration of where the dog should be homed following retirement also presents a challenge. Staying with the client potentially enables the human-animal bond to be maintained but often the client requires a new assistance dog and is unable to manage two dogs, especially an older dog with declining health. Equally, the dog may not adapt to no longer being needed or the presence of a replacement. Rehoming the dog means breaking the bond, which is emotionally distressing for both. A good compromise may be rehoming the dog to someone that the client knows, thus enabling the relationship to be maintained through visits.

Decisions regarding when to retire a dog require assessment of a number of factors – physical and cognitive health, age, and role-specific factors and expectations – and are made jointly between the assistance dog organization and client, with possible input from the veterinary team. It is quite subjective and no evidence-based standards are currently available.

Welfare considerations for AAT/AAA animals

Animals used for AAT or AAA are taken into a variety of environments and confronted with strangers. Although they have been assessed for their suitability to perform these roles, it should be acknowledged that certain situations can still provoke a stress response. Animals are very dependent on their handler's ability to identify this; it is important that there is always someone advocating for the animal. There is the potential for stress-related fatigue; consideration should be given to the duration of AAT/AAA sessions. It has been suggested that there should be a maximum duration of 1 hour for each session but this is dependent on the individual animal's response and needs. In addition to this, adequate opportunity for rest following each session should be provided.

Residential animals can be particularly at risk of stress-related fatigue if they do not receive adequate 'downtime'. They need a 'safe area' where they can retreat and residents/staff know that they cannot be disturbed. Again, having a designated person that can advocate for them is important. There is the potential for rough handling or abuse/cruelty if adequate supervision is not provided; this can be more of a concern in specific environments where there are behavioural or mental health concerns.

There is no doubt that the impact of assistance and therapy animals can be hugely positive and transformational for the recipients. However, as the scope of these roles continues to evolve, it becomes even more important that the welfare needs of these animals are taken into account. There are organizations seeking to achieve appropriate standardization and accreditation of assistance dog programmes, including the welfare of the animals, but this is currently not compulsory. Research on the benefits of these relationships for people is plentiful; future research needs a shift in focus to one that considers the animal.

Covid-19

This chapter was written as the world was in the middle of a novel coronavirus pandemic. The outbreak was first identified in Wuhan, China in December 2019. At the time of writing, evidence suggests that the origin of the virus was an animal source, with the wet markets and seafood markets under scrutiny. However, the evidence is not sufficient to identify the source or explain the original route of transmission to humans (i.e. the possible involvement of an intermediate host). The implication of the role of wildlife as a source and the subsequent detection of the virus in other species highlights the links between the human–animal–environment interface. It also emphasizes the complex relationship of the human–animal bond.

Despite a lack of convincing evidence of the involvement of animals in the spread of coronavirus to humans, reports of the detection of the virus in other animals were enough to cause initial panic, with reports of pet cruelty and abandonment. Other reasons for abandonment included people forced into evacuation from their homes in some countries, and unemployment. Conversely, there was also an increase in the number of people wanting to foster or adopt animals during the imposed lockdown of their country. The lockdown also meant that those with companion animals had more time to spend with them, strengthening their bond.

Wildlife also took the opportunity to benefit from a locked-down world, roaming urban areas freely. Not all wildlife appeared to benefit, however; protected species were left vulnerable to poaching and destruction of habitats through illegal deforestation due to the inability to maintain adequate surveillance of conservation areas. Animals in zoological collections that were forced to close demonstrated a range of behavioural changes, with some reports claiming they appeared to miss the attention of visitors, and their existence was under threat due to the costs associated with closures.

There were also benefits and consequences for the environment. Reduction in travel, resulted in significant reductions in air pollution and greenhouse gas emissions, and a vast improvement in air quality. Conversely, an increase in takeaways and online purchases, resulted in a rise in the production of unrecyclable waste. Vast quantities of used personal protective equipment have further contributed to this.

Healthcare providers for both people and animals were required to undergo a rapid transformation in response to the virus. Hospitals needed to divert all of their resources to coping with the volume of people affected by the virus, with new facilities rapidly being erected to provide enough beds. Veterinary practices needed to respond and adapt to new ways of providing services, for example via telemedicine. Guidelines and information required continuous writing and updating in response to the rapidly changing situation. The pandemic also gave rise to excellent examples of interdisciplinary collaboration; veterinary professionals shared personal protective equipment, medical equipment and laboratory equipment with the NHS, and utilized their knowledge and skills to support public health through disease modelling.

Since its emergence, coronavirus has caused a global state of instability – a cycle of lockdowns and rule changes. Even with the development of vaccines, the future remains uncertain. The veterinary profession, already in a recruitment and retention crisis, is now facing additional workload pressures due to the impact of the pandemic, self-isolation requirements and an unprecedented rise in pet ownership.

The coronavirus pandemic made clear the risk for an unknown pathogen to emerge at any time and has served as a stark reminder of the need for the interdisciplinary collaboration and communication of the One Health approach and that this cannot exist at just a global or national level. The response has demonstrated the capability to adopt this approach at a local level; veterinary and healthcare professionals should ensure that this is continued. We have a responsibility to embed a One Health approach in our daily work and to educate the wider community on their role within it, whether this is in response to another pandemic or tackling one of the many other issues under the One Health umbrella.

References and further reading

Association of Respiratory Nurse Specialists (2017) *ARNS leads with RCN & RCVS on One Health Project*. Available from: arns.co.uk

Bartges J, Kushner RF, Michel KE, Sallis R and Day MJ (2017) One Health Solutions to Obesity in People and Their Pets. *Journal of Comparative Pathology* **156**, 326–333

British Veterinary Association (2018) *UK's leading veterinary body debunks links between canine autism and vaccination*. Available from: www.bva.co.uk/news-and-blog/news-article/uk-s-leading-veterinary-body-debunks-link-between-canine-autism-and-vaccination/

Davidson S and Rossall P (2015) *Age UK Loneliness Evidence Review*. Available from: www.ageuk.org.uk

Day M (2017) One Health Approach to Preventing Obesity in People and Their Pets. *Journal of Comparative Pathology* **156**, 293–295

Destoumieux-Garzón D, Mavingui P, Boetsch G *et al.* (2018) The One Health Concept: 10 Years Old and a Long Road Ahead. *Frontiers in Veterinary Science* **5**, 14

Endenburg N and van Lith HA (2011) The influence of animals on the development of children. *The Veterinary Journal* **190**, 208–214

Knisely JS, Barker SB and Barker RT (2012) Research on benefits of canine-assisted therapy for adults in non-military settings. *US Army Medical Department Journal* **2012**, 30–37

Levine GN, Allen K, Braun LT *et al.* (2013) Pet Ownership and Cardiovascular Risk: A Scientific Statement From the American Heart Association. *Circulation* **127**, 2353–2363

McNicholas J, Gilbey A, Rennie A *et al.* (2005) Pet ownership and human health: a brief review of evidence and issues. *British Medical Journal* **331**, 1252

Paules CI, Eisinger RW, Marston HD and Fauci AS (2017) What Recent History Has Taught Us About Responding to Emerging Infectious Disease Threats. *Annals of Internal Medicine* **167**, 805–811

People's Dispensary for Sick Animals (2020) *PDSA Animal Wellbeing (PAW) Report 2020*. Available from: www.pdsa.org.uk

Prochaska J and DiClemente C (1983) Stages and processes of self-change in smoking: toward an integrative model of change. *Journal of Consulting and Clinical Psychology* **5**, 390–395

Public Health England (2018) *Turning the tide on tobacco: Smoking in England hits a new low*. Available from: publichealthmatters.blog.gov.uk/2018/07/03

Public Health England (2019) *Guidance – Emerging infections: how and why they arise*. Available from: www.gov.uk/government/publications

Rabinowitz PM, Odofin L and Dein FJ (2008) From "us *versus* them" to "shared risk": can animals help link environmental factors to human health? *EcoHealth* **5**, 224–229

Royal College of Nursing (2019) *Working with Dogs in Health Care Settings* – 2019 revision. Available from www.rcn.org.uk/professional-development/publications/

Rutstein DD, Mullan RJ, Frazier TM *et al.* (1983) Sentinel Health Events (occupational): a basis for physician recognition and public health surveillance. *American Journal of Public Health* **73**, 1054–1062

Wensley (2008) Animal welfare and the human–animal bond: considerations for veterinary faculty, students, and practitioners. *Journal of Veterinary Medicine Education* **35**, 532–539

Willis CM, Church SM, Guest CM *et al.* (2004) Olfactory Detection of Human Bladder Cancer by Dogs: Proof of Principle Study. *BMJ* **329**, 712

Wolfe ND, Dunavan CP and Diamond J (2007) Origins of major human infectious diseases. *Nature* **447**, 279–283

World Health Organization (2020) *Rabies factsheet*. Available from: www.who.int/news-room/fact-sheets/detail/rabies

Useful websites

Assistance Dogs International
assistancedogsinternational.org/

BSAVA/SAMSoc Guide to Responsible Use of Antibacterials: PROTECT ME
www.bsavalibrary.com/protectme

BVA Resources & support
www.bva.co.uk/resources-support

Centre for Disease Control and Prevention (CDC)
www.cdc.gov/

Guide Dogs for the Blind Association
www.guidedogs.org.uk/

Human Animal Bond Research Institute (HABRI)
habri.org/

International Guide Dog Federation
www.igdf.org.uk/

Links Group – raising awareness of the link between the abuse of people and animals
thelinksgroup.org.uk/

Pet Partners – therapy pets and animal-assisted activities
petpartners.org/

Small Animal Veterinary Surveillance Network (SAVSNET)
www.liverpool.ac.uk/savsnet/

Street Vet – veterinary care of the pets of the homeless
www.streetvet.co.uk/

The Blue Dog Project – safe relationships between children and dogs
www.thebluedog.org/en/

Vet Sustain – Championing sustainability in the veterinary professions
vetsustain.org/

Chapter 10

Veterinary team health and welfare

Carolyne Crowe, Amy Martin and Penny Barker

A good day in practice

- How was work today?
- Did you have a good day?

These are simple questions, but their answers run deeper than a simple yes or no. When teams in veterinary practices are asked 'what makes a good day in practice?', their answers encompass broad themes including job satisfaction, personal growth, supporting others, and physical and mental health (Figure 10.1).

As Figure 10.1 demonstrates, many different aspects of practice life are mentioned; some of these factors are directly within our control but many are not. We cannot control which animals or clients walk through the practice door, nor, to a large extent, how well they respond to our efforts to help them; we can simply do our best to positively influence outcomes.

The theme of 'control' is central to this chapter. When things are within our control, we can take action to change them; if they are not, we need to learn to manage our reactions to both situations and people. Therefore, whatever your position in practice, the authors would encourage you to reflect on what is within your control that will help you and your team to thrive at work.

- What can you do to help yourself?
- What can you do to help your team?

- Feeling I have made a difference
- Learning something new
- Comfortably busy
- Grateful clients
- Time for lunch
- Feeling supported
- Feeling refreshed
- Helping someone else
- Teaching students
- Time to exercise or socialize after work
- Interesting cases
- Not being overbooked
- Discussing cases with colleagues
- Time for a break
- Getting feedback from my manager
- Cake!
- Time to finish a cup of tea
- Good patient outcomes

10.1 Delegate thoughts on 'what makes a good day in practice?'

There is often more within our collective control than we think and, by working together as individuals, managers and practice owners, we can all have more good days in practice.

What is wellbeing?

At a basic level, psychological wellbeing is about feeling good. It is, however, more than just being in a good mood – it is *feeling good about yourself and your life*. The model described by psychologist Carol Ryff breaks wellbeing down into six categories:

- **Purpose in life** – Goal orientation and conviction that life holds meaning
- **Autonomy** – Lives in accordance with one's own personal convictions, independent of social pressures
- **Personal growth** – Continues to develop, welcomes new experiences and recognizes improvement in behaviour and self over time
- **Environmental mastery** – Makes effective use of opportunities and feels in control of environmental factors and activities, including managing everyday affairs and creating situations to benefit personal needs
- **Positive relationships** – Engages in meaningful relationships with others that involve reciprocal empathy, intimacy and affection
- **Self-acceptance** – A positive attitude about his or her self.

It is clear from this model that the practice has a key part to play in supporting the psychological wellbeing of its team members. This could be in small things such as enabling employees to manage their everyday affairs (e.g. attending a doctor's appointment), through to more actively supporting their personal and professional development.

Veterinary surgeon (veterinarian) David Bartram has expanded on these themes by describing four mechanisms that create conditions for teams to thrive in practice. These are:

- Providing discretion with regards to decision-making (autonomy)
- Sharing information
- Minimizing incivility
- Offering performance feedback.

These models are important to consider as they clearly differentiate between good physical health and good psychological wellbeing.

- An individual may have physical health problems but still feel good about themselves and their lives.
- An individual may have excellent physical health but low psychological wellbeing.

In the workplace, this highlights the need to support both the physical health and psychological wellbeing of the wider practice team, to reduce:

- Poor physical health, which can negatively impact psychological wellbeing, particularly over time or if the employee does not feel supported to recover
- Long-term psychological distress caused by workplace stress, leading to physical illness such as cardiovascular disease, diabetes and immune system malfunction.

Practices and teams that are thriving are often composed of happy, healthy individuals who feel connected to and satisfied by their work.

- Are you, your team and your practice thriving?

Psychological safety

Amy Edmondson, from the Harvard Business School, refers to psychological safety as a climate in which "people are comfortable being (and expressing) themselves". It encourages individuals to demonstrate both vulnerability and creativity without fear of recrimination, thus creating an open and supportive environment where individuals feel able to discuss mistakes and near misses, express opinions and engage in healthy debate about ideas and approaches. In this kind of environment, people feel confident that they are supported, can ask for and will receive help when in difficulty and are therefore willing to stretch themselves to learn and grow.

Within the veterinary profession, patient safety and quality improvement are driven by a culture where mistakes, learning and new ideas can be discussed openly. Creating a culture of psychological safety is therefore vital not just for the wellbeing of team members, but for the welfare of the animals under their care.

Workplace wellbeing – a business priority

There is a growing emphasis on workplace and employee wellbeing in business and with good reason – employee wellbeing impacts the bottom line. Research shows that high levels of employee wellbeing lead to increased:

- Productivity
- Client satisfaction
- Staff retention and recruitment.

In the veterinary profession, individuals who feel satisfied and supported in their work, and who have the mental and physical resources to cope with the demands they face, will make better clinical decisions and fewer mistakes. Making employee wellbeing a priority is therefore not just good business sense but a moral and ethical imperative; practices and larger organizations ignore it at their peril.

Who is responsible for wellbeing in practice?

Wellbeing is everyone's responsibility. Every team member in a practice is an individual with a life that extends beyond the practice walls. Some elements of wellbeing are solely within the control of the individual (e.g. what time they choose to go to bed) and some are solely within the control of the employer (e.g. ensuring the physical equipment is safe to use).

There are many elements, however, that are a shared responsibility between the team member and the practice. One example of this would be the management team actively encouraging and supporting employees to take adequate breaks through the implementation of policies and the modelling of behaviours, and the team member taking it upon themselves to not only take breaks but use them to rest, eat and recover rather than simply catching up on work.

If the responsibility for wellbeing is shared by engaged individuals, teams and the practice, it becomes embedded and sustainable. Everyone at every level makes wellbeing a priority and takes ownership and action for bringing it alive, thus creating a culture in which both individuals and the business can thrive (Figure 10.2). This is the essence of organizational culture; it is both top-down from the leaders and bottom-up from individuals and teams. Everyone has a part to play in building and shaping the practice culture.

In this chapter, strategies that enable individuals, teams and practices to put wellbeing at the heart of their culture are discussed. The nature of the profession is changing and not all practices or veterinary businesses are the same; however, the recommendations in this chapter can be adopted and adapted whatever the size or type of practice.

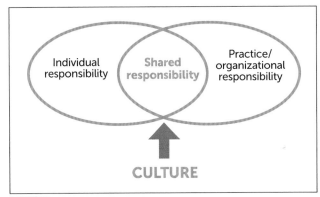

10.2 Sharing responsibility to create a wellbeing culture.

Environmental mastery

Workplace stress

The Health and Safety Executive (HSE) defines workplace stress as "the adverse reaction people have to excessive pressures or other types of demand placed on them" (HSE, 2022). It is the feeling of being out of control and unable to cope with the pressures and demands placed upon you.

Workplace stress affects everyone differently; what stresses one person may be a motivator for another. Therefore, it is essential not to make assumptions and presumptions but to identify the actual risks and challenges to those working within your team so that you are aware and can take appropriate action to prevent problems arising and escalating.

Historically, a reactive approach has been taken, with action only occurring as a direct response to a significant problem occurring in a practice, but the profession is now starting to reflect changes in wider society and taking a more proactive approach to identifying and mitigating the causes of workplace stress. Doing so will improve well-being at all levels, as well as improving outcomes for patients and practices alike.

Legal responsibility

There is also a legal responsibility to create safe places of work and to assess and minimize the risks of workplace stress. Workplace stress straddles several pieces of legislation (Acas, 2014). Those of note are:

- Health and Safety at Work etc. Act 1974
- Management of Health and Safety at Work Regulations 1999
- The Equality Act 2010
- The Management Standards 2004 (set of best practice standards not the law).

What influences workplace stress?

The HSE Management Standards identify six key areas:

- The **demands** people are under – workloads, work patterns and the work environment
- How much **control** people have over the way in which they work
- Their job **role** – do people know their role and have steps been taken to ensure job roles aren't conflicting?
- The quality of **relationships** within the team
- How **change** is managed and communicated at work
- The degree of **support** available, both in terms of people, systems and resources available.

Identifying the signs of stress

Stress is a normal physiological and emotional response to pressure and it therefore drives changes in our physiology and behaviour. This is helpful because it means that we can start to recognize and acknowledge the signs of stress in both ourselves and others. We can then try to identify the cause(s), discuss the challenges, review possible options and then implement potential solutions and review their impact. Identifying the signs of stress early on can help to prevent more serious mental and physical health problems, as well as preventing indirect issues for patient care through poor communication or impaired decision-making.

Individuals express a variety of signs and everyone may react differently. Some of the common signs of stress are listed in Figure 10.3.

- Which signs of stress do you recognize in yourself?
- What about the signs within your team?
- How long have they been going on for?
- What does this tell you?
- Have you ever discussed with your colleagues how you know that you are stressed?
- How can you work together to get to know each other's early signs to offer support when you spot them?

Physical signs

- Hyperventilating
- Heart palpitations
- Sweating
- Fatigue
- Disturbed sleep patterns
- Headaches
- Back aches, muscle tension
- Digestive disorders: stomach ache, nausea, ulcers, diarrhoea, 'butterflies in stomach'
- Frequent illness/colds
- Weight gain/loss
- Crying

Emotional signs

- Overwhelmed
- Upset
- Angry
- Out of control
- Worried
- On edge
- Lack of confidence
- Not able to relax
- Depressed
- Sad

Behavioural signs

- Quicker to anger
- Procrastinating
- More aggressive
- Use of drugs or alcohol to 'relax'
- Using food for comfort or control
- More nervous
- Impatient
- Mood swings
- Hyperexcitable/more fidgety
- Withdrawn
- Disinterested
- Lack of creativity
- Lack of concentration
- Distracted
- Defensive
- Passive
- Indecisive
- Unable to delegate
- Burying self in work
- Blaming self – 'It's all my fault', 'I should be able to cope', 'Everyone else can cope'

10.3 Common physical, emotional and behavioural signs of stress.

The 'Good Day in Practice' model in Figure 10.4 can be a useful starting point for thinking and talking with your team about challenges to wellbeing in practice.

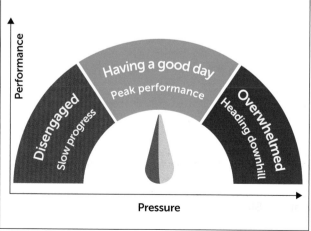

10.4 'Good Day in Practice' model.
(Adapted from Robertson Cooper)

Asking teams and individuals questions can raise awareness, stimulate discussion and generate ideas for resolutions. Such questions may include:

* What does a good day in practice look like for you?
* What tips you into the red/grey zones?
* What takes you back into the green zone?

What is under your control?

As individuals and teams, consideration should be given to the following questions:

* What about these situations is within your control?
* What can you influence?
* What action can you take?

In practice, as in life, there are things that we cannot control; these are the things that we have to accept. An example of this is a client being rude; we can do our best to influence the situation, but we cannot choose how the client speaks to us. Acceptance does not mean that we have to like the situation; we just have to give it space mentally and choose the response that is going to be most helpful to us and the situation going forwards.

For situations that are not within your control, the following questions should be considered:

* How would you like to respond to them?
* How can you help each other to deal with these situations?

When you have identified the challenges within your team on an individual, team and practice level, remember it is not the responsibility of the managers to 'fix' and provide solutions to the problems but rather it is an opportunity for everyone to openly discuss the facts, suggest ideas and have a collaborative approach to solutions that everyone buys in to and can be held accountable for.

Working together helps to empower individuals and generate buy-in from the team, in contrast to solutions simply generated and imposed by management. This collaborative approach significantly increases the likelihood that sustainable behavioural change will be achieved and a culture of wellbeing created.

Nurturing physical wellbeing

Whilst supporting the health of the animals under our care is at the heart of the veterinary profession, supporting our own health has historically been less of a priority. As individuals, teams and practices there are steps that we can all take to improve physical wellbeing.

Food, water and rest

These most basic human needs can easily be cast aside in a busy veterinary practice, but they are key to both health and performance. Team members may feel that their animal patients take priority over their own needs; however, there are several studies in human healthcare that show that taking breaks, even during procedures, enhances performance and is not detrimental to the patient. Studies also show that the productivity of team members per hour may decrease if they work long hours, making long hours counterproductive in both the short and long term.

Both management and team members can uphold the importance of taking breaks to rest and to eat and actively encourage each other to do so. This also applies to leaving shifts on time. In an organization that performs out-of-hours work, rest breaks and time off after a shift must be a priority.

The Working Time Regulations provide evidence-based guidance for employers and bearing these in mind when designing a rota is likely to make it more sustainable.

Being a veterinary team member is mentally and physically demanding and whilst individuals may want to eat healthily, practice life presents its own obstacles to this – early starts and late finishes, long hours in the car driving to calls and an abundance of chocolates from grateful owners being just the start.

* What are the challenges within your practice?
* What behaviours do you notice?
* What do people do for lunch?
* How could you discuss this with your team?

Consideration should be given to putting in place facilities that enable team members to eat, support their nutritional needs and have time away from both animals and computers. Whilst this is not logistically possible in all practices, the impact on wellbeing needs to be considered and mitigated.

Purpose and autonomy in practice

Team members should be encouraged to pay attention to their purpose (their motivation and the meaning they find from life and work). They should be encouraged to check that their values align with the job they are currently doing and encouraged to reflect on both purpose and values in their reviews. Useful questions to consider include:

* What is important to you?
* What is important to you about being a veterinary surgeon/nurse/receptionist?
* What motivates you?
* What gets you out of bed in the morning?

Clarifying and aligning your purpose as a team and a practice will build bonds and ensure everyone is working towards the same goal; Figure 10.5 suggests a few questions to help individuals and teams with this activity. Conducting exercises like this in team meetings helps to foster a shared sense of purpose, builds trust and encourages ownership of a common vision and goals. Practices can display their values and purpose for both clients and team members to see.

When purpose and values are aligned (Figure 10.6), there is a clear line of sight for all parties from the needs of the business to the needs of the individual team member. This provides a sense of security and environmental mastery as everyone can feel that their needs are being met and have awareness of the bigger picture.

* What is your organization's purpose?
* What is your job's purpose?
* How does your job's purpose support your organization's purpose?
* What is your personal purpose and how does work support this?
* Are all purposes aligned?

10.5 Aligning your purpose.
(From Donovan, 2016)

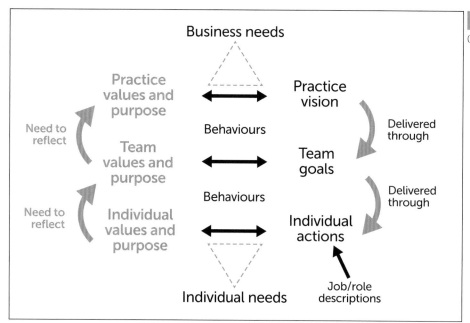

10.6 Aligning values, vision and purpose.
(Courtesy of VDS Training)

The importance of autonomy

In his 2018 book *Drive: The Surprising Truth About What Motivates Us,* Dan Pink highlights the importance of autonomy – the chance for employees to be self-directed – as a key driver for motivation, engagement and productivity. Autonomy promotes self-worth, provides a sense of control over the working day, and allows team members to work on their purpose.

- How can you give team members more autonomy?
- What would be the benefits:
  - For them?
  - For you?

Values and behaviours

Discussing values and behaviours with your team is a powerful way to enable and embed a positive wellbeing culture and create a sense of shared ownership. Questions could include:

- What is important to you as a team?
- What is important about how you work together?
- What do we stand for:
  - As a team?
  - As a practice?

Values are often abstract words such as openness, integrity or professionalism, or broad concepts such as 'clinical excellence' or 'outstanding customer service'. These can be worked into behaviours that can be seen day-to-day with questions such as:

- How do we know when we are acting this value?
- What does this look like day-to-day?
- What behaviours will we not stand for?

A 'behavioural contract' can be discussed and decisions made by everyone about what will and will not be tolerated within the workplace. Team members can then be responsible for ensuring that anyone displaying behaviour not in line with the agreed contract is held accountable, once again ensuring that the culture is supported and maintained by everyone.

Job descriptions

- Do team members know:
  - What is expected of them?
  - What is involved in their job role?
  - How their performance will be measured?
  - How they and their job role fit into the wider team and practice performance?
  - How all the teams fit together?
- Do you have a job/role description that matches what you do?
- Does each member of your team have a job/role description that matches what they do?
- Have job roles and descriptions been individually discussed and agreed?
- How often are job roles and descriptions agreed?

Job descriptions, with responsibilities clearly outlined, provide a line of sight from the business strategy to individual job roles. When discussed and agreed with team members, they support a sense of security for all parties and allow purposeful conversations to be had about performance and development. Regular review ensures they are relevant to both the individual and the wider team.

Discussing role descriptions and expectations across the team ensures everyone is clear about who is doing what. This prevents assumptions and therefore decreases the likelihood of miscommunication, misunderstanding and stress.

New starters

- What are your processes for bringing new team members on board?

New staff should have a job description and be subject to a thorough induction with initially regular weekly reviews, then at 1, 3 and 6 months. This will help to ensure that they understand all the requirements of their job and enhance their feeling of security in their position.

> • Have you considered a mentor or buddy system?

Mentors are typically more experienced people who can share their experience and knowledge and support the development of less experienced individuals. A buddy is someone who is working at the same level as the newcomer. This type of socialization gives new starters an increased sense of wellbeing and self-esteem and may enable them to feel engaged with work and part of the team at an earlier stage.

Performance feedback for personal growth

The value of feedback

> • How do your team know how they are performing?
> • How and when do you give feedback?

For people to be effective and fulfilled at work, they need to understand their impact on others (both colleagues and clients) and the extent to which they are achieving their goals in both their work itself and their working relationships. This is achieved by well-presented, timely and evidence-based feedback. This allows individuals to gather and reflect on the information and then to decide how they will respond to this insight. Genuine praise and feedback from the line manager also bolsters the team member's self-confidence, increases their sense of security in their role and provides a supportive environment in which they can stretch and develop.

Regular one-to-one meetings should be prioritized but feedback is not just about having a conversation on a particular day – make a point of doing it as part of normal practice life; a chat whilst waiting for the kettle to boil or at the end of a meeting is often better received and more effective than having a specific meeting days after the event.

A useful model for giving both positive feedback (praise) and developmental feedback is shown in Figure 10.7.

Situation	The context in which the behaviour occurred	This morning during ops…
Behaviour	The behaviour that was demonstrated	…. you were late getting everything set up…
Impact	The impact the behaviour had (on a person or situation)	…. as a result we were late getting started, which meant it was a rush getting finished before consults and all the lunchbreaks had to be rearranged
Questions	To gain further understanding, to raise awareness and to seek solutions	What stopped you getting set up on time?

10.7 Situation–Behaviour–Impact–Question model for feedback.

Appraisals

Appraisals are a forum for discussion of performance and future plans to allow the team member to realize their potential. Individuals should be encouraged to think about their own development and set 'SMART' (specific, measurable, achievable, relevant and time-bound) goals for self-improvement based on their strengths, weaknesses and areas of interest.

Appraisals should be used to discuss opportunities and to help team members to put in place action plans that will help them to achieve the next level in their career. This could be something they have been working towards or a change in direction. Collaboration should be sought to come up with creative solutions.

Appraisals should not be used to deliver negative feedback that team members have not heard before; constructive discussion on areas for improvement should be had but the focus of the meeting should be positive.

Training for the appraiser may be required to ensure these meetings are conducted well. Both the appraiser and the appraisee should have a number of skills to equip them for the discussion (Figure 10.8).

Follow-up after the appraisal is important; if this is not completed, the system is devalued and this can lead to an erosion of trust between individuals and their line managers.

- Preparation
- Encouragement
- Praise
- Interviewing skills
- Listening skills
- Empathy
- Basic counselling skills
- Negotiating skills
- Job analysis
- Effective use of data
- Discretion
- Objectivity
- Ability to constructively criticize

10.8 Appraisal skills.
(From Hunt, 2010)

Sharing information

Good communication is essential for every aspect of veterinary practice from patient experience and outcomes to client satisfaction. Done well, face-to-face communication through meetings creates a shared understanding and builds trust and relationships.

Meetings serve many different functions including:

- Information sharing
- Decision-making
- Discussion of ideas
- Problem-solving
- Team building
- Clinical governance.

'Huddles'

Huddles are short check-ins (<10 minutes) at the beginning of a day or shift with a member of each team. The purpose is to ensure that all teams are aware of key points or challenges for the day and are aligned and agreed on the plan. Huddles enable all teams, both clinical and non-clinical, to feel involved and empowered in the running of the day.

Team meetings

Each team in the practice (e.g. veterinary surgeons, nurses, receptionists, management) should hold regular meetings, enabling discussion of items relevant to that team.

Practice/inter-team meetings

It is important to bring teams together on a regular basis to encourage teamwork and allow problems and challenges to be seen and discussed from different perspectives. Morbidity and mortality rounds and clinical governance can be discussed in these wider forums to ensure that all factors are considered.

Meetings are also a great forum for disseminating continuing professional development (CPD) information or inviting an external speaker to the practice. The sharing of financial data with team members is also encouraged as it can motivate staff and provide real engagement in the business and ownership of the practice outcomes. Sharing information about the financial health of the practice with team members and discussing the effect of, for example, rising overheads, pay rises or Christmas bonuses, helps team members to understand the workings of the wider business. This approach also enables collaborative problem-solving from the team rather than top-down solutions from management, which are likely to be less well received.

Thought should be given to the purpose of each meeting and attendees should have their time protected so as not to waste unnecessary time away from practice.

The wider veterinary community

Engagement in the wider veterinary community, for example through group meetings in corporate practices, networks or relevant conferences and events, should be encouraged for all types of team members. This will engender self-esteem in colleagues and allow them to build a network of external contacts. Job swaps to other practices will also foster relationships and connections outside of the practice for support and ideas.

Fostering positive relationships in practice

Many interactions occur every day in practice, either face-to-face, by email, telephone or via social media. Whether team members are communicating amongst themselves or with clients or other external personnel, some of these interactions may be more challenging than others; some will lead to positive outcomes and others will lead to frustration, resentment or even complaints.

Everyone is different with different needs, motivations, fears and styles of communicating. If not discussed, these differences can lead to miscommunication, misunderstanding and a breakdown in relationships.

- What are the challenges with communication you see within your team?
- Which relationships are working well?
- Which interactions are more difficult?

Using a behavioural profiling tool such as DISC can be hugely beneficial for individuals and teams alike – it raises self-awareness and helps people identify their own and others' strengths, weaknesses and communication preferences. Different behavioural styles respond differently to conflict (real or perceived), stress and change, and understanding these responses enables individuals to communicate better, to work more effectively together and to understand the things that might trip them up.

The DISC system shown in Figure 10.9 considers four main behavioural types; 15% of people are one style, the rest are a blend of two or three. There is no right or wrong style; each has its strengths and weaknesses. It is not about labelling people or putting them into boxes – it is simply a way to think about how we interact with others and within situations, whether this helps or hinders us, and how we can flex our style to get the best from a situation.

Figure 10.10 shows the strengths of each of the different styles and how each of those styles can be perceived. Those colleagues or clients that we consider 'difficult' are usually a different style to us.

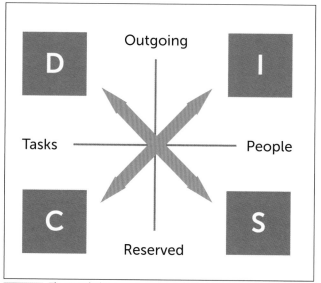

10.9 The DISC behavioural model. C = compliant; D = dominant; I = influencing; S = steady.

Style	Strengths	Can be perceived as...
Dominant	Drive for results, directness, courageous, competitive	Pushy, demanding, insensitive, reckless, ruthless
Influencing	Enthusiasm, optimism, spontaneous, imaginative, persuasive	Overpromising, 'showy', unrealistic, emotional, unfocused, manipulative
Steady	Teamwork, cautiousness, relaxed, stable, single-minded, good listener, amiable	Unwilling, slow, lacking initiative, resistant to change, uncommunicative, easy to manipulate
Compliant	Accuracy, high standards, data analysis, orderly, logical, cautious	Indecisive, critical, picky, compulsive, fearful, inflexible

10.10 DISC style strengths and perceptions.

Minimizing incivility: dealing with bullying and conflict

The Advisory, Conciliation and Arbitration Service (Acas) defines workplace bullying as behaviour that is "offensive, intimidating, malicious or insulting, or an abuse or misuse of power that undermines, humiliates, or causes physical or emotional harm to someone" (Acas, 2021). The HSE emphasizes this is a pattern of behaviour happening repeatedly and persistently over time, rather than isolated instances.

Harassment, on the other hand, may be persistent or an isolated incident and is when the unwanted behaviour is related to one of the following:

- Age
- Sex
- Disability
- Gender reassignment
- Marriage or civil partnership
- Pregnancy and maternity
- Race
- Religion or belief
- Sexual orientation.

Harassment is unlawful under the Equality Act 2010 and whilst bullying itself is not against the law, employers have a duty of care to protect their employees under the Health and Safety at Work etc. Act 1974.

Bullying or harassment may be by an individual against an individual or involve groups of people. They can also take many forms – written word, email, text or via social media, as well as through verbal communication and physical actions.

How common are bullying and harassment in practice?

There are no veterinary-specific statistics on workplace bullying simply because there have been no profession-wide surveys or research to capture these data. Anonymous surveys at practice level and anecdotal reports suggest that, unfortunately, bullying is still present within the veterinary profession. VDS Training are creating a cross-profession database through their Practice Culture Surveys that will in time provide a rich source of data about the health of our professional culture and the prevalence of bullying and harassment in practice.

In the absence of veterinary-specific data, the research on bullying within comparable professions such as medicine and dentistry can be reviewed. Research has shown that over a third of junior doctors and over a quarter of National Health Service (NHS) nurses identified themselves as being victims of bullying. In addition, a much greater proportion had experienced bullying behaviours despite not labelling themselves as being bullied. These numbers reflect the wider societal picture; a 2015 poll carried out by YouGov for the Trades Union Congress (TUC) revealed that nearly a third of people (29%) are bullied at work.

These statistics suggest that we need to face the uncomfortable truth that bullying is likely to be more widespread within the veterinary community than we would like to think. As a profession, we need to look inwards at what is happening in our own practices and ask ourselves:

- Is bullying happening here?
- What behaviour am I being subjected to?
- What is the impact of my own behaviour on others?

What does bullying look like in practice?

As anyone who has ever been bullied knows, bullying is not always physical or easy to spot. Whilst you can easily see those people who shout, throw things or become aggressive towards others, there are many more subtle behaviours that can constitute bullying, including:

- Unwarranted or invalid criticism
- Undermining work
- Excluding others from the decision-making process (e.g. within a partnership)
- Excessive monitoring or micromanaging
- Giving work with unrealistic deadlines
- Blocking another member of staff's progress or refusing training opportunities
- Assigning blame without factual justification
- Spreading malicious rumours
- Ridiculing or demeaning behaviour
- Practical jokes.

Do you recognize any of the following scenarios?

- A receptionist who sends one veterinary surgeon out on all the 'difficult' calls.
- A senior nurse repeatedly ignoring a junior practitioner's request to do something differently.
- Cliques within your team, with members making jokes at the expense of other team members.
- Emails sent last thing on a Friday or before you go on annual leave with complaints or issues that could have been dealt with sooner.

These can all be signs of bullying behaviour and over time they will have a detrimental effect on the performance and wellbeing of both the team and the individual.

Who are the bullies?

As the above scenarios and behaviours show, bullying can affect, and be carried out by, anyone at any level within the practice; it is not just from a senior member of staff to a more junior team member. The key thing to remember is that there is no such thing as a 'typical bully' and we need to keep watch for behaviours and be aware of the lenses that we observe ourselves and others through.

Is a 'bit of banter' okay?

In a word, no!

Colleagues will often speak jokingly to each other and banter (light-hearted teasing) is commonplace in veterinary practices. However, relaxed and 'humorous' conversations can easily lull you into a false sense of security and lead you into making more offensive comments. This is where a 'bit of banter' becomes harassment and bullying; it should be remembered that what one person thinks is teasing, someone else may consider offensive or hurtful. What may appear amusing to you, others may see very differently – so think before you speak.

Teamwork and effective communication are critical to deliver safe, effective working and a high standard of care. Studies in the human medical field have shown that rudeness and mild incivility significantly reduces both individual and team performance; creating an environment where communication is guarded leads to less sharing of information and people are less likely to ask for help. This is dangerous for both patients and team members.

Why does it matter?

Left unchecked, bullying and conflict will have a detrimental effect on everyone in practice (Figure 10.11). It is not just the team that suffers; little slip-ups, bigger mistakes and bad decisions will all start having an impact on the clinical outcomes for patients, which are sometimes obvious, but often less so. People no longer go the extra mile for clients and communication with them suffers, increasing the likelihood of complaints. 'People buy people' and clients also pick up on the team not being happy and the increased staff turnover. They no longer have the relationship they want with staff that they trust, and client retention may fall as a result.

As Figure 10.12 shows, this can become a vicious cycle.

Potential impact on the victim
• Shock • Anger • Feelings of frustration and/or helplessness • Increased sense of vulnerability • Loss of confidence and self-esteem • Altered eating and sleeping habits • Psychosomatic symptoms such as gastrointestinal problems or headaches • Panic or anxiety, especially about going to work • Family tension and stress • Inability to concentrate • Low morale and productivity
Potential impact on the team
• Witnesses to the bullying can experience feelings of isolation, helplessness and anxiety • Poor morale • Reduced motivation • Disrespect from others towards the bully • Seen as a cultural norm – bullying can spread • Reduced team productivity
Potential impact on the practice
• Increased absenteeism • Reduced engagement • Increased staff turnover • Decreased morale, motivation and productivity • Increased costs of recruitment • Difficulty replacing good staff as word spreads of the bullying culture • Increased workplace accidents/incidents • Poor client service

10.11 Bullying: impacts on the individual, team and practice.

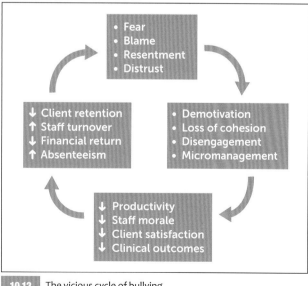

10.12 The vicious cycle of bullying.

We all have a role to play in stamping out bullying

Whenever bullying occurs, there is a recognized cycle that requires three parties to be involved: the bully, the victim and the bystander(s) (Figure 10.13). When bullying happens in secret, the bystander may only become involved when the issue is reported.

The role of the bystander (which could be you, other members of the team or management) is crucial – there can be no passive onlookers when dealing with bullying. It is everyone's responsibility to look out for it, report it and deal with it. The responsibility also extends to the victim who needs to act, either by confronting the bully or by reporting it. As discussed, the cost of allowing bullying to continue is deeper-reaching than simply to the individual, and if you are being bullied it will affect your ability to work effectively and have an impact on your patients and your team.

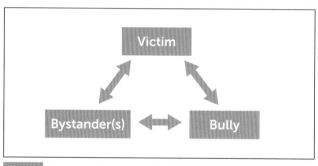

10.13 Three roles in the cycle of bullying.

Appropriately assertive or bullying?

As discussed in the section 'Fostering positive relationships', misunderstandings can easily happen due to differences in people's behavioural styles. If you are in a position of management or leadership, be aware of how you come across and flex your style with the different members of your team whilst being polite, fair and consistent at all times.

Assertive behaviour is being clear and direct about your needs, your wants and your opinions whilst being mindful of other people's needs, wants and opinions – in itself this does not constitute bullying or harassment even though it may feel hurtful, especially if clumsily done. Examples include:

- Expressing differences of opinion
- Offering constructive feedback, guidance or advice about work-related behaviour
- Saying 'no' to extra shifts or tasks
- Reasonable disciplinary action taken by an employer or manager.

If you are on the receiving end of any of these scenarios and feel hurt or offended, consider the intention behind the behaviour. Ask yourself if it is likely to be a difference in behavioural style, a lack of self-awareness or whether the offence was deliberate.

When bullying happens
If you are being bullied

The first step is to name the behaviour and to admit to yourself that you feel you are being bullied. At this point it is also important to recognize that it is not your fault.

Try talking: If you are offended or hurt by someone's behaviour, especially early on in the relationship, try talking to them as bullying may not be deliberate; the other person may lack self-awareness and be genuinely unaware of the effect that the behaviour is having on you.

- Choose a suitable time and place.
- Work out what to say beforehand.
- Stay calm and be polite.
- Use the feedback model in Figure 10.7 to describe what has been happening, the impact it has had on you and what you would like to happen instead.

Keep records: Keep a record of daily events; this is very important – recorded accounts will help you build your case against the bully.

- Note the date, time and what happened.
- Were there any witnesses and what was the outcome?
- Keep copies of any correspondence, including emails and text messages.
- Record who else you speak to about the bullying (e.g. colleagues or your manager).

Make a formal complaint:
- Report the behaviour to your direct team leader or line manager.
- Be very clear about what is happening and the impact that it is having on you – be specific and use the evidence you have gathered.
- If your concerns are not dealt with appropriately, take them to the next level of management.

If you are the boss and you are being bullied, either by a more junior member of staff or by a partner: Follow the above steps and seek legal advice from your practice solicitors, Acas or an employment law specialist such as Citation. British Veterinary Association (BVA), British Veterinary Nursing Association (BVNA) and BSAVA members have access to free legal helplines.

If you witness bullying

Do not be a passive bystander – this behaviour is as bad as that of the bully, so take action.

- Offer support to the victim – tell them that what is happening is not right and that you want to help them.
- Take responsibility – call out the behaviour by speaking to the bully and telling them that their behaviour is not right; chances are they are not doing it to just one person or have done it before to someone else.
- Consider reporting it to your line manager, ideally after talking to the victim.
- Remember, bullying affects everyone, and everyone is responsible for dealing with it.

If bullying is reported to you

If you find that you have a bully on your team, check your practice handbook for policies on how to deal with the situation. Talk to the victim to find out exactly what has happened, and communicate your support and commitment to dealing with the situation.

As a manager, if you receive a complaint of bullying and/or harassment, you should:

- Take the complaint seriously – listen and reassure the employee that it will be investigated
- Ask the employee how they would like their complaint to be handled

- Encourage the employee to detail what he or she believes has occurred
- Be supportive, and do not dismiss the person as being 'oversensitive'
- Ensure that events are handled confidentially and that others do not become aware of the allegations
- Try not to ask for repeated recounting of the events, as the victim may find this difficult and/or upsetting
- If you are implicated in any way, then pass the complaint on to a more senior (and uninvolved) manager.

Victims may feel that they invite the bullying – they may internalize their feelings and not tell others what is happening as they feel ashamed that they are letting it happen. It is thought that only 11% of victims report bullying to their managers and this is frequently after enduring it for a long time (commonly around 22 months).

Your personal reaction to the complaint is important – this may be another problem for you to deal with but it is vital that you are supportive and understanding, even if you wish they had said something earlier.

Next steps

Once a manager has received an allegation of bullying or harassment, the next stage will be to consider whether the allegations, if substantiated, could result in disciplinary action. If your practice is a client of a human resourcdes (HR) provider, speak to them or contact your practice legal advisors. BVA, BVNA and BSAVA members can access free legal helplines to speak to a team of specialist legal advisors about any professional or personal subject.

- Discuss with the individual concerned – get their side of the story.
- Explain that the practice will not tolerate bullying behaviour.
- Seek legal advice if necessary.
- Issue a formal warning if necessary.
- Take further steps to formal disciplinary action if required.

Fortunately, most minor incidents can often be resolved by obtaining a written commitment to change and making sure that the bully understands what will happen if they do not change. There is always guidance and support available and there are many different routes that, if taken promptly, can lead to a satisfactory conclusion; even steps that seem drastic, such as mediation, can end up having very positive outcomes.

Additional mitigators for workplace stress

Just as it is often the little things that make a good day at work, it can often be the small things that create frustration, friction and stress in the workplace.

- Which of these have you already thought about?

Holidays

Regular holiday planning is essential to wellbeing and a fair rota, published well in advance (including a duty rota for public holidays), will help team members to plan their activities outside of work. Flexibility will be welcomed where possible, especially if a big trip or family event is planned; it is usually returned by team members when someone is ill or resigns and work needs covering.

> • Do you have a procedure for booking holidays that is fair and clearly communicated?
> • Does it address:
>   • Guidelines for the number of team members that can be absent at any one time?
>   • When and how holiday should be booked?
>   • An expectation of when team members should hear whether their booking has been successful?

Flexible working

It should be remembered that work–life balance is not just an issue that affects those with families. Flexible working, job shares and part-time positions can all work extremely well; they keep skills within the practice, save additional recruitment costs and help to bond individuals to the practice as they feel their needs are being met. Certain roles may also benefit from the ability to work from home for some of their contracted hours.

Technology facilitates flexible working by allowing people to work and to be connected from (almost) anywhere, but this can present its own problems. As people can connect via email, social media and potentially practice systems, the boundaries between work and home can become eroded. This can present real challenges for wellbeing if not discussed and managed.

> • Have you discussed with your team how you all like to work?
> • What expectations do you have of each other regarding working and connecting outside of working hours?
> • Have you communicated these?
> • How can you use technology to enhance wellbeing?
> • How can you all maintain your boundaries?

Maternity/paternity leave

Maternity, paternity, adoption leave and pay is vital for new families and they need plenty of support at this time. Work–family conflict can be a source of distress for staff; therefore, having a culture that respects family life is likely to enhance wellbeing.

Disability and chronic illness

Under the Equality Act 2010, a disability is defined as a physical or mental impairment that has a 'substantial' or 'long-term' negative affect on the person's ability to do normal daily activities. Once a disability has been disclosed to an employer, they have an obligation to consider reasonable adjustments to that person's role. As discussed previously, it is of paramount importance to create a culture of psychological safety, where individuals feel able to disclose relevant health conditions without fear of discrimination.

Earlier in this chapter, the importance of work and being able to fulfil our purpose for psychological wellbeing was highlighted. It is important to recognize that both disability and chronic illness may have a negative impact on an individual's psychological wellbeing beyond the direct effects of their condition; they may have financial concerns, be worried about their future and, in a profession

that is physically and mentally challenging, they may feel stigmatized or guilty for not being able to work in the same manner as their colleagues. Taking the time to support a team member with a disability or chronic illness will not only enable them to thrive as part of the team, it will also create a culture within the team where individual wellbeing is valued.

The role of occupational health

Occupational health support can be used at any time during a person's employment to help team members continue to work whilst managing either short-term conditions (e.g. following injury or surgery) or chronic conditions. Using an occupational health service can greatly assist both employers and the individual by providing not only legal and practical advice on adjustments but also reassurance for both parties that the right steps are being taken.

Adjustments to working practices for individuals are best considered after a combination of thorough discussion with the team member and professional help from either an occupational therapist or the individual's medical professionals. It is important to discuss each case individually as conditions manifest themselves differently for different people.

Regular reviews of the team member's role and adjustments should be scheduled, as many chronic conditions can be progressive or fluctuating. Team members also have a responsibility to discuss changes in a chronic condition with their manager to enable any necessary adjustments to be made.

Leaving for absence/returning to work

For sabbaticals, maternity/paternity leave and longer term sickness absence, it is important that both the departure from and return to work are planned and handled well (wherever possible); this can mean the difference between retaining and losing talented staff. 'Keep in touch' (KIT) days can be utilized for the benefit of both the employee and the employer. Some organizations and CPD providers now offer 'return to work' courses to assist staff with their reintroduction.

> • What has worked well for both individuals and the practice with regards to returning to work?
> • What could be improved in the future?

Remuneration and reward

Financial and job security are more important to individual wellbeing than increased salary itself. Salary is also not a reliable motivator; as Dan Pink comments in his book *Drive: The Surprising Truth About What Motivates Us*, "the best use of money as a motivator is to pay people enough to take the issue of money off the table" (Pink, 2018). When money is removed from the equation, then purpose, autonomy and mastery become the intrinsic drivers for engagement and motivation.

Remuneration packages should be fair and reasonable for all team members. As well as basic salary and pension, other benefits to consider include:

* Medical insurance
* The Cycle to Work Scheme
* Gym membership
* Spending discount platforms
* Staff discounts.

Wherever possible, talk to your team and find out what would work best for them; give them some autonomy to choose how they are rewarded. What works for one person might not work for everyone and within the boundaries of what is fair and reasonable, some degree of flexibility will increase motivation.

Practice resources

Equipment maintenance should be a priority; difficult to use or poorly functioning equipment will make tasks more difficult and time-consuming, as will competition for resources such as computers, or basic items such as stethoscopes. This will lead to frustration and a decrease in both job satisfaction and productivity. The amount and location of equipment should be considered in relation to workload to ensure efficiency.

Tools and initiatives to facilitate wellbeing in practice

Workplace policies

HR and legal advice should be sought to establish specific practice or organizational policies around key areas that support wellbeing, including but not limited to:

- Workplace bullying
- Staff absence
- Workplace stress.

These policies should provide clear information to everyone involved about the practice's position, procedures to be followed and employee/employer rights. However, simply having them is not enough; it is crucial that team members read them and know where to find them, that they are followed when necessary, and that they are regularly reviewed and updated.

Practice Culture Surveys

Anonymous surveys, such as the Veterinary Defense Society (VDS) Practice Culture Survey, provide an invaluable source of data about workplace stress and the wellbeing of the practice team. They are a rich source of information about what is working within the practice and the areas where improvement is required, as well as being a benchmark against which progress can be measured. They also inform purposeful conversations with your team, allowing you to create ideas together and identify workable interventions to improve the workplace. There is often a worry that surveys will open the proverbial can of worms, but if acted upon the team feel listened to, motivated and engaged. The results and the solutions can be owned by the team and everyone is empowered to change things for the better. Surveys should be repeated every 6–12 months, even if everything seems fine, and consideration given to what interventions could be responsible for any changing results.

Schwartz rounds

Schwartz rounds are monthly multidisciplinary meetings for both clinical and non-clinical team members (Figure 10.14). Rather than focusing on problem-solving or discussing policies and procedures, Schwartz rounds address the

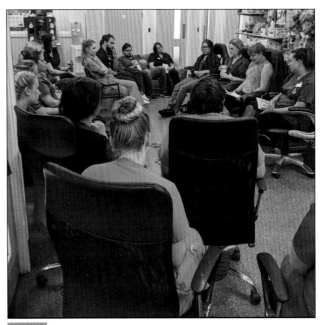

10.14 A Schwartz round in progress.

social and emotional impact that work has on individuals both personally and professionally. Team members discuss a particular patient care scenario, their involvement in it, how it made them feel and any challenges or issues it raised for them.

Trained facilitators ensure that the original model is adhered to, that staff wellbeing is supported and that full benefit from the meetings is realized. Through listening to colleagues describing their work and their challenges, team members who attend Schwartz rounds:

- Report lower levels of stress
- Experience less isolation at work
- Develop a shared understanding of one another's work
- Discover more senior employees have similar experiences to themselves, leading to flattened hierarchies
- Are more able to attend to a patient's (client's) emotional needs
- Have increased empathy for clients and colleagues.

Figure 10.15 details themes that explain how interventions such as Schwartz rounds work – the connection to a culture of wellbeing and psychological safety is clear.

The Schwartz rounds programme is provided in cooperation with the Schwartz Center for compassionate healthcare and with the support of the Point of Care Foundation. Although there is a cost involved in running the rounds, the Point of Care Foundation (2019) has produced a document to evidence the benefits and there is a huge amount of information that can be sourced by visiting the Point of Care Foundation website.

- Trust, emotional safety and containment
- Group interaction
- Countercultural/third space for staff
- Self-disclosure
- Storytelling
- Role-modelling vulnerability
- Contextualizing patients
- Contextualizing staff
- Reflection and resonance

10.15 Schwartz round themes.
(From Maben et al., 2018)

VetSafe

VetSafe is the VDS' confidential significant event reporting service to facilitate quality improvement and risk management in veterinary practice. It helps individuals and practices to learn from mistakes by capturing information about incidents in practice that result in patient harm or other losses, and near misses. It supports second victims – the clinicians and team members involved in mistakes – and provides a wider database for the profession about the nature of significant events in veterinary practice. VetSafe Contributory Factor cards are designed to help practices to talk about mistakes and can help the facilitation of effective mortality and morbidity rounds.

In-house training

In-house training by external facilitators can be a great way to get the practice together to discuss challenges, changes or general wellbeing topics. Using behavioural profiling tools such as DISC (see above) can help to raise awareness around relationships and interactions, build trust and enhance teamwork. There are many different options, from lunch-and-learns through to whole-day workshops, or evenings with pizza. Time invested in developing the team will pay off in all aspects of practice life and performance.

Health and Safety Executive

The HSE has a wealth of information relating to stress and mental health at work which can be found online. The HSE management indicator tool, which facilitates discussion about a person's wellbeing at work, may be particularly useful.

Wellness Action Plan

Mind (the mental health charity) has produced a Wellness Action Plan template, which can enable team members to discuss with their manager what keeps them mentally well at work, how they would like to be communicated with, and how their manager can help them, especially in times of crisis.

Health and wellbeing representatives

Championing team members within the practice, and allowing them to undertake training to support and signpost other team members, can create satisfaction for the team members selected (or self-selected). It also helps to encourage buy-in and provides another layer of support to team members who may not wish to speak with their manager.

Anti-stigma interventions, such as Mental Health First Aid (MHFA) training in the workplace, can lead to improved knowledge and supportive behaviour towards people with mental health problems.

Health and wellbeing champions can maintain a wellbeing notice board (Figure 10.16) with information on physical and mental health, email interesting blogs and websites to teams and take a slot in practice meetings to discuss any health and wellbeing initiatives which team members can become involved in.

External initiatives

There are many schemes within the wider veterinary community, such as those being explored by the Royal College of Veterinary Surgeons (RCVS) Mind Matters Initiative, which practices can become involved in. This includes the Society of Practising Veterinary Surgeons (SPVS) Wellbeing Awards, which provide a handy checklist of things to consider when promoting wellbeing in practice. It may be a good idea to involve the team in filling in the checklist and entering the awards.

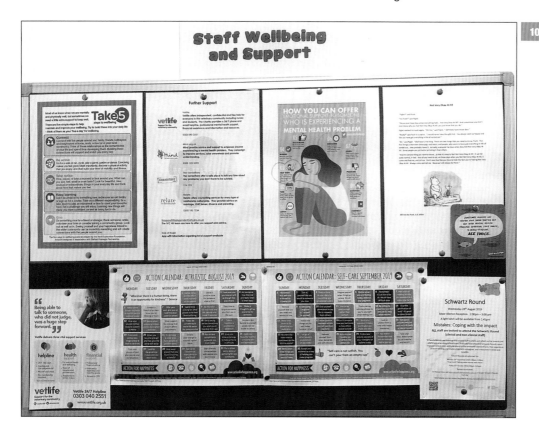

10.16 Wellbeing noticeboard.

Personal strategies for thriving in practice

Being responsibly selfish

"Fit your own oxygen mask before helping other people."

Whilst caring for ourselves may seem selfish, it is the responsible thing to do. It is up to you to decide that you need a break, a drink, something to eat or to take a walk outside, and it is up to you to make this happen whilst being mindful of other people. You will be a more effective, more productive and safer veterinary professional if you take time to care for yourself – building a culture of wellbeing is everyone's responsibility.

Wellbeing toolkit

Our wellbeing requires constant attention; we need to be mindful of what is going on for us, what has changed and what we need to do differently as a result. There will always be areas that need a little more focus or a different strategy.

Figure 10.17 is a toolkit of questions to help you reflect on and maintain your own wellbeing; what can you to do help yourself to thrive?

1	Eat and hydrate	A healthy, nutrient-rich diet is essential to fuel our bodies and minds • On a scale of 1–10, how would you score your nutrition day-to-day? • What one change could you make that would increase this score? • What would be the benefit if you did?
2	Exercise	Take a look at the NHS Physical Activity Guidelines for Adults • How are you doing in comparison? • What could be better? • What would help you to prioritize exercise?
3	Sleep	Research shows that we need between 7 and 9 hours of sleep a night • Out of the last 14 nights, how many nights have you achieved this? • What could you do to improve the quality or quantity of your sleep? • What would be the benefits of doing this?
4	Switch off	Actively engaging our parasympathetic system helps to combat the negative effects of cortisol and boost our restorative hormones • What do you do to switch off? • When do you have 'tech-free time'? • How do you spend time in nature?
5	Breathe	When you feel your stress response being triggered and you feel yourself moving into the red zone, this is your cue to hit the 'pause' button and to breathe • Take some slow, deep breaths in through the nose and out through the mouth • Do not try to control your breath, just focus on it and allow it to deepen naturally • Centre yourself and bring your mind into the present; right here, right now • Notice what is going on in your body • As you breathe, feel your mind quietening and your heart rate slowing • How will you now approach the situation? • What do you need to do next?
6	Reframe	The meaning of a situation is determined by what we choose to focus on. There will always be something positive, however small, in any situation. Focusing on these changes our mindset: • What was good about today? • What did you do well today? • What did you learn?
7	Set and manage expectations	Not having your expectations met or not knowing what others expect from you can be a source of frustration, anxiety and conflict • What do you expect from others? • Have you communicated these expectations? • What is expected of you? • What conversations do you need to have?
8	Build positive relationships	It is important to be aware of the effect that people around you have on you and to purposefully choose who you spend your time with, both physically and online • Who are the people in your life who give you positive energy, who make you feel good about yourself and about life? • Who are the people who are your 'dementors' personally and professionally, the ones who drain your mental battery? • Who would you like to spend more time with? • Who would you like to spend less time with? • Who would you like to meet?
9	Be curious	Curiosity cultivates personal growth, a key element of wellbeing • What would you like to learn? • How would you like to grow, personally and professionally? • Where could you be more curious?
10	Be purposeful	Knowing what gives you meaning and fulfilment in life enables you to take proactive steps towards working on your purpose • How fulfilled on a scale of 1–10 are you personally and professionally? • What is important to you personally and professionally? • What changes can you make that will enable you to act with purpose?

10.17 Personal wellbeing toolkit.

Leadership of a wellbeing culture

Lead by example

It should be remembered that 55% of our communication is through body language, and therefore what you do is more important than what you say. This is crucial, particularly when asking people to change behaviour.

Be open, fair and consistent in your behaviour towards others and be aware of your own triggers, weaknesses and challenges. Treat everyone with respect and dignity. Operate a zero-tolerance attitude to bullying; act on it if it occurs and be seen to be doing so.

Empower, educate and communicate

Empower your team to discuss challenges and to report bullying behaviour they witness. Educate everyone in the importance of wellbeing and explain the importance of creating a safe and just culture in practice. Equip leaders and managers with the skills and support they need to have difficult conversations, deal with bullying and identify the signs of poor wellbeing. Encourage open and honest conversations and bring people together to discuss challenges.

Conclusion

To build a sustainable profession, capable of delivering the full remit of its services, we need individuals who are healthy, happy and fulfilled at work. Working as a motivated, effective, engaged team in practice is essential to enable everyone to perform at their best, whatever their role.

Ultimately, working in veterinary practice is an extremely rewarding career; providing the basic needs are looked after, the work that we do every day can sustain us. Whatever our role or position in the profession, we all have our part to play in creating a safe, healthy workplace culture and a motivating environment that enables people to thrive at work.

References and further reading

Acas (2021) *Bullying and harassment at work: a guide for managers and employers.* Acas, London

Acas (2015) *Seeking better solutions: tackling bullying and ill-treatment in Britain's workplaces.* Acas, London

Bartram D, Curwen A and Hardy B (2012) Building a thriving workforce. *In Practice* **34(6)**, 355–361

Black C (2008) *Working for a healthier tomorrow.* Available from: www.gov.uk/government/publications

Black C (2012) Why healthcare organisations must look after their staff. *Nursing Management* **19(6)**, 27–30

Cake MA, Bell MA, Bickley N and Bartram DJ (2015) The life of meaning: a model of the positive contributions to well-being from veterinary work. *Journal of Veterinary Medical Education* **43(3)**, 184–193

Diener E and Seligman MEP (2004) Beyond money: toward an economy of well-being. *Psychological Science in the Public Interest* **5(1)**, 1–31

Donovan M (2016) *The Golden Apple: Redefining Work-Life Balance for a Diverse Workforce.* Routledge, London

Engleman C, Schneider M, Grote G *et al.* (2012) Work breaks during minimally invasive surgery in children: patient benefits and surgeon's perceptions. *European Journal of Paediatric Surgery* **22(6)**, 439–444

Engleman C, Schneider M, Kirschbaum C *et al.* (2001) Effects of intraoperative breaks on mental and somatic operator fatigue: a randomised clinical trial. *Surgical Endoscopy* **25(4)**, 1245–1250

Equality Act 2010. Available from:www.legislation.gov.uk

Goodrich J (2012) Supporting hospital staff to provide compassionate care: Do Schwartz Center Rounds work in English hospitals? *Journal of the Royal Society of Medicine* **105**, 117–122

Hanisch SE, Twomey CD, Szeto ACH *et al.* (2016) The effectiveness of interventions targeting the stigma of mental illness at the workplace: a systematic review. *BMC Psychiatry* **16(1)**, 1–11

Health and Safety at Work etc. Act 1974. Available from: www.hse.gov.uk/legislation

Health and Safety Executive (2006) *Bullying at work: a review of the literature.* HSE, Buxton

Health and Safety Executive (2022) *Stress and mental health at work.* Available from: www.hse.gov.uk/stress

Hunt NC (2010) *Setting Up and Running Effective Staff Appraisals and Feedback Review Meetings.* How To Books Ltd, Oxford

Maben J, Taylor C, Dawson J *et al.* (2018) A realist informed mixed methods evaluation of Schwartz Center Rounds® in England. *Health Services and Delivery Research* **6(37)**

Mind (2020) *Guide for employees: Wellness Action Plans (WAPs): How to support your mental health at work.* Available from: www.mind.org.uk

National Health Service (2019) *Guidelines for Physical Activity in Adults.* Available from: www.nhs.uk/live-well/exercise/

Nigah N, Davis AJ and Hurrell SA (2012) The impact of buddying on psychological capital and work engagement: an empirical study of socialization in the professional services sector. *Thunderbird International Business Review* **54**, 891–905

Pink DH (2018) *Drive: The Surprising Truth About What Motivates Us.* Canongate, London

Point of Care Foundation (2019) *Evidence to demonstrate the impact of Schwartz Rounds.* Available from: www.pointofcarefoundation.org.uk/resource-library

Quine L (2001) Workplace bullying in nurses. *Journal of Health Psychology* **6(1)**, 73–84

Quine L (2002) Workplace bullying in junior doctors: questionnaire survey. *British Medical Journal* **324**, 878–879

Riskin A, Erez A, Foulk TA *et al.* (2015) The impact of rudeness on medical team performance: a randomized trial. *Pediatrics* **136(3)**, 487–495

Robertson Cooper and the Bank Workers Charity (2016) *What is a good day at work? Wellbeing, expectations and experiences of work.* Available from: www.robertsoncooper.com/resources

Robertson Cooper and the Bank Workers Charity (2018) *Creating well workplaces.* Available from: www.robertsoncooper.com/resources

Ryff CD (2014) Psychological well-being revisited: advances in science and practice. *Psychotherapy and Psychosomatics* **83(1)**, 10–28

Steadman L, Quine L, Jack K, Felix DH and Waumsley J (2009) Experience of workplace bullying behaviours in postgraduate hospital dentists: questionnaire survey. *British Dental Journal* **207(8)**, 379–380

Trades Union Congress (2015) *Nearly a third of people are bullied at work, says TUC.* Available from: www.tuc.org.uk

UNISON (2013) *Tackling bullying at work. A UNISON guide for safety reps.* UNISON Communications, London

Walker M (2018) *Why we sleep.* Penguin, London

Wax R (2013) *Sane New World – Taming the Mind.* Hodder, London

Working Time Regulations 1998. Available from: www.legislation.gov.uk

Useful websites

There is assistance available for anyone experiencing difficulty. Contact your community mental health crisis team if you have an urgent mental health crisis. You can also contact your GP or visit A&E and ask to be seen by the duty psychologist. Call 999 if you are worried about immediate risk of harm.

Campaign Against Living Miserably (CALM)
0800 58 58 58
www.thecalmzone.net

IAPT services
www.nhs.uk/service-search/find-a-psychological-therapies-service

IMALIVE
www.imalive.org
Online crisis chat

Mind
0300 123 3393
www.mind.org.uk
info@mind.org

NHS
www.nhs.uk/oneyou/every-mind-matters/urgent-support

RCVS Mind Matters Initiative
Offers mental health awareness training
www.vetmindmatters.org

Relate
www.relate.org.uk/relationship-help/talk-someone

Samaritans
116 123
www.samaritans.org
jo@samaritans.org

SANEline
0300 304 7000
07984 967 708
www.sane.org.uk
support@sane.org.uk

VDS Training
Providing training for you, your team, your practice
www.vds-training.co.uk

Vetlife – For all of the veterinary team
0303 040 2551
www.vetlife.org.uk
Register to send anonymous emails to Vetlife

Index

Note: page numbers in *italics* refer to figures
(●) indicates downloadable content in the BSAVA Library